PEDIATRIC CCRN CERTIFICATION REVIEW

MW01156722

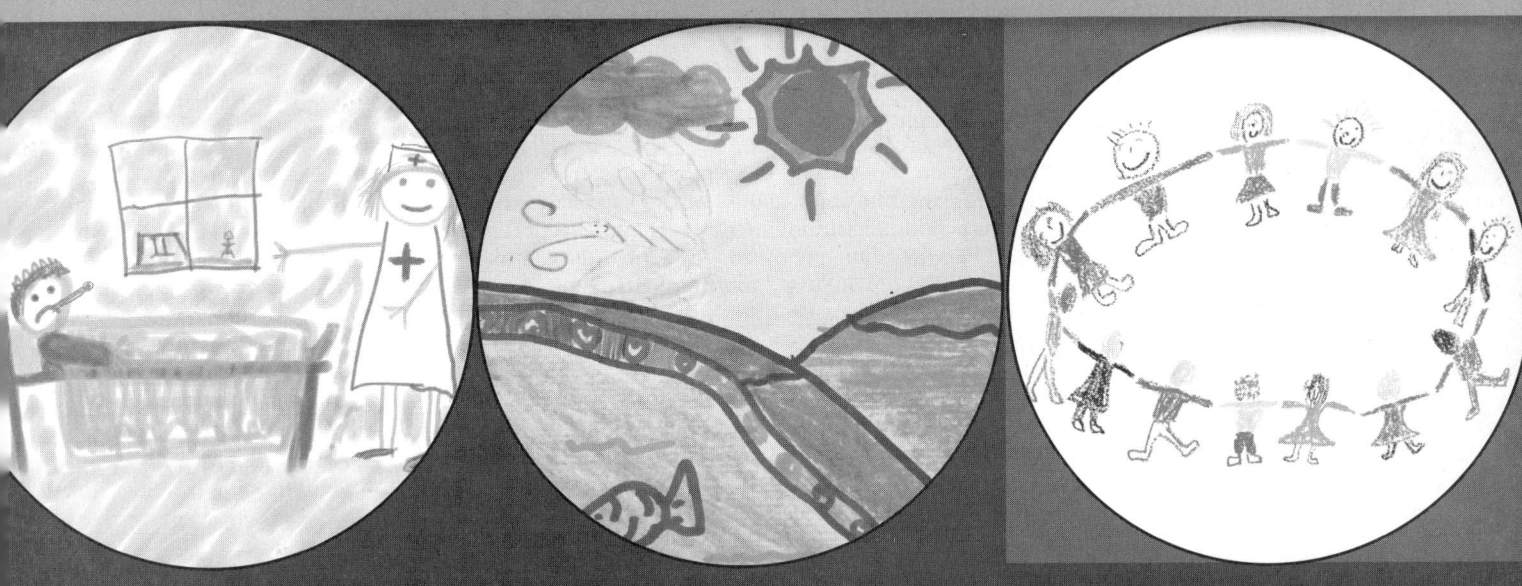

Ann J. Brorsen, MSN, RN, CCRN, CEN
COO and Director of Clinical Applications
Pro Ed
Menifee, California

Keri R. Rogelet, MSN, MBA/HCM, RN, CCRN
CFO and Director of Clinical Development
Pro Ed
Menifee, California

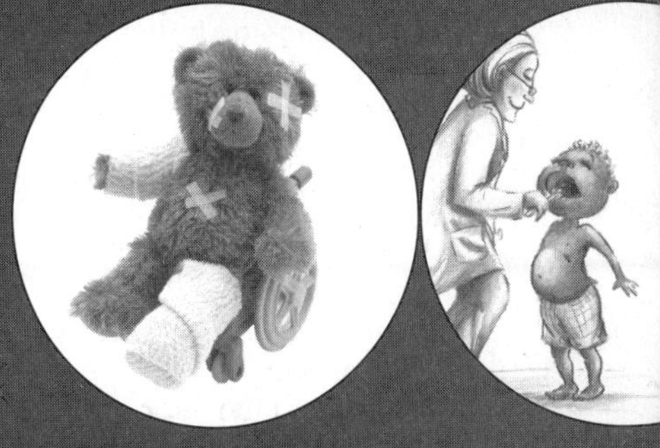

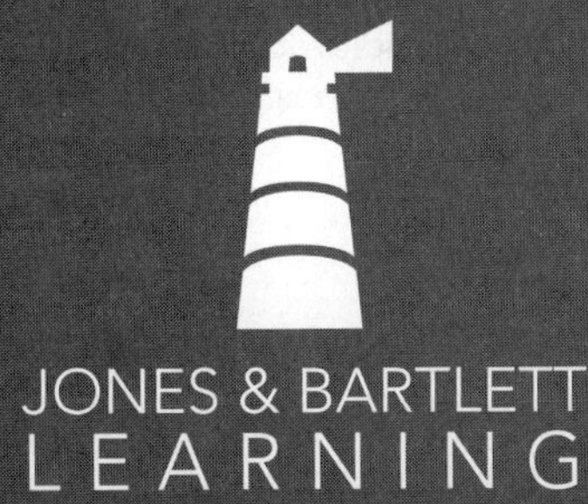

JONES & BARTLETT
LEARNING

World Headquarters
Jones & Bartlett Learning
5 Wall Street
Burlington, MA 01803
978-443-5000
info@jblearning.com
www.jblearning.com

Jones & Bartlett Learning books and products are available through most bookstores and online booksellers. To contact Jones & Bartlett Learning directly, call 800-832-0034, fax 978-443-8000, or visit our website, www.jblearning.com.

Substantial discounts on bulk quantities of Jones & Bartlett Learning publications are available to corporations, professional associations, and other qualified organizations. For details and specific discount information, contact the special sales department at Jones & Bartlett Learning via the above contact information or send an email to specialsales@jblearning.com.

Copyright © 2012 by Jones & Bartlett Learning, LLC, an Ascend Learning Company

All rights reserved. No part of the material protected by this copyright may be reproduced or utilized in any form, electronic or mechanical, including photocopying, recording, or by any information storage and retrieval system, without written permission from the copyright owner.

The authors, editor, and publisher have made every effort to provide accurate information. However, they are not responsible for errors, omissions, or for any outcomes related to the use of the contents of this book and take no responsibility for the use of the products and procedures described. Treatments and side effects described in this book may not be applicable to all people; likewise, some people may require a dose or experience a side effect that is not described herein. Drugs and medical devices are discussed that may have limited availability controlled by the Food and Drug Administration (FDA) for use only in a research study or clinical trial. Research, clinical practice, and government regulations often change the accepted standard in this field. When consideration is being given to use of any drug in the clinical setting, the health care provider or reader is responsible for determining FDA status of the drug, reading the package insert, and reviewing prescribing information for the most up-to-date recommendations on dose, precautions, and contraindications, and determining the appropriate usage for the product. This is especially important in the case of drugs that are new or seldom used.

Production Credits
Publisher: Kevin Sullivan
Acquisitions Editor: Amanda Harvey
Editorial Assistant: Rachel Shuster
Production Assistant: Sara Fowles
Marketing Manager: Meagan Norlund
V.P., Manufacturing and Inventory Control: Therese Connell
Composition: Auburn Associates, Inc.
Cover Design: Kristin E. Parker
Cover Images: (Clockwise from upper left) © Matthew Jacques/ShutterStock, Inc.; © Tungphoto/ShutterStock, Inc.; © Tupungato/ShutterStock, Inc.; © DeepGreen/ShutterStock, Inc.; © c.byatt-norman/ShutterStock, Inc.
Printing and Binding: Edwards Brothers Malloy
Cover Printing: Edwards Brothers Malloy

To order this product, use ISBN: 978-1-4496-2916-8

Library of Congress Cataloging-in-Publication Data
Brorsen, Ann J.
Pediatric CCRN certification review / Ann J. Brorsen, Keri R. Rogelet.
p. ; cm.
Includes bibliographical references.
ISBN 978-1-4496-1579-6(pbk.)
1. Pediatric nursing—Examinations, questions, etc. 2. Critical care nursing—Examinations, questions, etc. I. Rogelet, Keri R. II. Title.
[DNLM: 1. Critical Care—Examination Questions. 2. Pediatric Nursing—methods—Examination Questions. 3. Child. 4. Critical Illness—nursing—Examination Questions. 5. Nursing Assessment—Examination Questions. WY 18.2]
RJ245.B77 2011
618.92'00231076—dc22

2010052811

6048
Printed in the United States of America
18 17 16 15 10 9 8 7 6 5 4 3

Contents

About the Authors v

Contributor vii

Reviewers ix

Acknowledgments xi

Preface xiii

Section 1: The CCRN Credential and Registering for the Exam 1

Section 2: Test-Taking Strategies 7

Section 3: Cardiovascular 11

Section 4: Pulmonary 81

Section 5: Endocrine 141

Section 6: Hematology/Immunology 171

Section 7: Neurology 203

Section 8: Gastrointestinal 247

Section 9: Renal 291

Section 10: Multisystem 333

Section 11: Behavioral 383

About the Authors

ANN J. BRORSEN, MSN, RN, CCRN, CEN

Ann is a nationally known speaker and has presented certification review courses for the Adult and Pediatric CCRN, PCCN, and CEN. Ann has presented programs as diverse as advanced hemodynamics to best practice models for hospital corporations. Ann is a member of Sigma Theta Tau, the American Association of Critical-Care Nurses, the Society of Critical Care Medicine, and the Emergency Nurses Association. Ann also works as a consultant for educational program development and management training for healthcare facilities. She is currently the COO and Director of Clinical Applications for Pro Ed in Menifee, California.

KERI R. ROGELET, MSN, MBA/HCM, RN, CCRN

Keri has presented national programs for adult health issues, the Neonatal CCRN, Pediatric CCRN, and developmental care. Keri is a regional NRP trainer for the American Academy of Pediatrics and a lead instructor for the S.T.A.B.L.E. program. Keri's professional associations include Sigma Theta Tau, the American Association of Critical-Care Nurses, and the Academy of Neonatal Nurses. In addition, she works as a consultant for pediatric and neonatal product applications. She is currently the CFO and Director of Clinical Development for Pro Ed in Menifee, California.

CONTACT INFORMATION

Website: www.forproed.com
Email: proedcertify@yahoo.com

Contributor

MELISSA R. CHRISTIANSEN, MSN, RN, NP-C, CCRN, CNRN

Melissa has more than 23 years of experience as a critical care nurse in neurological, cardiac, and trauma ICUs. She is currently working as a family nurse practitioner in Southern California. Melissa has presented programs on neurological and neuroscience topics, adult critical care certification reviews, and courses in postanesthesia nursing. Melissa is a member of Sigma Theta Tau, the American Association of Critical-Care Nurses, the American Association of Neuroscience Nurses, and the American Academy of Nurse Practitioners. Melissa is also on the faculty for the BSN, MSN, and Nurse Practitioner programs at the University of Phoenix.

Reviewers

Mary A. Cowett, RN, RNC-BC
Riverside Community Hospital
Riverside, California

Susan Skelly, BSN, RN, CCRN
Palmetto Health Children's Hospital
Columbia, South Carolina

Acknowledgments

Mary Margaret Forsythe, RN, and Nancy O. Roberts, RN

Mary Margaret and Nancy were two instructors who were ultimate professionals and who believed in their students and the profession of nursing. These women were incredible individuals and will live in the hearts of hundreds of nurses. They passed before their time and are desperately missed.

Karen S. Ehrat, RN, PhD

Karen saw potential in a new grad and made education a joy and a privilege. Her untimely death stole a piece from every soul she touched.

Damien, Minerva, and M'Leah: Angels that taught me every life touches another and reminds me why I do what I do.

We are grateful to all the nurses who provided suggestions for content of this book. We are indebted to Melissa Christiansen for her dedication and long hours toward making this work a success. Thank you to the reviewers who gave their time, effort, and suggestions to enhance the content of this manuscript. We would also like to express our gratitude to the editorial and production staff at Jones & Bartlett Learning.

A.J.B. and K.R.R.

Preface

Congratulations! You are one step closer to achieving certification as a pediatric critical care nurse. Even if you plan to use this book as a study guide for pediatric critical care nursing, this will be an invaluable resource. This book will present an introduction to the Pediatric CCRN credential. We will guide you through the process of registering for the Pediatric CCRN exam and offer some test-taking strategies. We will even provide you with the resources you will need to complete the process.

This book contains test questions with rationales that will cover a broad range of topics and will be representative of the types of questions you will find on the actual examination. With this book purchase you will have access to an online version that allows you to create your own practice tests. The questions online will be randomly selected and will enable you to time yourself and practice as if you were taking the actual examination.

We are dedicated to helping you successfully pass this exam and achieve certification as a pediatric critical care nurse. Please feel free to contact us if you have any questions or you would like to schedule a Pediatric CCRN review course for your facility or group.

Ann and Keri

SECTION 1

The CCRN Credential

Traditionally, nurses have worked in a variety of roles and environments. For most of the twentieth century, by the time nurses graduated from their programs, they had spent many hours in clinical situations and were prepared to practice in any area. Nursing eventually had to adjust from the general practitioner to a nurse who would concentrate practice in one area. Nurses worked in emergency rooms, operating rooms, recovery rooms, obstetrics, and medical–surgical units. Only those nurses who worked in operating rooms or who administered anesthesia were considered specialized.

With the advent of emerging technology, the post–World War II population boom, and a trend toward increasingly more acute patients, nursing and hospitals adjusted by placing patients in more subspecialized areas.

One critical issue that arose in the twentieth century related to patients with poliomyelitis, who were increasing both in number and in special needs. The "iron lung" had been around for years. In the 1930s, the machine cost $1500, which was also the median cost for a home at that time. Patients who could afford such treatment began to recover, only to develop sequelae that required specialized care. Tilt beds and hot pack treatments were initiated to care for them. At one time, even curare was used to combat the severe muscle spasms suffered by polio victims. All of these treatments required time and resources, including larger numbers of nurses.

In 1931, the American Association of Nurse Anesthetist (no "s" on the end) formed. On June 4, 1945, the organization held the first-ever certification examination for a nursing specialty. In 1952, the first accredited program for nurse anesthetists was started.

In 1955, Jonas Salk announced the discovery of a vaccine for polio. The vaccine would help prevent spread of the disease, but thousands of victims still required care. Technology in general was improving and becoming more broadly available. Although the first EKG machines were available in the United States as early as 1909, they were not widely used until the late 1950s.

In the 1960s, many patients required around-the-clock specialized care that required resources and practitioners who were experts or who had a great deal of experience with the particular condition or disease process. Veterans of previous wars and the escalating Vietnam War required increasingly more medical resources. Hospitals began placing cardiac, trauma, burn, and acute medical patients in areas of the hospital designated as providing more "intensive" care. Patient survival rates improved, so the numbers of specialized areas increased.

In 1967, nurses from Nashville Baptist Hospital were frustrated at the lack of educational opportunities for continuing education for intensive care nurses, so they sent inquiries to other nurses to see if interest existed to form an association or some type of national association to provide education to other intensive care nurses. At that time, most of the ICUs served cardiac patients. A year later, more than 400 nurses attended a symposium and affirmed the need for an organization. In 1969, the American Association of Cardiovascular Nurses was formed. In 1971, the name was changed to the American Association of Critical-Care Nurses (AACN) in recognition of the broad area covered by critical care.

AACN is now the largest specialty nursing organization in the world. In 1975, the AACN Certification Corporation was established and began offering the CCRN examination.

We invite you to visit the AACN website at www.aacn.org to learn more about the CCRN credential. Thousands of nurses have successfully attained the CCRN credential, and we are here to help you become successful. The next section will explain the registration procedure for the examination. You can do it!

REFERENCES

http://www.aacn.org (accessed June 15, 2010).

http://www.aacn.org/AACN/mrkt.nsf/vwdoc/HistoryofAACN?opendocument (accessed July 19, 2010).

http://americanhistory.si.edu/polio/howpolio/index.htm (accessed July 20, 2010).

http://www.anesthesia-nursing.com/wina.html (accessed July 20, 2010).

Registering for the Pediatric CCRN Examination

The first thing you must do is determine if you are eligible for the exam. To be able to take the pediatric CCRN exam, you must not have any encumbrances on your current registered nursing license in any state—in other words, no restrictions, disciplinary actions, attached conditions, or provisions of any kind that would affect your ability to practice as a nurse. You need to have completed 1750 hours of direct bedside care for a critically ill pediatric patient population during the past 2 years. For you to qualify for the pediatric CCRN exam, all of your practice hours must involve care of pediatric patients. You may not split the hours between, say, a neonatal ICU and a pediatric ICU.

Of the 1750 hours of direct care, 875 hours must have been completed in the past year. If you are an educator, a CNS, or a manager, you can still qualify for the exam. If you directly supervise students or nurses at the bedside, you will qualify. You must, however, participate in the care of the patient. For example, if you demonstrate a procedure or supervise a nurse or student performing the procedure, that activity would be acceptable.

Nurses must have a certain level of experience to qualify for the CCRN exam. Many questions require integration of knowledge and critical thinking, and the test covers advanced concepts such as hemodynamics and ventilator management. It would be difficult, though not impossible, to pass the test if you have not had experience with either of these clinical situations.

Other questions test your familiarity with technology such as central lines and ECMO. Passing the test would certainly be easier if you have experience with this technology, but not every critical care area utilizes these therapies. For example, some nurses do not have direct experience with patients undergoing open heart surgery or neurosurgery. In such cases, the relevant concepts can be learned from reading appropriate critical care texts or by consulting another nurse with experience in the particular area. Nursing is a mobile profession, and quite often a person you work with may have experiences and qualifications unknown to you. Some nurses have the opportunity to work via registries or as travelers and have a wide base of experience. Other nurses will seek out new experiences within their own facility or work part time in other facilities. We are not trying to scare you. Thousands of nurses have passed this exam, and it is certainly feasible to do so even without experience in certain areas. Candidates for the CCRN come from various levels of pediatric ICUs.

To see what the CCRN exam covers, you can download a copy of the pediatric CCRN Test Plan from AACN at www.aacn.org. The test plan is an outline, or blueprint, of the major areas to be tested. The test plan also indicates the percentage of questions tested in that particular section or system. Specific conditions and pathophysiology to be tested are listed on the test plan, allowing you to better focus your study time and resources. In addition, a list of testable nursing actions is available with the test plan. You can obtain these materials and register for the exam and membership online at aacn.org.

When you sign up for the CCRN exam, you can sign up as either a member or a nonmember of AACN. The cost is lower if you are a member. You can join AACN at the time you register to receive the member discount. Just email us if you have any questions. After your documents are received by AACN, you must allow several weeks for processing. You will then be sent a postcard stating that, from that date, you will have 90 days to complete the exam.

Once you register for the exam, you will be provided with a list of examination locations near you, based on your ZIP code. The test is administered at Applied Measurement Professional (AMP) sites around the United States, and you may take the exam at any AMP testing center.

Your next step is to call the AMP testing center you select and make an appointment for the exam. The testing center will authorize the time and day when you will take the test. Visit the AACN website or the AMP website for updated information. Please note: You will be sent a specific authorization code to access the AMP website to register for the exam. Specific rules apply when you want to change an appointment, so make sure you have the most current information on this process.

The CCRN exam is now computer based and given year round. You may also take the CCRN exam the old-fashioned way, by pencil and paper. These written exams are given only a couple times a year and require special registrations and arrangements. Please contact AACN directly if you wish to test in this manner.

Remember, thousands of nurses have passed this examination and you can, too!

SECTION 2

Test-Taking Strategies

When preparing for the pediatric CCRN exam, the first thing to do is be absolutely honest with yourself about how you study. If you have good study habits and plenty of time, you are very fortunate. If you are a procrastinator, studying a little bit at a time might help. Nurses have to juggle so many roles that take up their time: parent, child, employee, student, teacher, and on and on. One of the biggest struggles is simply finding time and a place to study. Discovering your learning style will help you find a better way to absorb information.

Three types of learners are commonly identified: visual, auditory, and kinesthetic. There is no perfect strategy for learning, because every person is unique. Not everyone has a single style of learning; you may use a mix of styles depending on your situation.

Visual learners learn better from reading and writing than from hearing and talking about information. Background noise, such as music or television, is distracting to these types of learners. Finding a quiet space is a problem for some people. You may have to stay awake after family members have gone to bed. Flashcards often work and some people use colored markers to highlight important information.

Auditory learners learn information effectively by listening and talking. Playing music, listening to audiotapes, or being part of a study group often works.

Kinesthetic learners prefer to learn via a "hands-on" approach. Nurses often learn this way because we have to listen to lectures and then demonstrate skills. This approach focuses on the use of models, manikins, or patients, and works well for many healthcare providers. Kinesthetic people are often "antsy" and cannot sit still for long periods of time, so lectures may be difficult for them without frequent breaks. If you are a kinesthetic learner, some of the things that might help while studying include taking frequent breaks, walking around, or riding a stationary cycle.

No matter what your personal learning style, your test-taking skills can be improved.

How? Practice! That is why we wrote this book in a question-and-answer format. Keep practicing the questions until you can answer at least 80% correctly. Research has shown that two-thirds of study time should be spent taking sample tests, and only one-third of study time should be spent reviewing content.

Studying, like regular exercise, is good for the brain. As nurses, we must always keep abreast of the professional literature and spend time studying to keep our knowledge and skills up-to-date. In addition, many states require continuing education to renew a professional license. The CCRN requires 100 hours of continuing education to be obtained within a 3-year period. Anything worthwhile studying takes time, effort, and sacrifice.

There is no way around studying for this certification. There are no shortcuts!

If you have been out of school for a while, don't despair! It may be slow going at first, so take things a little at a time. Just like going to the gym, you should make a plan to study in one particular place and at the same time, if possible. This is your space and your time—claim it. Have all your books, tapes, and other study materials handy. If you need snack food, make sure it is not all sugar, and include some salty food. Caffeine tends to make people jittery, but if you need it, it may be right for you.

The pediatric CCRN Test Plan is a blueprint of the exam's content. The major sections are broken down into subheadings and topics. If you study only a little at a time, you will be fine. One day you may feel like studying cardiomyopathy; the next day, you may focus on chest tubes. You may download the current pediatric CCRN Test Plan from AACN at www.aacn.org. We did not include the test plan in this book because the exam changes frequently, and you should have a copy of the current information.

If you study with a group, you can save a lot of time and effort by breaking up the topics for that study period and having each person present his or her topic(s), and provide handouts and practice questions for the rest of the group. When you can make up a test question about a subject, you really will be prepared. Study for short periods of time—say, 30 to 45 minutes—and then take a break. Set small goals, and after you have accomplished each one, reward yourself!

EXAM CONTENT

The pediatric CCRN certification exam consists of 150 multiple-choice test questions. Twenty-five of those questions do not count; they are there to be validated. In other words, every question is tried first to see if it is written well and if a certain percentage of people answer it correctly. At this point in the process, a question can still be "tweaked" for use on future exams.

Your results are determined by how many answers you get correct. Some answers are a bit harder than others. The final score usually indicates a pass if you get at least 70% correct. If you do not know an answer, take your best guess, because you have at least a chance of guessing correctly. You get points only for questions answered correctly.

The test plan shows the breakdown of questions by topic and section. AACN uses the Synergy Model as a basis for practice. Here is the good news: There are no questions on the test that deal specifically with the terminology of the Synergy Model. Instead, the answers to questions are based on best practice that utilizes and synthesizes the Synergy Model.

STUDY TIPS

A multiple-choice test question consists of three parts: an introductory statement, a stem (question), and options, from which you must select the correct answer. The introductory statement provides information about a clinical issue, pathophysiology, or a nursing action or duty.

Stems are worded in different ways. Some stems are in the form of a question; others are in the form of an incomplete statement. Additionally, a stem will usually request one of two types of responses: a positive response or a negative response. More good news: The test was recently changed so that it does not include negative stem questions! This means stems such as "all of the following except" are no longer part of the exam. (The questions you will practice from in this book may have an occasional negative stem to facilitate learning.) More good news: There are no longer any multiple-multiple-choice questions on the exam!

Key words are important words or phrases that help focus your attention on what the question is asking. Examples of key words include *always, most, first response, earliest, priority, first, on admission, common, best, least, not, immediately,* and *initial.*

You should always be looking for a *therapeutic response.* The nurse is *always* therapeutic. In other words, your *initial response* as a nurse is *always* the therapeutic response—you must acknowledge and validate the patient's feelings. Communication skills learned in Nursing 101 are important components of successful test-taking strategies. More than one option may contain a therapeutic response. When in doubt, validate, validate, validate. Always validate the feelings before you present information. A medical emergency would, of course, take precedence.

Who is actually the focus of the question? You need to be able to identify this person.

Sometimes questions are asked about a friend, a relative, or a significant other instead of a patient. A lot of information in the question may be deliberately distracting. Also, you must, when applicable, validate that person's feelings first.

WHEN IN DOUBT

When answering questions, remember Maslow's hierarchy of needs and the ABCs (airway, breathing, circulation). When these goals are met, then safety is the priority. After safety, the psychological needs are a priority. Assessment always comes before diagnosis and treatment (intervention). Learning takes place only if the learner is motivated.

Eliminate incorrect options. This gives you a 50% chance of guessing the correct answer. Here are some hints:

- Select the most general, all-encompassing option.
- Eliminate similar options. If two options say essentially the same thing, then neither is correct. If three of the four options sound similar, choose the one that sounds different.
- Eliminate any options that contain the words "always" or "never."
- Look for the longest option. It is usually the correct answer.
- Watch for grammatical inconsistencies between the stem and options.

IT'S TIME TO TAKE YOUR CERTIFICATION EXAM!

Well, you are finally ready! The night before the exam, get a good night's sleep. Do not cram the night before, although that is easier said than done. Do something relaxing and enjoyable, such as going to a movie or out to dinner. Try to avoid caffeine or any other stimulant. Please let us know when you pass the exam so we may congratulate you.

REFERENCES

Kobel Lamonte, M. (2007). Test-taking strategies for CNOR certification. *Association of Operating Room Nurses: AORN Journal, 85*(2), 315–332.

Ludwig, C. (2004). Preparing for certification: Test-taking strategies. *Medsurg Nursing, 13*(2), 127–128.

PRACTICE QUESTIONS

The next sections will contain over 1,200 practice questions. The questions are written with four responses, like you will find on the CCRN examination.

Even though questions are divided into systems and issues, many topics will cross over to another section. For example, even though there is a section on endocrinology, you will find questions about endocrine problems in several sections.

The questions will have a variety of complexity. Some will be quite easy to answer, and some will be quite difficult to answer and require critical thinking and integration of practices. On occasion, we ask information previously covered within the context of another patient situation. We have included material on drug dosages and medications commonly in use at time of publication.

Keep practicing until you can routinely answer 80% of these questions correctly. At this point, you should be ready to take the certification examination.

SECTION 3

Cardiovascular

1. **Your pediatric patient has the following parameters**

   HR 80

   BP 100/60

   SV 40

   BSA 0.9 m^2

   The cardiac index (CI) for this patient is

   A. 4.4 L/min

   B. 3.2 L/min/m^2

   C. 3.5 L/min/m^2

   D. 3200 mL/m^2

2. **Calculate the cardiac output for a 16 year old patient with a heart rate of 72 and a stroke volume of 70 mL**

   A. 55%

   B. 5.04 L/min

   C. 504 mL/min

   D. 1.02 L/min

3. **What is the mean arterial pressure for a patient with a blood pressure of 110/50 and a heart rate of 80?**

   A. 80

   B. 70

   C. 50

   D. 60

4. **Which of the following percentages would be considered a normal value for an ejection fraction (EF)?**

   A. 25%

   B. 35%

   C. 40%

   D. 60%

5. **The ejection fraction (EF) most closely represents which of the following hemodynamic parameters?**

   A. RVEDP

   B. PAOP

   C. RVP

   D. LVEDP

6. **Tetralogy of Fallot manifests itself by which of the following combinations of defects?**
   A. VSD, overriding aorta, pulmonary stenosis, and right ventricular hypertrophy
   B. Aortic stenosis, atrial septal defect, coarctation of the aorta, and PDA
   C. ASD, mitral prolapse, PDA, and pulmonary stenosis
   D. Mitral stenosis, PDA, ASD, and coarctation of the aorta

7. **Which of the following statements is true about events that occur during a normal cardiac cycle?**
   A. Metabolism in the heart is unchanged during diastole
   B. Metabolism of the heart is decreased during diastole
   C. An increase in cardiac output increases diastole
   D. Diastole comprises about 40% of the cardiac cycle

8. **A reflex tachycardia caused by stretch of right atrial receptors is known as**
   A. The Herring-Sines law
   B. The Bainbridge reflex
   C. Starling's law
   D. The renin–angiotensin system

9. **Pressures in the left side of the heart and pulmonary filling pressures are represented by the**
   A. PAOP
   B. PAD
   C. CI
   D. SVR

10. **Your patient required placement of a left atrial pressure monitoring line. The pressure reads 18 mmHg. This value might indicate**
    A. Pulmonary embolus
    B. Pulmonic stenosis
    C. Tricuspid regurgitation
    D. Mitral valve dysfunction

11. **Which of the following statements is true regarding the fourth heart sound (S_4)?**
    A. S_4 occurs just after the first heart sound
    B. The fourth heart sound occurs with ventricular contraction
    C. The fourth heart sound is benign
    D. The fourth heart sound is always pathologic after 24 hours of life

12. **The mean pressure difference in the systemic vascular bed divided by blood flow is known as**
    A. LAP
    B. SVR
    C. PCW
    D. PVRI

13. **A heart murmur associated with acute valvular regurgitation is called**
    A. S_3
    B. S_2
    C. S_1
    D. S_4

14. **Stroke volume is comprised of which of the following factors?**
    A. Viscosity, blood volume, and impedance
    B. Cardiac output, heart rate, and compliance
    C. Contractility, preload, and afterload
    D. Systemic impedance, heart rate, and compliance

15. **Your patient was admitted for severe dyspnea, dysphagia, palpitations, and an intractable cough. On auscultation, you hear a loud S_1 and a right-sided S_3 and S_4. A pulmonary artery catheter is placed and large A waves are seen in the PAOP tracing. The patient probably has**
    A. Mitral stenosis
    B. Myocarditis
    C. Atrial stenosis
    D. Mitral insufficiency

16. **Patrick was admitted to the PICU with aortic insufficiency. During his initial assessment, you note the popliteal BP is higher than the brachial BP by at least 30 mmHg. This phenomenon is known as**
    A. DeRoge's sign
    B. Hill's sign
    C. Holmes' sign
    D. Rochelle's sign

17. **Pulsus alternans is most often noted with**
    A. Mitral stenosis
    B. Constrictive pericarditis
    C. Left ventricular failure
    D. Aortic stenosis

18. **Susan has been consuming large quantities of power drinks and has been having intermittent episodes of SVT. Today she was admitted to the PICU because she had a syncopal episode at school and requires therapy for the SVT. Which of the following medications is specific to the treatment of sustained supraventricular tachycardia?**
    A. Atropine
    B. Theophylline
    C. Amiodarone
    D. Adenosine

19. **Stimulation of the vasomotor center in the medulla occurs when the partial pressure of oxygen changes. This is initiated by**
    A. Chemoreceptors
    B. The Bainbridge reflex
    C. The Purkinje system
    D. Baroreceptors

20. **Symptoms of right-sided heart failure include**
    A. Orthopnea
    B. Elevated PAD and PAOP
    C. Hepatomegaly
    D. Pulmonary edema

21. **On an EKG, left-sided heart failure results in**
    A. Tall, peaked P waves
    B. Wide, notched P waves
    C. Changes in ST segments
    D. A prolonged Q wave

22. **Your patient has been diagnosed with an AV canal defect. Defects closely associated with this condition would be**
    A. ASD, PDA, ostium primum, a cleft in the anterior mitral valve leaflet, and a VSD in the inlet portion of the ventricle septum
    B. PDA, a cleft in the anterior mitral valve leaflet, pulmonary stenosis, and a cleft in the septal leaflet of the tricuspid valve
    C. ASD, a cleft in the anterior mitral valve leaflet, ostium primum, a VSD in the inlet portion of the ventricle septum, and a cleft in the septal leaflet of the tricuspid valve
    D. VSD, ostium secundum, mitral stenosis, and a cleft in the septal leaflet of the tricuspid valve

23. **A moderate-sized ventricular septal defect results in**
    A. A right-to-left shunt
    B. A left-to-right shunt
    C. Decreased systemic vascular resistance
    D. A decrease in pulmonary vascular edema

24. **Bobby, age 3, was admitted to the PICU to help control his increasing tet spells. Tet spells may be treated with which of the following medications?**
    A. Dilantin
    B. Gentamycin
    C. Morphine
    D. Digoxin

25. **The resistance against which the right ventricle must eject its volume is known as**
    A. SVR
    B. PVR
    C. PAOP
    D. LVEDP

26. Alpha-adrenergic effects of norepinephrine include
A. Increased force of myocardial contraction
B. Peripheral arteriolar vasoconstriction
C. Increased AV conduction time
D. Central venous vasodilation

27. While auscultating heart sounds on your new patient, you hear an S_3 heart sound. The third heart sound occurs as a result of
A. Active atrial contraction
B. Aortic stenosis
C. Closure of the aortic and pulmonic valves
D. Increased blood flow across the AV valves

28. Infants with CHF are at high risk during interventional procedures because of
A. Transcatheter defect occlusion
B. Prolonged testing times
C. Balloon atrial septostomy
D. Contrast dye

29. Intravenous hydralazine is incompatible with
A. Furosemide
B. Hydrocortisone
C. Potassium chloride
D. Heparin

30. If infiltration of a dopamine infusion occurs, the suggested treatment is to inject which of the following medications into the affected area?
A. Epinephrine
B. Phentolamine
C. Lidocaine
D. Atropine

31. Surgical management of hypoplastic left heart syndrome includes staged procedures. The second stage is a bidirectional Glenn procedure. Which of the following statements is true regarding this procedure?
A. A single right ventricle supplies systemic circulation after the procedure
B. The ductus is ligated and the pulmonary artery is divided
C. The superior vena cava is anastomosed to the right pulmonary artery
D. The ductus is left open until the third stage is completed

32. Which of the following heart defects would be classified as a cyanotic heart defect?
A. An atrial septal defect
B. Aortic valve stenosis
C. Coarctation of the aorta
D. Pulmonary atresia

33. **An example of an acyanotic congenital heart defect would be**
    A. Tricuspid stenosis
    B. Mitral stenosis
    C. Pulmonary valve stenosis
    D. Tetralogy of Fallot

34. **The type of heart murmur commonly heard in patients with tricuspid atresia is**
    A. A diastolic murmur
    B. A holosystolic murmur
    C. A systolic murmur
    D. A pansystolic murmur

35. **Which of the following hemodynamic changes will occur with cardiac tamponade?**
    A. Increased contractility
    B. Decreased heart rate
    C. Decreased stroke volume
    D. Increased cardiac output

36. **Your patient has developed diffuse chest pain and tachycardia. Upon auscultation, you hear muffled heart sounds and note an increased JVD. You suspect the patient has developed a cardiac tamponade. If your patient does have a cardiac tamponade, which of the following findings would you expect on a chest X-ray?**
    A. A dilated superior vena cava
    B. Pneumothorax
    C. Narrowed mediastinum
    D. Delineation of the pericardium and epicardium

37. **Beck's triad is a combination of symptoms useful in diagnosing tamponade. These symptoms include**
    A. Increased pulse pressure, increased JVD, and tachycardia
    B. Pericardial friction rub, hypertension, and RV failure
    C. LV failure, tachycardia, and hypertension
    D. Distended neck veins, muffled heart sounds, and hypotension

38. **During evaluation of CVP pressure monitoring, the c wave represents**
    A. Mechanical atrial diastole
    B. The decrease in RA volume during relaxation
    C. Emptying of the right atrium into the RV
    D. The increase in RA pressure from closure of the tricuspid valve

39. **When evaluating the CVP pressure waves, the v wave represents**
    A. Mechanical atrial diastole
    B. The increase in RA pressure from closure of the tricuspid valve
    C. Emptying of the right atrium into the RV
    D. The decrease in RA volume during relaxation

40. A low CVP reading may represent

A. Pulmonary hypertension
B. Increased contractility
C. Biventricular failure
D. Cardiac tamponade

41. A patient with tricuspid atresia may exhibit

A. Polycythemia
B. A smaller than normal heart
C. Sinus tachycardia
D. Small, inverted P waves

42. Quincke's sign is usually observed in patients who have a diagnosis of

A. Mitral stenosis
B. Endocarditis
C. Aortic insufficiency
D. Pericarditis

43. If the inferior wall of the heart is infarcted, the leads that will most directly reflect the injury are

A. I and aVL
B. II, III, and aVF
C. V_1–V_2
D. V_5–V_6

44. An anterior wall infarction may be seen in leads

A. V_4 and R
B. V_5–V_6
C. V_7–V_9
D. V_2–V_4

45. An example of a pansystolic murmur is

A. Pulmonic insufficiency
B. Tricuspid insufficiency
C. Atrial stenosis
D. Mitral stenosis

46. Increased afterload would be present in a patient with which of the following conditions?

A. Polycythemia
B. Aortic insufficiency
C. Hypovolemia
D. Sepsis

47. Roxanne had a pulmonary artery catheter placed. When a wedge pressure was initially obtained, large V waves were noted and the PAOP was 27. The probable cause of this reading is

A. Equipment malfunction
B. Left heart failure
C. Papillary muscle rupture
D. Right heart failure

48. A definitive diagnosis of myocarditis can be made via

A. Transmural catheterization
B. Transesophageal ultrasound
C. Transcutaneous ultrasound
D. Endomyocardial biopsy

49. Ebstein anomaly has been associated with maternal use of

A. Caffeine
B. Lithium
C. Cigarettes
D. Thalidomide

50. Twelve-lead EKG findings for a patient with Ebstein anomaly could include

A. Junctional tachycardia
B. Wenckebach phenomenon
C. Sinus rhythm with paroxysmal SVT
D. Prolonged PR intervals

51. Cardiac glycosides are often used in the treatment of Ebstein anomaly. A major effect of this class of medications is

A. Increased conductivity
B. Positive chronotropism
C. Its usefulness as a ventricular antiarrhythmic
D. Inotropism

52. Which of the heart valves is most rarely affected by infective endocarditis?

A. Tricuspid
B. Pulmonic
C. Mitral
D. Aortic

53. Francine, age 13, has been experimenting with multiple drugs. She was admitted to your PICU after a cocaine overdose. Francine has had an anterolateral myocardial infarction. Where do you expect to see changes on the 12-lead EKG?

A. V_1, V_2, I, and AVL
B. V_2, V_3, V_4, I, and AVL
C. V_2, V_3, V_4, II, III, and AVF
D. V_1, V_2, II, III, and AVF

54. What do abnormal Q waves signify on a 12-lead EKG?

A. Partial-thickness death of myocardium
B. Complete thickness infarction of myocardium
C. They are of no significance
D. Repolarization of the myocardium

55. Which of the following drugs contains a high concentration of iodine?

A. Lidocaine
B. Amiodarone
C. Aminophylline
D. Digoxin

56. Milrinone lactate exerts which of the following actions?

A. Decreased cardiac contractility
B. Decreased PVR
C. Increased SVR
D. Potentiation of cyclic AMP

57. Which of the following drugs would be used for a hypercyanotic spell often seen with tetralogy of Fallot?

A. Digoxin
B. Epinephrine
C. Norepinephrine
D. Neo-Synephrine

58. An infant was born at 39 weeks gestation via cesarean section because of persistent fetal tachycardia. At day 2 of life, severe tachypnea developed. Blood cultures were obtained and all labs were normal. The tachypnea resolved. The infant was discharged home on day 4 of life. That evening, the infant became apneic and bradycardic and was admitted to the PICU. Antibiotics were started. The next morning, the infant developed a fever, DIC, jaundice, slight hepatomegaly, and hepatitis. Labs showed high numbers of bands and an elevated platelet count. A diagnosis of myocarditis was made. A likely causative agent for this condition is

A. Group B *Streptococcus*
B. *Escherichia coli*
C. Coxsackie B1 virus
D. Halothane toxicity

59. Right ventricular afterload may be reduced by

A. A hypoxic state
B. Hypoventilation
C. Inhaled nitric oxide
D. Administration of epinephrine

60. Mast cell degranulation with resultant histamine release and vasodilation would be an appropriate definition of

A. Septic shock
B. A pleural effusion
C. Anaphylaxis
D. MODS

61. **Systemic inflammatory response syndrome (SIRS) can best be defined as**
    A. Sepsis with cardiovascular failure
    B. Sepsis with accompanying organ failure
    C. Tachycardia or tachypnea with a fever
    D. Systemic organ dysfunction

62. **Sandra is a cheerleader at her middle school. Today Sandra was admitted for increased exercise intolerance, syncope, severe edema, dyspnea at rest, and decreased LOC. A pulmonary artery catheter was placed and the following pressures were obtained: RAP = 20, PA = 65/32, RV = 64/28, PAOP = 13. You would suspect Sandra is suffering from**
    A. Cardiac tamponade
    B. Pulmonary hypertension
    C. A pulmonary embolus
    D. Congestive heart failure

63. **Sharon and her family just returned from a vacation in Europe. Sharon has been complaining to her parents about leg cramping for the past three days. Her pediatrician admitted her to the hospital two days ago for management of a deep vein thrombosis. During your initial assessment this morning, you found Sharon sitting on the side of the bed and leaning forward. She states that this position relieved her newly developed chest pain. She also states that the pain is worse on inspiration. You notify the physician, who orders a CXR and lab work. The sed rate and WBCs are elevated. Sharon most likely is suffering from**
    A. A thoracic aneurysm
    B. Pericarditis
    C. Pulmonary hypertension
    D. A pulmonary embolus

64. **Theo received 3 mg of morphine IV. He is now unresponsive and his respiratory rate and depth are diminished. The antagonist for morphine is**
    A. Naloxone
    B. Atropine
    C. Regitine
    D. Bicarbonate

65. **Which of the following medications should be monitored for cyanide toxicity and avoided in patients with renal problems?**
    A. Propranolol
    B. Sodium nitroprusside
    C. Dopamine
    D. Verapamil

66. **Julie is 15 years old and just gave birth to Charlie. Julie has lupus, so Charlie is at risk for cardiomyopathy and**
    A. Myocarditis
    B. Blisters on the skin
    C. Congenital heart block
    D. Weight gain

67. Adverse effects of procainamide include

A. Depression of the excitability of cardiac muscle
B. Junctional tachycardia
C. Slowing conduction in the atria
D. Severe hypotension

68. Which of the following statements is true about pericardial effusion?

A. Diastolic filling is increased
B. On CXR, a "water bottle" silhouette is noted
C. The voltage of the QRS complex is increased
D. This is a painless, hard to diagnose condition

69. Which of the following pulmonary artery pressures would be considered in the normal range for a 14 year old?

A. PAP = 40/24, PAOP = 15
B. PAP = 14/8, PAOP = 4
C. PAP = 24/12, PAOP = 9
D. PAP = 36/30, PAOP = 22

70. You are mentoring a new nurse in the PICU. The patient you will be caring for is receiving lidocaine via a continuous infusion. The new PICU nurse must know that lidocaine may cause adverse effects such as

A. Hyperexcitability
B. CNS toxicity
C. Ventricular tachycardia
D. Premature atrial complexes

71. Jane is 9 years old and has a PAOP (PCWP) of 4. She is restless and mildly tachycardic. Absent any specific cardiac issue, you anticipate which of the following interventions?

A. Administration of an inotrope
B. Volume replacement
C. Administration of a vasoconstrictor to increase afterload
D. Administration of nitroprusside to decrease preload

72. Micah is a 15 year old Jehovah's Witness who has just undergone a cardiac surgical procedure. His Hgb and Hct are falling and are now Hgb 6.5 and the Hct 24. Micah's chest tubes have drained 960 mL in the last four hours. The anticipated treatment would be to

A. Administer 500 cc of albumin
B. Administer one unit of type specific whole blood
C. Administer 250 mL of fresh frozen plasma
D. Administer continuous circuit autotransfusion

73. Stimulation of the right vagus nerve in turn stimulates the

A. Sinoatrial (SA) node
B. Mandibular branch of the trigeminal nerve
C. Acetylcholine reabsorption
D. Chemoreceptors in the carotid arch

74. If a $beta_2$ receptor in the heart is stimulated, it may cause

A. A reflex bradycardia
B. Arterial vasoconstriction
C. Bronchodilation
D. Increased SVR

75. Nick was admitted to the PICU with cough, fever, chills, anorexia, malaise, and headache. He currently has a pericardial friction rub and has a history of rheumatic fever. While examining Nick, you note fine, dark lines in his nail beds and some flat lesions on his palms. These flat lesions are known as

A. Janeway lesions
B. Osler's nodes
C. Roth spots
D. Pella's sign

76. Fiona is 8 years old and is in cardiogenic shock. At this time she is awaiting placement of an intra-aortic balloon pump. In any patient with cardiogenic shock, an undesirable outcome would produce

A. Increased cardiac output
B. Increased systemic vascular resistance
C. Decreased ventricular preload
D. Decreased pulmonary artery pressures

77. Jayden was diagnosed with left ventricular failure. Early signs of left ventricular failure are

A. Hypoxemia and peripheral cyanosis
B. Tachypnea and tachycardia
C. Dyspnea and profuse sweating
D. Central cyanosis and paradoxical respirations

78. Cyanotic heart defects may cause cyanosis of the skin, mucous membranes, and nail beds that can occur when deoxygenated hemoglobin is present within the circulation. This cyanosis may be observed when which of the following levels of deoxygenated hemoglobin is reached?

A. 5 g/100 mL
B. 50 g/500 mL
C. 50 g/250 mL
D. 15 g/200 mL

79. Which of the following statements is true about lidocaine?

A. Lidocaine may cause hypotension
B. Lidocaine administration may cause a moderate gastrointestinal intolerance
C. Lidocaine does not impair normal contractility
D. Lidocaine can cause nystagmus

80. Calcium channel blockers act primarily on

A. Serotonin uptake
B. Arteriolar tissue
C. Lung receptors only
D. Reduction of cardiac output

81. You have been selected to present a cardiac assessment class at your facility. You are asked the location of the PMI in an infant. As a PICU nurse, you know newborns and infants usually demonstrate right ventricular dominance. The location of the PMI in this case would be

A. At the lower left sternal border
B. At the right midclavicular line
C. At the second right intercostal space
D. At the right lower sternal border

82. The S_2 heart sound is created by

A. Opening of the aortic and mitral valves
B. Closure of the pulmonic and aortic valves
C. Opening of the pulmonic and mitral valves
D. Closure of the pulmonic and tricuspid valves

83. Regurgitation systolic murmurs are associated with

A. Aortic stenosis
B. Pulmonic valve disease
C. Ventricular septal defects
D. Atrial septal defects

84. Mariah has been diagnosed with acquired valvular heart disease. The primary cause of acquired valvular heart disease is

A. Heredity
B. Drug abuse
C. Rheumatic fever
D. Fetal alcohol syndrome

85. Indications for use of a ventricular assist device include

A. Extensive organ damage
B. As destination therapy
C. Prolonged cardiac arrest
D. Dysrhythmias

86. The most commonly used type of ventricular assist device used is the

A. RVAD
B. VAD
C. BIVAD
D. LVAD

87. The most common infection in patients with a ventricular assist device is

A. Septicemia
B. Pericarditis
C. Pneumonia
D. Pericardial effusion

88. In patients with normal cardiac anatomy, right atrial pressure equals

A. Right ventricular end diastolic pressure
B. Left atrial pressure
C. Right ventricular systolic pressure
D. Right ventricular diastolic pressure

89. Gretchen was diagnosed with refractive SVT that did not respond to either adenosine or cardioversion. She was admitted to your PICU for monitoring prior to ablation therapy. Tachyarrhythmias that are refractive to conventional therapies may have to be treated with radio-frequency ablation. This treatment is usually successful on reentry tachyarrhythmias. The radio-frequency destroys myocardial tissue via

A. Radiation
B. Heat
C. Cold
D. An overriding signal to ablate the pacemaker

90. Michael is 4 years old and was sent home from kindergarten because of dyspnea. His physician discovered a heart murmur and admitted Michael to the PICU. Michael required a pulmonary artery catheter placement to help monitor fluid and oxygenation. While the catheter was being inserted, blood gas samples were obtained from the right atrium (O_2 sat 75%), right ventricle (92%), and pulmonary artery (92%). These results probably indicate

A. Pericarditis
B. A monitor or catheter malfunction
C. A ventricular septal defect
D. Pneumonia

91. Mary has Wolff-Parkinson-White syndrome. She has been having increasing bouts of tachycardia over the past few weeks. Mary's cardiologist has decided to utilize overdrive pacing. How do you explain this type of pacemaker to a new orientee you are precepting in the PICU?

A. The pacemaker or AICD is set on demand mode and is asynchronous
B. The pacemaker is set at a constant rate of 80 bpm and is synchronized
C. The pacemaker or AICD is set on demand mode and is synchronous
D. The pacemaker or AICD is set on inhibit mode and is synchronous

92. Which type of pacemaker/AICD program code would you expect for a patient with complete heart block?

A. VVT
B. DDI
C. VVI
D. DDD

93. Skyler has had an AICD for 8 months. He has been admitted to the pediatric intensive care unit for a syncopal episode during school today. You note that his pulse is very irregular and he is complaining of getting "zapped" often. Skyler says he is exhausted from the repeated shocks and asks for pain medication. His EKG shows sinus bradycardia with numerous pacemaker spikes. As a PICU nurse, you suspect

A. Skyler's AICD has a faulty lead
B. Skyler has been in the proximity of a large magnetic field
C. The battery in Skyler's AICD is losing power
D. Skyler has a generator failure of his AICD

94. Troy had a DDD pacemaker inserted 3 years ago. His schoolwork has been declining and he has not been participating in activities with his friends. He has been admitted for pacemaker syndrome. Which symptoms do you expect to see with this condition?

A. Fatigue, agitation, and forgetfulness
B. Fatigue, dizziness, and confusion
C. Fatigue, agitation, and dyspnea
D. Fatigue, dizziness, and syncope

95. Mort is 14 years old and took his brother's motorcycle out for a ride. Mort lost control of the motorcycle in the rain. He was wearing a helmet and protective gear. Mort suffered a fractured left femur, left flail chest, a cervical sprain, and road rash on his face and neck. He is admitted with a blood pressure of 82/42, HR 102, RR 26 and shallow, and T 98.2 °F. His 12-lead EKG shows ST elevation in the anterior leads. His CXR shows a normal cardiac silhouette and no infiltrates. His Hgb is 9.0, Hct is 31. MB is 18%. Mort is restless and complains of pain in his chest and left leg. He is probably suffering from

A. Pulmonary edema
B. Hypovolemic shock
C. Systolic dysfunction
D. Pulmonary hypertension

96. What are the most valuable pieces of information evaluated with a 12-lead EKG?

A. Rate, rhythm, and arrhythmias
B. Rate, rhythm, axis, hypertrophy, and infarction
C. Rate, arrhythmias, and infarction
D. Rate, bundle branch block, and hypertrophy

97. On an EKG, leads V_1 and V_2 indicate which of the following types of bundle branch block?

A. Right
B. Left
C. Dual bundle
D. V_1 and V_2 do not show bundle branch blocks

98. Monica has an arterial line and is being mechanically ventilated. You note very pronounced phasic variations in the arterial line and suspect that

A. Monica's ETT is becoming dislodged
B. Monica has tricuspid regurgitation
C. Monica is suffering from heart failure
D. Monica's arterial line is kinked

99. In patients with normal cardiac anatomy, pulmonary artery wedge pressure equals

A. Aortic stenosis
B. RVEDP
C. Pulmonary artery occlusion pressure
D. Central venous pressure

100. Monte returned from cardiac surgery for a mitral valve dysfunction 2 hours ago. A pulmonary artery catheter was placed during surgery. Initial pulmonary artery wedge pressures have been holding at 8–12 mmHg. Over the past 15 minutes, the PAOP acutely rose to 24–26 mmHg. This rise in pressure probably indicates

A. Misplaced mediastinal wires
B. Postpericardial effusions
C. Impending right heart failure
D. A tension pneumothorax

101. Kent is an 8 year old with Wolff-Parkinson-White syndrome. He was admitted via the emergency room in SVT and treated x1 with adenosine. He is admitted to the PICU because he may need to receive additional doses of adenosine. Which of the following foods should Kent avoid when receiving adenosine?

A. Broccoli
B. Apple juice
C. Cola
D. Pineapple

102. You are preparing to give adenosine to a 3 year old in SVT. It is important that adenosine be given rapidly. Why?

A. If given slowly, the adenosine will probably fail to convert the SVT
B. Adenosine is incompatible with adrenalin
C. If given slowly, adenosine may cause systemic vasodilation and reflex tachycardia
D. If given slowly, adenosine may cause blurred vision

103. Nifedipine is classified as a

A. Calcium channel blocker
B. Beta blocker
C. MAO inhibitor
D. Catecholamine

104. Dobutamine is used to improve cardiac output primarily by

A. Causing profound peripheral vasodilation
B. Acting on alpha-adrenergic receptors in the heart
C. Acting on $beta_1$-adrenergic receptors in the heart
D. Acting on both alpha- and beta-adrenergic receptors in the cardiovascular tissue

105. Your 10 year old patient is in decompensated shock. You have dobutamine infusing via a peripheral IV line with TPN and intralipids. You have just received an order to give sodium bicarbonate intravenously and to give ampicillin intravenously as well. As a PICU nurse, you know the most appropriate actions to take would be to

A. Stop the intralipids and infuse the sodium bicarbonate while waiting for the pharmacy to send the ampicillin
B. Start a peripheral heparin lock to infuse the sodium bicarbonate and follow with the ampicillin infusion
C. Ask the physician to place a central line or PICC line for additional venous access ports
D. Piggyback the ampicillin on the main IV line and start another peripheral line on the other arm

106. Your patient has been on dobutamine for blood pressure support three days. Which of the following lab results should you monitor closely for life-threatening effects from the dobutamine?

A. Calcium levels
B. Potassium levels
C. Magnesium levels
D. Chloride levels

107. You are admitting a 6 year old to the PICU with suspected sepsis. His blood pressure is 72/54, heart rate is 140, respiratory rate is 20, and O_2 saturation is 82% in room air. Prior to initiating an infusion of dopamine, which of the following actions is a priority for the nurse?

A. Obtain consent for placement of a central line from the parents
B. Prepare to infuse dobutamine and dopamine together
C. Verify the number of isotonic crystalloid boluses given in the ED
D. Ensure phentolamine mesylate is available at the bedside

108. You are mentoring a new nurse in the PICU who is caring for a 4 year old receiving a dopamine drip. The order is to titrate the dopamine to keep the systolic blood pressure greater than 68 mmHg. You note that the nurse is titrating the drip every 2–3 minutes. You should

A. Praise the nurse for her diligence
B. Verify the order for systolic blood pressure, because it should be > 80 mmHg for a 4 year old
C. Contact the physician for a new blood pressure order because 78 mmHg may be too high for the patient's age
D. Advise the nurse to wait at least 5 minutes between titrations

109. High-dose epinephrine was started for your 7 year old patient post cardiac arrest due to beta blocker overdose. Which of the following lab results should you monitor closely?

A. Glucose levels
B. Calcium levels
C. Chloride levels
D. Sodium levels

110. Heather has asthma and is in decompensated shock. You are preparing to begin vasoactive support. Which of the following is the most appropriate vasoactive drug of choice in this case?

A. Isuprel
B. Dopamine
C. Vasopressin
D. Neo-Synephrine

111. Vasopressin was started for your 12 year old patient who is suffering from diabetes insipidus. Which of the following side effects warrants immediate intervention?

A. Unexplained weight loss
B. Hyperactivity
C. Abdominal cramping
D. Confusion

112. Adam is a 10 year old patient with severe hypotension. Norepinephrine bitartrate (Levophed) is infusing via his central line. Which of the following orders should you question?

A. Monitor blood pressure every 30 minutes
B. Administer with dopamine
C. Dilute in D_5W
D. Titrate off over a period of 6 to 24 hours

113. Emma is a 2 year old with tetralogy of Fallot. She has phenylephrine hydrochloride infusing via a central line. You note that her systolic blood pressure is 100 mmHg and heart rate has been steadily decreasing and is now 65. As a PICU nurse, you should take which of the following actions?

A. Increase the titration because her blood pressure is too low
B. Call the physician and prepare to stop the infusion
C. Administer atropine to increase her heart rate
D. Provide additional oxygen and continue to monitor

114. Harry is a 5 year old patient who was started on digoxin for paroxysmal atrial tachycardia. He will be going home today, where he will continue taking the digoxin. What would you teach the parents regarding the safe administration of this drug?

A. Contact the physician immediately if Harry experiences an increase in appetite
B. It is acceptable to use a regular teaspoon to administer liquid digoxin at home
C. Have Harry's parents return demonstrate how to take a pulse and withhold the drug for any heart rate under 80
D. Stress the importance of taking digoxin at the same time each day and not doubling up on any doses if a dose is skipped

115. Atropine was given to Marco, 8 years old, during an episode of bradycardia that resulted in a heart rate in the 20s. Marco had just been deeply suctioned. The low heart rate was unresponsive to oxygen support, so assisted ventilation via a bag-valve mask was provided. Marco's heart rate improved to prebradycardic levels. Which of the following potential complications of atropine administration may now occur?

A. Diuresis
B. Hypertension
C. Rebound bradycardia
D. Headache

116. Jose is a 16 year old football player who was brought to the hospital with chest pain. The EKG monitor now reveals PVCs and runs of tachycardia. Lidocaine is ordered. Which of the following symptoms of lidocaine toxicity requires immediate intervention?

A. A respiratory rate of 7
B. A narrowing QRS
C. A heart rate of 70
D. Hypertonicity

117. Maria is a 6 month old admitted for recurring SVT due to Wolff-Parkinson-White syndrome. She was started on procainamide five days ago and has had no episodes of SVT during that time. While assisting the parents with feeding, you notice Maria's heart rate suddenly increase to 300 and she becomes irritable and restless. Adenosine is given, and her rhythm converts back to her baseline rhythm. Twelve hours later, she goes into SVT again and is converted with adenosine. What is the probable explanation for Maria's repeated dysrhythmias after successful treatment for five days?

A. Maria is developing a tolerance to the procainamide
B. Maria was vagally stimulated during the feeding
C. Maria needs to have her dosage adjusted for weight gain
D. Maria's Wolff-Parkinson-White syndrome is getting worse

118. Dominick is receiving propranolol IV for SVT and hypertension. Which of the following are life-threatening side effects of propranolol administration?

A. Laryngospasm and bronchospasm
B. Complete heart block and dizziness
C. Respiratory depression and cardiovascular collapse
D. Polymorphic VT and dyspnea

119. Brian was started on esmolol for severe hypertension refractive to other drug regimens. Esmolol is incompatible with which of the following medications?

A. Cimetidine
B. Furosemide
C. Penicillin G potassium
D. Midazolam

120. The chest radiograph for a 4 month old infant shows enlargement of the right atrium, right ventricle, and pulmonary artery. The heart also exhibits a "snow-man" appearance. These findings are indicative of

A. A cardiac effusion
B. Aspiration pneumonitis
C. Total anomalous pulmonary venous return
D. An atrial septal defect

121. Which of the following places the patient at an increased risk for an allergic reaction to protamine sulfate?

A. Influenza vaccine
B. Type 2 diabetes
C. A history of PKU
D. Allergy to fish

122. Your patient has been scheduled for a modified Blalock-Taussig shunt. This procedure will connect

A. The superior vena cava and pulmonary artery
B. The subclavian and pulmonary arteries
C. The aorta and pulmonary artery
D. The subclavian artery and aorta

123. Severe cyanosis usually occurs with

A. Atrial septal defects
B. Patent ductus arteriosus
C. Tricuspid atresia
D. A left to right shunt

124. What are some common reasons for pacemaker insertion?

A. Tachycardia, Wenckebach phenomenon, and bradycardia
B. Symptomatic bradycardia, overdrive pacing, and acute MI with sinus dysfunction
C. Complete heart block, Wenckebach phenomenon, and tachycardia
D. Bundle branch block, Wenckebach phenomenon, and tachycardia

125. Alpha-adrenergic effects of norepinephrine include

A. Peripheral arteriolar vasoconstriction
B. Increased SA node firing
C. Norepinephrine has only beta-adrenergic effects
D. Increased force of myocardial contraction

126. Treatment for malignant hyperthermia consists of the administration of

A. Dantrolene sodium
B. Regitine
C. Opioids
D. Calcium chloride

127. Right-sided congestive heart failure signs and symptoms include

A. Respiratory distress and hepatomegaly
B. Rapid capillary refill and absent jugular venous distention
C. Weak femoral pulses and abdominal tenderness
D. Increased SVR and strong femoral pulses

128. Quinidine and hypomagnesemia can both lead to which of the following conditions?

A. Monomorphic ventricular tachycardia
B. Torsades de pointes
C. Ventricular fibrillation
D. Atrial tachycardia

129. Why is Lasix given slowly?

A. Lasix may cause nausea
B. A rash may develop
C. Hyperkalemia may occur
D. A rapid infusion can lead to hearing loss

130. Calcium channel blockers act primarily on

A. Arteries to arterioles
B. Reduction of cardiac output
C. Lung receptors only
D. Arterioles to capillaries

131. The type of echocardiography that shows the quantity of flow across an obstruction is called

A. Two-dimensional echocardiography
B. Continuous-wave Doppler echocardiography
C. M-mode echocardiography
D. Contrast echocardiography

132. The type of echocardiography used to evaluate the motion of the cardiac valves and detect pericardial fluid is ____________ echocardiography

A. M-mode
B. Two-dimensional
C. Contrast
D. Continuous-wave Doppler

133. Your patient is 14 years old and is being discharged home following treatment for a pulmonary embolus. He will continue to take anticoagulant therapy after his discharge. You are reinforcing previous teaching about his medication. The patient takes numerous herbal remedies daily. Which ones should he avoid while he is taking an anticoagulant?

A. Dong quai, gingko biloba, and ginseng
B. Aloe extract, bilberry, and broccoli
C. Calendula, clove, and allspice
D. Fenugreek, licorice, and leeks

134. A potential complication with the high-contrast media used for cardiac catheterizations is

A. Hypoglycemia
B. A high sodium content
C. Polycythemia
D. Seizures

135. Joseph is a 10 year old with recurrent VT who was started on intravenous amiodarone today. Which of the following signs should the nurse monitor closely during administration of the initial loading dose?

A. Urine output and parathyroid levels
B. Urine output and liver function tests
C. Thyroid levels and hypertonicity
D. Observe for greenish discoloration of the skin and monitor thyroid levels

136. Clara is a 7 year old with SVT. She will be discharged today with amiodarone to control her SVT. Which of the following discharge instructions is appropriate?

A. Continue normal outside activities without restrictions
B. Continue the original theophylline regimen
C. Avoid grapefruit
D. Dark urine is normal during the first three months of treatment

137. Which of the following medications is contraindicated for use in children younger than 1 year of age?

A. Verapamil
B. Adenosine
C. Procainamide
D. Esmolol

138. Isoptin was ordered for a 4 year old who is suffering from paroxysmal atrial tachycardia. Which of the following medications should be kept at bedside to mitigate the possible side effect of hypotension?

A. Potassium
B. Normal saline
C. Regitine
D. Calcium chloride

139. In addition to heart rate and urine output, which of the following laboratory values should be monitored closely for a patient taking diazoxide and furosemide for hypertension?

A. Glucose levels
B. Bilirubin levels
C. Calcium levels
D. Copper levels

140. Erik is a 15 year old admitted to the PICU for treatment of chest pain and severe hypertension. A nitroglycerin drip was ordered. Which of the following statements is true regarding nitroglycerin administration?

A. Use polyvinyl chloride tubing
B. Nitroglycerin may be piggybacked to Isolyte P
C. Nitroglycerin should be filtered prior to delivery
D. Have normal saline or other volume expander available at the bedside

141. Alisa was born at home 2 weeks ago with a midwife in attendance. She presented to the PICU with respiratory distress, crackles, edema, hepatomegaly, JVD, and a soft systolic murmur at the left sternal border. Over the last week, she has had poor intake and does not cry. Alisa is cyanotic, tachypneic, and tachycardic. As a PICU nurse, which of the following orders would you anticipate receiving?

A. Administer three boluses of normal saline at 20 mL/kg over 5 minutes each
B. Administer prostaglandin E_1
C. Administer PGE_2 intravenously
D. Start a dopamine infusion

142. You are teaching 9 year old Kayla and her parents about her Coumadin (warfarin) therapy. Part of your teaching must include foods to avoid. Which of the following should be avoided?

A. Broccoli, soybean oil, and spinach
B. Olive oil, peanut butter, and kale
C. Avocado, broccoli, and peas
D. Broccoli, green beans, and spinach

143. Luis is an 11 year old patient with a history of type 2 diabetes. He was admitted for multiple syncopal episodes, dyspnea, and tachycardia. A pulmonary artery catheter was placed and the following pressures obtained: wedge pressure (PAOP) of 20 mmHg, pulmonary artery pressure of 52/22 mmHg and a right atrial pressure (RAP) of 4 mmHg. The least likely diagnostic possibility would be

A. Pulmonary embolism
B. Aortic stenosis
C. Mitral regurgitation
D. Aortic insufficiency

144. A complete obstruction of the pulmonic valve resulting in a hypoplastic right ventricle and tricuspid valve is the definition of

A. Pulmonary embolus
B. Pulmonary stenosis
C. Persistent pulmonary hypertension
D. Pulmonary atresia

145. **Steven had a pulmonary artery catheter placed because he was being evaluated for lung function. His initial readings show a wedge pressure of 7 mmHg, pulmonary artery pressure of 40/12 mmHg and right atrial pressure of 19 mmHg. The cardiac index is 2.0 L/min/m^2. Which of the following conditions would be the least likely cause of these symptoms?**
   A. Pulmonary stenosis
   B. Right ventricular dysfunction
   C. Right ventricular infarction
   D. LAD obstruction

146. **Gregory, age 7, had a coronary bypass procedure and was admitted to the PICU approximately an hour ago. On admission, he was borderline ST with PVCs, for which he is receiving potassium replacement. His art line BP is 106/70, cuff correlated, PAD 12 mmHg, and RAP 6 mmHg. His mediastinal tubes have ceased draining, the PAOP has increased to 20 mmHg, and the RAP is now 14 mmHg. His heart rate is 92 with isolated PVCs and the art line BP is 124/72. The changes in his cardiac index are negligible. The most likely cause of these changes is**
   A. Pericardial tamponade
   B. A change in the transducer position or level
   C. Tension pneumothorax
   D. Increased auto-PEEP

147. **You are attempting to use a pulmonary artery wedge pressure (PAWP) to estimate the LVEDP. Which of the following conditions might make this measurement more difficult?**
   A. Mitral regurgitation
   B. Aortic stenosis
   C. A heart rate of 160
   D. Tricuspid regurgitation

148. **The most common new-onset dysrhythmia seen in a patient with a diagnosis of pulmonary edema is**
   A. Paroxysmal atrial tachycardia
   B. Supraventricular tachycardia
   C. Sinus rhythm with a RBBB
   D. Atrial fibrillation

149. **Simone will be having an LVAD placed this evening. She will be cared for in your unit. Family members are quite anxious to learn more about the device and to participate in the patient's care. An important point when teaching caregivers is to make certain they understand which changes in the patient's condition should be reported immediately to the staff. A complication that should be reported immediately would be**
   A. Irritation or redness at the incision site
   B. A temperature of 100.6 °F
   C. A rise in blood pressure over 10 mmHg
   D. Any change in the mentation of the patient

150. **Matthew is 6 years old and was seen in the ED after falling from the monkey bars while at school. He sustained a fractured left tibia and fibula and a fractured left clavicle. Matthew required a splenectomy and was just admitted to your care. Your initial assessment results are as follows:**

EKG: ST at 110 with isolated PVCs
Art line BP 70/50
Cuff BP 76/50
Skin pale, cool, clammy
RR 26, breath sounds clear, slightly diminished RLL
O_2 2 L/min via NC
Mentation: responds to questions slowly, oriented to self and time
Pulmonary artery catheter readings:
PAP 24/8
PAOP 5
RAP 4
Cardiac output 3.3
Cardiac index 1.7

Which of the following conditions do you believe Matthew is developing?

A. Cardiogenic shock
B. Hypovolemic shock
C. Septic shock
D. Left ventricular failure

151. **Jeffrey is a 14 year old freshman football player. When he returned home from school this afternoon, he was short of breath and overly fatigued. His mother mentioned that his ankles were quite swollen at that time. Jeffrey uncharacteristically went to bed; when his mother could not arouse him, she called paramedics. Jeffrey arrived in your PICU approximately 30 minutes ago. He is being mechanically ventilated at TV 650, FiO_2 .80, and AMV 14. He remains unresponsive. A pulmonary artery catheter was placed. His assessment findings are as follows:**

EKG: ST at 124
Art line BP 68/42
Cuff BP 64/46
Doppler only to dorsalis pedis, no pressure obtained
Skin pale, cool, clammy
RR 15, breath sounds = crackles LLL, RLL
Marked pretibial and pedal edema
Mentation: unresponsive to painful stimuli
Pulmonary artery catheter readings:
PAP 46/28
PAOP 26
RAP 18
Cardiac output 3.2
Cardiac index 1.2

Jeffrey is probably developing

A. Pulmonary hypertension
B. Cardiac tamponade
C. Cardiogenic shock
D. Right heart failure

152. **Which of the following is an end effect of CHF?**
A. Atrial fibrillation
B. Increased renal perfusion
C. Pulmonary venous shrinkage
D. Systemic venous engorgement

153. **Diuretics are used in the treatment of CHF. A diuretic that reduces urinary calcium losses is**
A. Diamox
B. Chlorothiazide
C. Furosemide
D. Spironolactone

154. **Aida was initially admitted to your PICU with a diagnosis of congestive heart failure. After further study, it was determined that she has restrictive cardiomyopathy. A common cause of restrictive cardiomyopathy is**
A. Unknown viral infection
B. Glycogen storage disease
C. History of diabetes
D. Unknown

155. **The type of cardiomyopathy that is characterized by replacement of normal cells with fatty tissue is known as**
A. Restrictive cardiomyopathy
B. Hypertrophic cardiomyopathy
C. Arrhythmogenic cardiomyopathy
D. Dilated cardiomyopathy

156. **Carl was admitted with a diagnosis of hypertrophic cardiomyopathy. Which of the following hemodynamic effects would be seen in a patient with hypertrophic cardiomyopathy?**
A. Increased CO and increased ejection fraction
B. Normal CO and increased ejection fraction
C. Increased CO and decreased ejection fraction
D. Decreased CO and increased ejection fraction

157. **Dilated cardiomyopathy is characterized by dilation of the ventricles and impaired systolic function. Common causes are valvular heart disease and ischemic heart disease. Other causes are idiopathic. The most common cause of idiopathic dilated cardiomyopathy is**
A. Autoimmune
B. Alcohol
C. Genetic
D. Familial

158. Harold was admitted to the PICU for changes in mentation, development of ascites, orthopnea, paroxysmal nocturnal dyspnea, and excessive fatigue. On physical examination, you note S_3 and S_4 gallops, basilar crackles, and the EKG shows sinus tachycardia. These symptoms are usually indicative of which type of cardiomyopathy?

A. Restrictive cardiomyopathy
B. Dilated cardiomyopathy
C. Alcohol-induced cardiomyopathy
D. Hypertrophic cardiomyopathy

159. Dottie is Kirk's mother. Kirk was diagnosed with pulmonary stenosis. During parent education, you discuss physical limitations for Kirk and note that he should be allowed breaks during physical activity to present fatigue. You know that the mother understands the teaching when she states that she intends to

A. Keep Kirk home and away from all sports
B. Take Kirk to physical therapy
C. Enroll Kirk in touch football
D. Stop Kirk from activity if she thinks he is tiring

160. Increased pulmonary blood flow is associated with which of the following cyanotic congenital heart defects?

A. Transposition of the great vessels
B. Pulmonary atresia
C. Ostium primum
D. Tetralogy of Fallot

161. Your patient requires an infusion of dobutamine. Dobutamine improves cardiac output primarily by

A. Increasing afterload
B. Increasing heart rate
C. Decreasing preload
D. Improving contractility

162. Bart is 13 years old and has been huffing freon and experimenting with crack cocaine. Yesterday, Bart was snorting cocaine when he became short of breath and felt diffuse chest discomfort. When he went inside for lunch, the pain disappeared. Bart tried watching TV but he felt more fatigued than ever. Today, Bart was admitted to your unit with orthopnea and profound dyspnea. Bart's parents agreed to placement of a pulmonary artery catheter and the following information was obtained:

EKG: Borderline ST at 100 with rare PACs
Cuff BP 142/74
Skin warm, pale
Capillary refill 4 seconds
2+ pitting edema (pretibial)
RR 20, breath sounds: crackles in posterior lobes
O_2 2 L/min via NC
ABGs were drawn, but results are unavailable

Mentation: alert, oriented ×4

Pulmonary artery catheter readings:

PAP 40/20

PAOP 20

RAP 5

Cardiac output 3.6

Cardiac index 2.0

Bart probably has developed

A. Chylothorax

B. Mild pericarditis

C. Pulmonary edema (noncardiac)

D. Left ventricular failure

163. Carlos had a VVI pacemaker inserted. What does the first "V" in this acronym indicate?

A. Paced, ventricular

B. Paced, inhibited

C. Ventricular inhibited

D. Ventricular

164. What does the second "V" in the acronym for a VVI pacemaker indicate?

A. Ventricular paced

B. Ventricular inhibited

C. Ventricular sensed

D. Ventricular programmed

165. Graciana, who is 11 years old, was alert and active last evening while she was playing with her friends. This morning, her mother found Graciana just sitting on the side of her bed, hardly able to move. At first, the paramedics and the personnel in the ED thought Graciana had suffered a stroke, but she was admitted to the PICU because her EKG showed large R waves in leads V_1 and V_2. A pulmonary artery catheter was placed without incident. Physical parameters include:

EKG: SR at 92, no ectopy

Cuff BP 94/62

Skin pale, cool, clammy

RR 18, breath sounds clear, slightly diminished LLL

O_2 2 L/min via NC

Moderate jugular venous distention, no bruits

Mentation: lethargic

Pulmonary artery catheter readings:

PAP 24/10

PAOP 9

RAP 20

Cardiac output 4.9

Cardiac index 2.4

An expected diagnosis for Graciana would be
A. Pericarditis
B. LV hypertrophy
C. RV infarction
D. Aortic insufficiency

166. **Carla was traveling home with her softball team on the school bus when she ate a snack that the coach provided. After about five minutes, she began to wheeze and her respirations became labored. The coach administered epinephrine via an Epi-Pen and her symptoms abated. Carla was taken by her parents that afternoon to her family physician. This physician did not explain the reason for the reaction to Carla. Two days later, Carla was sharing some of her snack mix with her nephew and again began wheezing. She became severely tachypneic and was transported to the ED. She required treatment with epinephrine and steroids. She was intubated and sent to your unit. After admission, it was determined that Carla was 6 months pregnant. She is currently exhibiting the following signs and symptoms:**
EKG: ST at 128 without ectopy
Cuff BP 88/58
Skin cool, pale
Capillary refill 4 seconds
Ventilator settings: AMV 14, TV 600, FiO2 100%
RR 30, breath sounds: clear
Temp 99.4 (rectal)
Mentation: awake, restless
Pulmonary artery catheter readings:
PAP 30/18
PAOP 17
RAP 8
SVR 816
Cardiac output 3.4
Cardiac index 2.2
Carla is probably developing
A. Anaphylactic shock
B. Cardiogenic shock
C. Hypovolemic shock
D. Distributive shock

167. **Brandon, who is 6 years old, was climbing on his neighbor's second story deck yesterday when he slipped and fell, impaling himself on an old board. The piece of board was removed and he is now in your PICU. Today, you note the following parameters and symptoms:**
EKG: ST at 120 without ectopy
Arterial line BP 90/60
Cuff BP 88/54
Skin warm, dry

Capillary refill 2 seconds
RR 26, breath sounds: clear
O_2 3L/min via NC
Temp 100.8 °F
Mentation: alert, oriented ×4
Pulmonary artery catheter readings:
- PAP 20/8
- PAOP 6
- RAP 4
- SVR 820

Cardiac output 7.6
Cardiac index 4.0
Brandon is probably developing
A. Pericardial tamponade
B. Left heart failure
C. Distributive shock
D. Septic shock

168. **Luigi is a 10 year old who was admitted following an open heart repair of a lacerated pulmonary artery. He is complaining of upper left anterior chest pain and is becoming dyspneic. During the past hour, his mediastinal tubes have drained 30 cc. Luigi has the following vital signs and parameters:**
EKG: ST at 126 without ectopy
Heart sounds somewhat muffled, no shift in PMI, noticeable JVD
Art line BP 82/70
Cuff BP 78/70
Skin pale, cool, clammy
RR 26, breath sounds: diminished
O_2 2 L/min via NC
BSA 1.9
Mentation: alert, oriented ×4
Pulmonary artery catheter readings:
- PAP 30/22
- PAOP 20
- RAP 20

Cardiac output 3.2
Cardiac index not calculated
Which of the following conditions does Luigi probably have?
A. Left ventricular failure
B. Pericardial tamponade
C. Right ventricular failure
D. Pericarditis

169. **Daniel is a 15 year old hockey player. He was admitted for cardiomyopathy. His initial ejection fraction was 24%, and he has been confused most of the time since admission yesterday. On admission, his EKG showed ST depression in leads V_1–V_4. Since then, he has become more dyspneic and is getting restless. Current vital signs and parameters are as follows:**

EKG: ST at 116
Art line BP 110/64
Cuff BP 102/70
Skin pale, cool
Bilateral pretibial and pedal edema
Sacral edema
Temp 99 °F
RR 30, breath sounds clear, slightly diminished RLL
O_2 4 L/min via mask
Mentation: oriented to self, confused at times
Pulmonary artery catheter readings:
  PAP 48/22
  PAOP 20
  RAP 16
Cardiac output 3.4
Cardiac index 2.0

Which condition does Daniel appear to be suffering from at this time?

A. Anterior MI
B. Inferior wall MI
C. Biventricular failure
D. Right ventricular failure

170. **Use the chart below to select the correct hemodynamic effects of epinephrine.**

	HR	MAP	CVP	SVR	CO
A.	↑	↓	↑	↓	↑
B.	↑/↓	↓	↑	↓	↑
C.	↑	↑	↑	↑	↑
D.	↑/↓	↑	↓	↑	↑

171. **Use the chart below to select the correct hemodynamic effects of milrinone.**

	HR	MAP	CVP	SVR	CO
A.	↑	↑	↓	↑	↑
B.	↑/↓	↑	↓	↑	↓
C.	0/↑	↓	0/↓	↓	↑
D.	↑	↓	↑/↓	↓	↓

172. **What is the preferred route of insertion for a left atrial catheter?**
   A. Percutaneously via the left chest wall directly into the left atrium
   B. Placed via the right superior pulmonary vein into the left atrium
   C. Placed into the ascending aorta and threaded to the left atrium
   D. Placed into the right atrium and threaded to the left atrium

173. **The a wave on a left atrial catheter tracing represents**
   A. The slight increase in intra-atrial pressure associated with opening of the aorta
   B. The pressure rise produced with atrial systole
   C. Contraction of the ventricles
   D. Mitral valve closure with a decrease in atrial pressure

174. **The x wave on a left atrial catheter tracing represents**
   A. Mitral valve closure with a decrease in atrial pressure
   B. Contraction of the ventricles
   C. The slight increase in intra-atrial pressure associated with opening of the aorta
   D. The a wave is present only in right atrial pressure catheter tracings

175. **Which of the following statements is true about the waves generated by a left atrial catheter?**
   A. Exaggerated a waves may indicate mitral regurgitation
   B. Exaggerated v waves may indicate pulmonary hypertension
   C. Elevated a waves rule out cardiac tamponade
   D. Missing a waves may occur with atrial fibrillation

176. **Rory has required placement of an intra-aortic balloon pump prior to surgery for a VSD. The IABP will have which of the following benefits for Rory's condition?**
   A. A decreased right-to-left shunt
   B. Increased afterload
   C. Increased pulmonary pressures
   D. Increased PVR

177. A relative contraindication for the use of an IABP would be

A. An aortic dissection
B. An abdominal aortic aneurysm
C. Thrombocytopenia
D. Aortic insufficiency

178. Which of the following waves will follow the dicrotic notch of an assisted beat on the IABP?

A. Systolic augmentation
B. Diastolic augmentation
C. The arterial waveform
D. The assisted end-diastolic pressure

179. On the IABP, balloon deflation is optimal when

A. A V is noted at the dicrotic notch
B. The assisted end-diastolic pressure is less than the unassisted systolic pressure
C. After the dicrotic notch, the augmented diastolic equals the previous systolic blood pressure
D. The assisted end-diastolic pressure equals the unassisted systolic pressure

180. If an early IABP balloon inflation occurs, the balloon inflates

A. Prior to closure of the aortic valve
B. Prior to opening of the pulmonic valve
C. Prior to closure of the mitral valve
D. Prior to opening of the tricuspid valve

181. Your patient is being treated with an IABP. While performing an assessment, you note that the patient no longer has a palpable left radial pulse. What is the probable cause of the loss of this pulse?

A. A malfunctioning arterial line
B. The patient's position
C. Hypovolemia
D. The IABP balloon catheter has migrated upward

182. The most common complication of IABP therapy is

A. Stroke
B. Infection
C. Lower limb ischemia
D. Anemia

183. An absolute contraindication to the use of IABP therapy is

A. An aortic dissection
B. Thrombocytopenia
C. Peripheral vascular disease
D. Femur fracture

184. In which of the following conditions is the PAOP less than the LVEDP?
A. Tachycardia
B. COPD
C. Mitral valve disease
D. Pulmonary embolism

185. The pressure in the area between the pulmonic and aortic valves is reflected by which of the following parameters on a pulmonary artery catheter?
A. RAP
B. PAD
C. PAS
D. RVEDP

186. Malignant hyperthermia is most likely to occur after the administration of
A. Morphine
B. Tetracycline
C. Halothane
D. Lidocaine

187. A late sign of malignant hyperthermia is
A. Jaw rigidity
B. Rhabdomyolysis
C. Tachycardia
D. Metabolic acidosis

188. An early sign of malignant hyperthermia is
A. Rhabdomyolysis
B. Bleeding from venipuncture sites
C. Increased temperature
D. Elevated serum creatinine phosphokinase

189. Your patient has transposition of the great arteries and requires an arterial switch procedure. The most difficult part of this surgery is
A. Correction of the coronary arteries
B. Hemodynamic instability
C. Postoperative return to normal function
D. The pulmonary artery

190. Which of the following is the first functional organ during embryonic development?
A. Heart
B. Lungs
C. Kidneys
D. Liver

191. Marge is a 10 year old who was initially diagnosed with VSD when she was 3 years old. She will undergo surgery in the morning. Which of the following factors may increase Marge's stress related to the surgery?

A. Body image fear
B. Introducing her to another patient with same surgery
C. Explaining the procedure
D. Family conferences

192. Daniel has been scheduled for an aortic valve replacement because of severe aortic stenosis—a rare condition at his young age. Which other treatment or procedure is available to treat his condition?

A. An AICD
B. An amiodarone infusion
C. Aortic valve replacement
D. Milrinone

193. New-onset atrial fibrillation frequently develops as a sequelae to

A. Pulmonary edema
B. Left heart failure
C. Use of PPIs
D. Tricuspid regurgitation

194. Which of the following statements is true regarding aortic regurgitation?

A. Aortic regurgitation will decrease preload in the left ventricle
B. Aortic regurgitation will increase LVEDP
C. Aortic regurgitation will result in a systolic blowing murmur
D. Aortic regurgitation will increase cardiac output

195. Mitral valve regurgitation will result in

A. Decreased LVEDP
B. Increased afterload
C. Decreased cardiac output
D. Ventricular tachycardia

196. Primary tricuspid regurgitation may be caused by

A. Dilated cardiomyopathy
B. A pulmonary embolism
C. Aortic valve disease
D. Rheumatic fever

197. According to American Heart Association 2010 guidelines, when providing chest compressions to infants and children, recommendations are to compress one-third the anterior–posterior depth of the chest. What approximate chest depth is this?

A. ½ inch for infants, 1 inch for older children
B. 1 inch for infants, 1.5 inches for older children
C. 1.5 inches for infants, 2 inches for older children
D. 2 inches for infants, 2.5 inches for older children

198. Which of the following is true regarding management of a child who has died after a sudden and unexpected cardiac arrest?

A. Provide grief counseling for staff members
B. Do not allow anyone to touch the body until after a clergy member has spoken with the family
C. Remove all tubes, treatment devices, and monitors prior to allowing the family to see the patient
D. Notify the family that a complete, unrestricted autopsy should be done

199. According to the American Heart Association 2010 guidelines, healthcare providers should begin chest compressions immediately on infants and children if they cannot palpate a pulse within how many seconds?

A. 3
B. 6
C. 10
D. 15

200. Per the American Heart Association 2010 guidelines, which of the following statements is true regarding calculation of pediatric emergency drugs?

A. If the patient is obese, calculate the drug dosage based on the ideal weight using the patient's body length as measured on a resuscitation tape
B. If the patient is obese, calculate the drug dosage based on the actual weight minus half the ideal weight based on body length
C. If the patient is obese, calculate the drug dosage based on the actual body weight
D. If the patient is obese, administer the recommended adult dosage

SECTION 3

Cardiovascular Answers

1. **Correct answer: C**
   The cardiac index for this patient is 3.5. First, you must calculate the cardiac output (HR × SV or 80 × 40 = 3200 = 3.2 L/min). Then, use the following equation:

   $$CI = CO/BSA\ (3.2/0.9 = 3.55\ L/min/m^2)$$

   The CI is a more specific indicator of hemodynamic status than cardiac output. The CO has a broader range of 4 to 8 L/min. To make the numbers specific to an individual, the person's body surface area is included in the equation. Then the normal range becomes 2.5–4.0 L/min/m^2. The *Pediatric CCRN Core Curriculum* lists the preceding value for the CI as correct. However, the *Procedure Manual for Pediatric Acute Critical Care* says the CI ranges from 3.3 to 6 L/min/m^2. If you have questions, contact AACN—they oversee publication of both books. The standard for years has been the value of 2.5–4.0 L/min/m^2.

2. **Correct answer: B**
   Normal cardiac output for a 16 year old should be in the range of 4 to 8 L/min. The formula for calculating this value is CO = HR × SV. In this case, 72(HR) × 70 (SV) = 5040mL/min. Converted to liters, the answer would equal 5.04 L/min.

   It is unlikely that you will be asked a question about cardiac output calculations for a specific age, but you should know the formula. Younger children tend to have a higher cardiac output because the heart rate is faster. It is more likely that you will need to know the formula for calculating the cardiac index.

3. **Correct answer: B**
   The MAP is a mean pressure that takes into account the fact that the diastolic phase represents two-thirds of the cardiac cycle. It is calculated as follows: MAP = 2(DBP) + (SBP)/3. If you took the average of the two pressures, it would not account for the importance of the diastolic phase. The heart rate is not entered into this calculation. Patients should maintain a MAP of at least 60 mmHg to ensure adequate perfusion to the brain and kidneys.

4. **Correct answer: D**
   The ejection fraction should be over 50%. This is the amount of blood ejected from the left ventricle compared to the total amount available. This amount is expressed as a percentage. For example, if the ventricle contains 90 mL of blood and 50 mL is ejected, the amount would be represented as a percentage—in this case, 55%. An ejection fraction of 35% or less indicates a problem with contractility, outflow, or filling.

5. **Correct answer: D**
   The ejection fraction (EF) most closely represents left ventricular end-diastolic pressure (LVEDP). EF and LVEDP are closely related. The LVEDP is the volume of blood under pressure left at the end of the contraction.

6. **Correct answer: A**
   Tetralogy of Fallot manifests itself by the following combinations of defects: VSD, overriding aorta, pulmonary stenosis, and right ventricular hypertrophy. This condition results in low oxygenation of blood due to the mixing of oxygenated and deoxygenated blood in the left ventricle via the VSD and mixing of blood from both ventricles through the aorta because of the obstruction to flow through the pulmonary valve. The end result is a right-to-left shunt. The primary symptom of tetralogy of Fallot is low blood oxygen saturation, with or without cyanosis, from birth or developing in the first year of life. If the baby is not cyanotic, then the condition is sometimes referred to as "pink tet." Other symptoms include a harsh grade II to IV systolic murmur with a thrill, difficulty in feeding, failure to gain weight, retarded growth, and physical development. Polycythemia may be present with dyspnea on exertion, along with clubbing of the fingers and toes.

   Children with tetralogy of Fallot may exhibit "tet spells." The precise mechanism of these episodes is unknown, but they may result from a transient increase in resistance to blood flow to the lungs along with increased flow of desaturated blood to the body. Tet spells may be precipitated by activity and are characterized by paroxysms of hyperpnea, irritability, prolonged crying, increasing cyanosis, and decreasing intensity of the heart murmur. Tet spells may result in hypoxic brain injury and death. Older children may squat during a tet spell, which cuts off circulation to the legs. The squatting position raises intrathoracic pressure and systemic vascular resistance, thereby improving blood flow to the brain and vital organs.

7. **Correct answer: B**
   Metabolism of the heart is decreased during diastole, which accounts for approximately half of the cardiac cycle at birth. Shortly after birth, the diastolic phase lengthens so that it represents two-thirds of the cardiac cycle. An increase in cardiac output decreases diastole.

8. **Correct answer: B**
   A reflex tachycardia caused by stretch of right atrial receptors is known as the Bainbridge reflex. The Bainbridge reflex is believed to occur to speed up the heart rate if the right side becomes overloaded and help equalize pressures in both sides.

9. **Correct answer: A**
   Pressures in the left side of the heart and pulmonary filling pressures are represented by the PAOP. When the balloon of a pulmonary artery catheter is inflated, it eventually "wedges" in the pulmonary artery. The turbulence behind the balloon is blocked, and it senses what is in front of it—is the pulmonary vascular bed and left side of the heart. This pressure was formerly known as pulmonary artery wedge pressure (PAWP). It is now known as pulmonary artery occlusive pressure (PAOP) and is sometimes called pulmonary capillary wedge pressure (PCWP). The normal value should be in the range of 5–12 mmHg.

10. **Correct answer: D**
    A left atrial pressure of 18 mmHg should indicate a mitral valve dysfunction. The mitral valve dysfunction is often seen with a postendocardial cushion repair. The LAP is usually approximately 8 mmHg, so the pressure of 18 mmHg is high. The right atrial pressures would be increased by either pulmonic stenosis or tricuspid regurgitation.

11. **Correct answer: D**
    The fourth heart sound, S_4, is always pathologic after the first 24 hours of life and indicates a decreased ventricular compliance. This heart sound is produced when an atrial contraction fills up the ventricle. S_4 is rarely heard in the newborn and occurs just before the S_1 heart sound. During the first 24 hours of life, S_4 may be heard just after S_1 and sounds like a clicking noise.

12. **Correct answer: B**
    The mean pressure difference in the systemic vascular bed divided by blood flow is known as systemic vascular resistance (SVR). It indicates the resistance the left ventricle must pump against.

13. **Correct answer: D**
    A heart murmur associated with acute valvular regurgitation is called S_4. S_1 and S_2 are normal sounds. S_3 is associated with fluid status, S_4 is associated with ventricular compliance.

14. **Correct answer: C**
    Stroke volume is comprised of contractility, preload, and afterload. Viscosity, blood volume, and impedance represent the components of afterload. The myocardium is sensitive to changes, especially increased afterload. With only minute changes in afterload, the stroke volume can fall significantly.

15. **Correct answer: A**
    On a pulmonary catheter tracing, large A waves may be seen with increased pressure during atrial contraction. This pattern could be caused by mitral stenosis, an ischemic left ventricle, or failure of a left ventricle.

16. **Correct answer: B**
    A popliteal blood pressure that is at least 20 mmHg higher than the brachial blood pressure is known as Hill's sign. Hill's sign reflects the rapid rise in pulsation found in patients with aortic insufficiency. DeMusset's sign is also found in aortic insufficiency (the bobbing of the head in time with the forceful pulse).

17. **Correct answer: C**
    Pulsus alternans occurs in left ventricular failure when the weakened myocardium cannot maintain an even pressure with each contraction. The pulses alternate between strong and weak. Pulsus alternans is also seen in CHF.

18. **Correct answer: D**
    Adenosine is used for the suppression or elimination of sustained supraventricular tachycardia. It can also be used in diagnostic studies to establish the cause of SVT. Adverse effects may include transient arrhythmias, flushing, dyspnea, and (rarely) apnea. It is important to note that in approximately 30% of patients, SVT recurs. Caffeine and theophylline act by competitive antagonism to diminish the effects of adenosine.

19. **Correct answer: A**
    Minute changes in the partial pressure of oxygen, pH, and the partial pressure of carbon dioxide result in changes in the heart and respiratory rates. These changes are initiated by the chemoreceptors located in the carotid and aortic bodies.

20. **Correct answer: C**
    When the right side of the heart fails, the cause is often left-sided failure. The right ventricle cannot adequately pump blood out, so filling pressures rise and the blood backs up, resulting in hepatomegaly. Thus the CVP and RV pressures are elevated. Additional symptoms may include splenomegaly, ascites, abdominal pain, S_3, S_4, and weight gain. Pulmonary edema, an elevated PAD and PAOP, and orthopnea are symptoms of left-sided heart failure.

21. **Correct answer: B**
    On an EKG, left-sided heart failure results in wide, notched P waves. Tall, peaked P waves are indicative of right-sided heart failure. Changes in ST segments (or T waves) usually indicate myocardial ischemia.

22. **Correct answer: C**
    Atrioventricular canal defect is a condition that is often associated with an ostium primum ASD. This defect is also associated with a cleft in the anterior mitral valve leaflet, a VSD in the inlet portion of the ventricle septum, and a cleft in the septal leaflet of the tricuspid valve.

23. **Correct answer: B**
    A moderate-sized ventricular septal defect causes the pulmonary vascular resistance (PVR) to be less than the systemic vascular resistance (SVR). This imbalance will cause a left-to-right shunt. With this condition, too much blood may enter the lungs, increasing edema and possibly preventing or delaying development and maturation of arterioles. A pansystolic murmur can be heard over the left sternal border.

24. **Correct answer: C**
    Tet spells may be treated with morphine to promote venous dilation. IV fluids are used for volume expansion with an increase in systemic BP. If this strategy does not control the spell, systemic BP can be increased with phenylephrine or ketamine (both of which have the added benefit of sedation). Propranolol may prevent or mitigate tet spells.

25. **Correct answer: B**
    The resistance against which the right ventricle must eject its volume is known as pulmonary vascular resistance (PVR). PVR is calculated as a mean pressure in the pulmonary vasculature that is divided by the blood flow. Another way to think of it is the pressure against which the right ventricle must pump.

26. **Correct answer: B**
    Alpha-adrenergic effects of norepinephrine include peripheral arteriolar vasoconstriction. Increased force of myocardial contraction and increased AV conduction time are effects of beta-adrenergic sympathetic stimulation.

27. **Correct answer: D**
    The third heart sound, S_3, occurs when increased blood flow travels across the AV valves secondary to rapid passive ventricular filling from the atria. This is easy to

remember if you associate the S_3 sound with fluid. It will be prominent in CHF, mitral valve insufficiency, anemia, and left-to-right shunts such as ASD, VSD, and PDA.

28. **Correct answer: D**
Infants with CHF are at high risk during interventional procedures because of the use of contrast dye. Contrast dye has high sodium content. Sodium contributes to myocardial depression and creates an osmotic effect that temporarily increases intravascular volume. Transcatheter defect occlusion and balloon atrial septostomy are procedures, not risks.

29. **Correct answer: A**
Hydralazine is incompatible with furosemide, phenobarbital, aminophylline, and ampicillin. Hydralazine is compatible with heparin, dobutamine, hydrocortisone, potassium chloride, prostaglandin E_1, and Dex/AA.

30. **Correct answer: B**
Phentolamine (Regitine) 1 mg/mL solution should be injected into the affected area if infiltration of dopamine occurs. It may take as much as 5 mL to treat the affected area.

31. **Correct answer: C**
The bidirectional Glenn procedure, where the superior vena cava is anastomosed to the right pulmonary artery, is usually performed prior to the child reaching 6 months of age, to specifically reduce volume overload to the right ventricle. The first stage, known as the Norwood procedure, consists of ligation of the ductus and division of the pulmonary artery. The end result of the staged procedures—and a disadvantage associated with them—is systemic circulation supplied by a single right ventricle.

32. **Correct answer: D**
All of the following heart defects would be classified as cyanotic heart defects: pulmonary atresia, tetralogy of Fallot, transposition of the great vessels, total anomalous pulmonary venous return, truncus arteriosus, hypoplastic left heart syndrome, and tricuspid valve abnormalities.

33. **Correct answer: C**
Acyanotic congenital heart defects include pulmonary valve stenosis, ventricular septal defect (VSD), atrial septal defect (ASD), patent ductus arteriosus (PDA), aortic valve stenosis, and coarctation of the aorta.

34. **Correct answer: B**
Cardiac murmurs are present in 80% of patients with tricuspid atresia. A holosystolic murmur that may have a crescendo and decrescendo quality is heard, suggestive of blood flow through the ventricular septal defect. A continuous murmur may be present. Systemic-to-pulmonary arterial collaterals or arterial-to-pulmonary arterial anastomoses surgically created to improve pulmonary blood flow may cause this finding. A murmur of mitral insufficiency may also be present.

35. **Correct answer: C**
Because the heart cannot adequately fill or eject its contents, stroke volume decreases, which leads to decreased cardiac output. Contractility decreases because the muscle cannot adequately stretch and, therefore, cannot contract effectively.

36. **Correct answer: A**
A dilated superior vena cava would appear on a chest X-ray if the patient had a cardiac tamponade. The vena cava is dilated because blood cannot empty into the right atrium. The mediastinum would be widened. A CXR will not show delineation of the pericardium or epicardium. A pneumothorax may exist, but would not be an expected finding on X-ray.

37. **Correct answer: D**
Beck's triad consists of distended neck veins, muffled heart sounds, and hypotension. In tamponade, tachycardia is an early sign. A narrowed pulse pressure occurs; fluid cannot be ejected from the heart. The muffled heart sounds occur because the fluid in the pericardial sac minimizes the transmission of sound waves.

38. **Correct answer: D**
During CVP pressure monitoring, the c wave represents the increase in RA pressure from closure of the tricuspid valve.

39. **Correct answer: A**
When evaluating the CVP pressure waves, the v wave represents mechanical atrial diastole.

40. **Correct answer: B**
A low CVP reading may indicate increased contractility or hypovolemia. A high reading may indicate LV, RV, biventricular failure, tricuspid regurgitation or stenosis, hypertension, hypervolemia, or cardiac tamponade.

41. **Correct answer: A**
A patient with tricuspid atresia may exhibit polycythemia. Because of hypoxia in patients with tricuspid atresia, polycythemia may be present. Prothrombin time and activated partial thromboplastin time may be abnormal secondary to the polycythemia. Cardiomegaly is usually present, along with a prominent right heart border that reflects enlargement of the right atrium. Sinus rhythm is generally present, with tall P waves indicative of atrial enlargement. First-degree atrioventricular block may be observed. Because of the origin of the left bundle branch from a common bundle, the frontal plane QRS axis may be either leftward or superior.

42. **Correct answer: C**
Patients who have aortic insufficiency often exhibit Quincke's sign. This sign is elicited by pressing down on the fingertip. A visible pulsation is seen in the nail bed. This results from a pulse characterized by a rapid initial hard pulsation followed by a sudden collapse as blood flows back through an incompetent valve.

43. **Correct answer: B**
Leads II, III, and aVF will show damage to the inferior wall of the heart. Leads I and aVL will show damage to the higher areas of the lateral wall. Leads V_1 and V_2 will show septal wall damage. Leads V_5 and V_6 will show damage to the apical area.

44. **Correct answer: D**
Leads V_2–V_4 indicate damage to the anterior wall of the heart. Leads V_4 and R indicate right ventricular damage. Leads V_5 and V_6 indicate apical injury. Leads V_7–V_9 are specific to the posterior wall.

45. Correct answer: B

By definition, "pansystolic" means the murmur is heard throughout systole. The only systolic murmur listed as an option here is tricuspid insufficiency; all of the other answers are diastolic murmurs.

46. Correct answer: A

Polycythemia would increase afterload due to the excess circulation red blood cells. Both hypovolemia and sepsis decrease afterload, as does aortic insufficiency. Aortic stenosis increases afterload, as do peripheral vasoconstriction and hypertension.

47. Correct answer: C

When the wedge pressure was initially obtained, large V waves were noted and the PAOP was 27. The probable cause of this reading was papillary muscle rupture. The most important thing to do in this case is to determine the source of the waveform. The large V wave may sometimes be mistaken for the right ventricular tracing or even a pulmonary artery tracing. Large V waves usually occur with a papillary muscle rupture (sometimes ischemia) secondary to mitral regurgitation or an acute lateral wall MI.

48. Correct answer: D

The only definitive way to diagnose myocarditis is via an endomyocardial biopsy.

49. Correct answer: B

Environmental factors implicated in the etiology of Ebstein anomaly include maternal ingestion of lithium in the first trimester of pregnancy. Some researchers have reported a teratogenic potential with high doses of lithium, and a 400-fold increase in the occurrence of Ebstein anomaly has been noted in association with lithium exposure in utero. In patients with bipolar disorder, the benefits of lithium may outweigh the small risk of Ebstein anomaly. Other possible causes of Ebstein anomaly include maternal rubella, maternal benzodiazepine use, maternal exposure to varnishing substances, and maternal history of previous fetal loss.

50. Correct answer: C

Twelve-lead EKG findings for a patient with Ebstein anomaly could include sinus rhythm with paroxysmal SVT. Usually, normal sinus rhythm with intermittent SVT, paroxysmal SVT, atrial flutter, atrial fibrillation, and ventricular tachycardia are present. The PR is usually prolonged, accompanied by abnormal P waves consistent with right atrial enlargement. However, the PR interval may be normal or short in patients with Wolff-Parkinson-White syndrome.

51. Correct answer: D

Cardiac glycosides possess positive inotropic activity, which is mediated by inhibition of sodium–potassium adenosine triphosphatase. Also, cardiac glycosides reduce conductivity in the heart, particularly through the atrioventricular node, and therefore have a negative chronotropic effect. The cardiac glycosides have very similar pharmacological effects but differ considerably in terms of their speed of onset and duration of action. They are used to slow the heart rate in supraventricular arrhythmias, especially atrial fibrillation, and also are used in patients with chronic heart failure.

52. Correct answer: B

The pulmonic valve is rarely affected by infective endocarditis. The mitral valve is the site most commonly affected by infective endocarditis; the aortic valve is the next most common valve affected. The tricuspid valve is often involved secondarily as a result of IV drug abuse.

53. **Correct answer: B**
Changes in leads V_2, V_3, V_4, I, and AVL are indicative of an anterolateral MI. The MI could also include changes in V_5, and V_6, which are also lateral leads.

54. **Correct answer: B**
Abnormal Q waves on an EKG signify a complete thickness infarction of the myocardium. When the tissue dies due to myocardial infarction it becomes electrically dead, causing the opposing energy to become the dominant feature on the EKG. Partial-thickness myocardial death would be evidenced as a non-Q-wave MI.

55. **Correct answer: B**
The high iodine content of amiodarone can actually exert an effect on the thyroid, thereby producing an antiarrhythmic action.

56. **Correct answer: B**
Milrinone decreases PVR and SVR, improves contractility, and inhibits cyclic AMP.

57. **Correct answer: D**
Neo-Synephrine is used as a treatment for hypercyanotic tet spells. It is also used to treat SVT and severe hypotension.

58. **Correct answer: C**
Myocarditis is clinically defined as inflammation of the myocardium. Coxsackie B1 virus has emerged as a more prevalent cause of myocarditis in recent years. In addition, numerous infections, systemic diseases, drugs, and toxins are associated with the development of myocarditis. Viruses, bacteria, protozoa, and even worms have been implicated as infectious agents. The normal WBC count in neonates varies, but a value of less than 4000 WBCs/μL or more than 25,000 WBCs/μL is considered abnormal. The absolute band count is not sensitive enough to predict the development of sepsis, but a ratio of immature to total polymorphonuclear leukocytes of less than 0.2 has a very high negative predictive value. A rapid fall in a known absolute eosinophil count and morphologic changes in neutrophils may indicate sepsis.

59. **Correct answer: C**
Right ventricular afterload may be reduced by inhaled nitric oxide. Use of epinephrine will increase systemic afterload due to vasoconstriction and promote increased PVR because of the increased left heart pressures. Hypoventilation and subsequent hypoxia will also increase right heart afterload. Use of inhaled nitric oxide, nitroglycerin, nitroprusside, PGE_1, or hyperventilation will reduce right ventricular afterload.

60. **Correct answer: C**
Anaphylaxis—a form of distributive shock—involves mast cell degranulation with resultant histamine release and vasodilation. The histamine release may cause normal peripheral vascular tone to become inappropriately relaxed. Vasodilation results in increased venous capacitance, leading to a relative hypovolemia even if the patient has not actually lost any net fluid. The common physiologic disturbance in all forms of distributive shock is a decrease in preload.

61. **Correct answer: C**
The international consensus conference in 2002 standardized the definition of systemic inflammatory response syndrome (SIRS) as tachycardia or tachypnea with fever or high leukocyte count. Sepsis is defined as SIRS in the presence of suspected or proven infection. Severe sepsis is defined as sepsis with accompanying organ dysfunction. When cardiovascular failure occurs in the setting of severe sepsis, then it is classified as septic shock.

62. **Correct answer: B**
The elevated right ventricular pressure and the elevated right atrial pressure indicate pulmonary hypertension. The wedge pressure is normal. The wedge pressure reflects the status of the left side of the heart. Fluid cannot clear the lungs, so pressure builds and the right-side pressures become elevated due to the increased workload. Edema results from the fluid accumulation. The patient's dyspnea and exercise intolerance are due to excess fluid in the lungs.

63. **Correct answer: B**
Sharon is probably suffering from pericarditis. The CXR will probably show a pericardial effusion. The elevated sed rate and WBC count indicate infection. With pericarditis, leaning forward often relieves chest pain, whereas lying supine makes it worse. The pain may worsen on inspiration when the lungs expand and come in contact with the pericardium. The patient will probably also have a fever. The nurse should monitor the patient for any sign of cardiac tamponade and make certain that anticoagulants are discontinued.

64. **Correct answer: A**
The antagonist for morphine and other opioids is Narcan (naloxone). Generally, the naloxone dose is 0.4 mg IV. This dose can be repeated about every 3 to 4 minutes, for a total of three times. When you give naloxone, you must always be alert for the patient's potential relapse once the dose wears off. Administering multiple follow-up doses is not uncommon.

65. **Correct answer: B**
Patients receiving sodium nitroprusside should be monitored for cyanide toxicity, and sodium nitroprusside should be avoided in patients with renal problems. Cyanide toxicity may result in tachycardia and severe hypotension. Monitor the patient's venous O_2 concentration and acid–base balance. If nitroprusside extravasates from an IV, it will cause tissue sloughing and necrosis. The RBC cyanide level should be less than 50 mcg/mL.

66. **Correct answer: C**
Charlie is at risk for cardiomyopathy and congenital heart block. Neonatal congenital heart block is thought to occur when maternal antibodies pass through the placenta into the fetal circulation. Some infants with congenital heart block are treated with corticosteroids and have limited mediation of symptoms; these symptoms may include thrombocytopenia, skin rash, and hepatitis. Even if the symptoms resolve, some research has shown that affected infants often develop a variety of autoimmune disorders later in life. If the congenital complete heart block does not resolve, it will become permanent. In approximately two-thirds of all infants with complete heart block, a pacemaker is required.

67. **Correct answer: D**
Procainamide's adverse effects include severe hypotension (usually because of a rapid infusion) and A-V block. Procainamide may also widen the QRS complex due to slow impulse conduction through the Purkinje fibers and ventricular myocardium. If the QRS complex widens more than 35% to 50%, use of procainamide should be discontinued. Adverse effects usually disappear when the drug is discontinued. Two of procainamide's actions are depression of the excitability of cardiac muscle and slowing of the conduction in the atria.

68. **Correct answer: B**
The classic description of an X-ray showing a pericardial effusion is the "water bottle" silhouette. In patients with a pericardial effusion, QRS amplitude is decreased. Diastolic filling is decreased as well.

69. **Correct answer: C**
Normal pulmonary artery pressures are as follows:
PAS = 20–30 / 6–10 mmHg
PAD = 5–12 mmHg
PAM = 10–20 mmHg
PAOP (PCWP) = 4–12 mmHg

70. **Correct answer: B**
Signs of CNS toxicity from lidocaine may include agitation, vomiting, drowsiness, and muscle twitching. Later signs may include loss of consciousness, seizures, respiratory depression, and apnea. Cardiac toxicity may develop and cause hypotension, bradycardia, and heart block, ultimately leading to cardiovascular collapse.

71. **Correct answer: B**
The low wedge pressure of 4 indicates hypovolemia. This patient will require volume replacement.

72. **Correct answer: D**
The religious preferences of the patient must be respected. The only acceptable form of transfusion in this case is autotransfusion.

73. **Correct answer: A**
When the parasympathetic and sympathetic nervous systems stimulate the right vagus nerve, the SA node is affected, which slows the heart rate. Acetylcholine is a neurotransmitter.

74. **Correct answer: C**
Stimulation of a $beta_2$ receptor in the heart may cause vasodilation (lowered SVR), bronchodilation, and smooth muscle relaxation.

75. **Correct answer: A**
Nick has endocarditis. Janeway lesions are flat and painless erythematous areas found predominantly on the palms and soles of the feet. Osler's nodes are small painful nodules that are also associated with endocarditis and found on the fingers and toes. Roth spots are seen when examining the retina. These rounded, white spots are associated with endocarditis. It is thought that microvascular clots form in the heart and pass through the microcirculation and impede peripheral circulation, sometimes causing necrosis. Pella's sign is not a medical term.

76. **Correct answer: B**
A primary goal in cardiogenic shock is to improve the pumping action of the heart (improve myocardial contractility), reduce the workload, reduce oxygen demand, and improve cardiac output. If possible, systemic vascular resistance should be decreased and the left ventricle augmented with an inotrope. Administration of nitroprusside will reduce both preload and afterload. The cardiac workload will be decreased as is the myocardial oxygen demand.

77. **Correct answer: B**
Early signs of left ventricular failure include tachypnea and tachycardia. Severe left ventricular failure also causes dyspnea and retractions (seen in infants predominantly).

78. **Correct answer: A**
Cyanosis may be observed when at least 5 g/100 mL of deoxygenated hemoglobin is present in the circulation.

79. **Correct answer: C**
Lidocaine does not impair normal contractility. Lidocaine may shorten the QT interval, however, and its side effects usually involve the CNS (i.e., slurred speech, drowsiness, confusion, paresthesias, seizures, and convulsions). Hypotension, nystagmus, and gastrointestinal intolerance are effects of phenytoin, another class 1B drug.

80. **Correct answer: B**
Calcium channel blockers act primarily on arteriolar tissue. Large lumen vessels in the arterial system are affected. The advantage of this action is that both systolic and diastolic pressures are reduced, so the patient will not have a drop in blood pressure. The blood pressure may be lowered slightly and cause a reflex baroreceptor response to speed up the heart rate to maintain cardiac output.

81. **Correct answer: A**
The PMI in a newborn is usually located at the lower left sternal border. The apical impulse of a newborn is usually felt at the fourth intercostal space, just to the left of the midclavicular line.

82. **Correct answer: B**
The S_2 heart sound is created by closure of the pulmonic and aortic valves. S_2 is best heard in the upper left sternal border or pulmonic area.

83. **Correct answer: C**
Regurgitation systolic murmurs are associated with VSD, tricuspid regurgitation, and mitral valve regurgitation. These murmurs are caused by blood flow from an area of higher pressure throughout systole to an area of lower pressure.

84. **Correct answer: C**
Rheumatic fever is the most common cause of acquired valvular disease. The valves are a perfect place for bacteria to colonize, and blood is a perfect medium for bacterial growth. The causative organism is beta hemolytic *Streptococcus*.

85. **Correct answer: B**
Ventricular assist devices are used as destination therapy as well as a bridge to transplant. Other indications for VADs include cardiogenic shock and inability to wean from cardiopulmonary bypass. VADs are not indicated for dysrhythmias. Prolonged cardiac arrest, especially when accompanied by neurological damage, is a contraindication to

use of a VAD. Extensive organ damage is another contraindication. Always be aware of the possibility of device failure.

86. **Correct answer: D**
The left ventricular assist device is the most commonly used because left heart failure is more common and usually precedes right ventricular failure.

87. **Correct answer: C**
Pneumonia secondary to immobility is the primary reason for infection in patients with VADs. Such patients may also require some type of ventilatory support. Placement of any kind of tube into the body serves as a potential source of infection, but this risk is usually minimized by good hand washing and aseptic technique.

88. **Correct answer: A**
In patients with normal cardiac anatomy, right atrial pressure equals right ventricular end-diastolic pressure, which equals central venous pressure.

89. **Correct answer: B**
Radio-frequency waves destroy myocardial tissue with heat. These waves actually heat the tissue around the active sites and prevent the occurrence of a reentry loop. Once the temperature reaches 50 °C, cell damage and death occur. The continuing heat and creates a lesion approximately 2 to 5 mm in diameter. This "burned" area is characterized by necrosis and will not conduct electricity.

90. **Correct answer: C**
Deoxygenated blood returns from the body with an O_2 saturation of approximately 75%. The right atrial value is normal. The right ventricle and pulmonary artery should also exhibit this saturation level. The high level means that some of the oxygenated blood from the left side of the heart has mixed with the deoxygenated blood through a ventricular septal defect. This effect would be called a left-to-right shunt, because the blood flows from an area of high pressure to an area of low pressure.

91. **Correct answer: A**
The nurse should explain that Mary needs a pacemaker or AICD that can deliver a more powerful impulse. The asynchronous mode will override Mary's internal pacemaker.

92. **Correct answer: D**
A dual lead pacemaker/AICD is necessary to maintain the atrial kick. Single-chamber pacing can lead to pacemaker syndrome. The letters on pacemaker modes are as follows:

Chamber Paced	Chamber Sensed	Mode of Response	Programmability, Rate Modulation	Antiatachy-arrhythmia Function
V = Ventricle	V = Ventricle	I = Inhibit	P = Simple programmable	P = Pacing
A = Atrium	A = Atrium	T = Triggered	M = Multi-programmable	S = Shock
D = Dual chamber	D = Dual chamber	D = Dual (T & I)	R = Rate modulation	Dual = Dual (P & S)

93. **Correct answer: A**
Skyler has probably dislodged a lead, or the lead may have been damaged on insertion. Either way, Skyler needs a new AICD or new leads.

94. **Correct answer: A**
Pacemaker syndrome is caused by a loss of atrial kick or regurgitation against a closed A-V valve. Fatigue, agitation, and forgetfulness are primary symptoms of this condition. It is possible that Troy's atrial lead has become damaged or has failed.

95. **Correct answer: C**
Mort is in the first stage of cardiogenic shock secondary to systolic dysfunction. The injuries to his chest may have caused a pulmonary artery laceration or a cardiac contusion (the latter is more likely). His blood pressure is low, and the EKG shows ST-segment elevation in the anterior leads. If the myocardium is contused, it will react the same way as if an MI had occurred. The ST elevation may be the result of a physiologic insult to a coronary artery, with an area of the myocardium becoming ischemic as a result. The pumping function of the myocardium is compromised and may need additional support with inotropes and possibly an intra-aortic balloon pump (IABP). Mort may undergo angiography and/or surgery. Volume replacement may be necessary.

96. **Correct answer: B**
Rate, rhythm, axis, hypertrophy, and infarction are the most valuable areas examined in a 12-lead EKG.

97. **Correct answer: A**
Leads V_1 and V_2 show right bundle branch blocks. A simple way to remember which type of bundle branch block occurs with a QRS complex wider than 0.12 seconds is to think of the turn signals on your car. To signal a right turn, you push the lever up; to signal a left turn, you push the lever down. Analogously, looking at leads V_1 and V_2, if the QRS complex is upright, then there is a right bundle branch block. If the QRS complex goes downward in V_1, and V_2, then it is a left bundle branch block.

98. **Correct answer: C**
Phasic variations in an arterial pressure waveform during mechanical ventilation usually indicate hypovolemia or heart failure.

99. **Correct answer: C**
In patients with normal cardiac anatomy, pulmonary artery wedge pressure equals pulmonary artery occlusion pressure, which equals left ventricular end-diastolic pressure, which equals left atrial pressure.

100. **Correct answer: C**
An acute rise in a pulmonary wedge pressure (pulmonary artery occlusion pressure) indicates a pulmonary artery hypertensive crisis and right heart failure.

101. **Correct answer: C**
Kent should avoid cola that contains caffeine. Caffeine is a central nervous system stimulant and a natural antagonist to adenosine. In addition, Kent should avoid methylxanthines such as theophylline, which acts as an antagonist to adenosine.

102. Correct answer: C
If adenosine is given slowly, it may cause systemic vasodilation and reflex tachycardia, further compromising cardiac output. Blurred vision is an expected adverse reaction. The patient should be monitored for development of atrial fibrillation, bradycardia, and heart blocks. Withhold adenosine if the patient experiences atrial fibrillation, atrial flutter, second-degree type II heart block, or complete heart block. Adenosine slows conduction via the AV node, and these rhythms may degrade to ventricular fibrillation.

103. Correct answer: A
Nifedipine is a calcium channel blocker. When beginning or discontinuing nifedipine, it must be titrated over a period of 7 to 14 days.

104. Correct answer: C
Dobutamine improves cardiac output by acting on beta$_1$-adrenergic receptors in the heart. It may cause minimal peripheral vasodilation, but primarily acts to increase contractility, coronary blood flow, and heart rate, thereby improving cardiac output. Dopamine acts on alpha-adrenergic receptors in the heart. Norepinephrine is a catecholamine that acts on both alpha- and beta-adrenergic receptors in the cardiovascular tissue.

105. Correct answer: B
Dobutamine is not compatible with either sodium bicarbonate or ampicillin, so the nurse cannot infuse the medications together. The appropriate choice would be to start another peripheral line to administer sodium bicarbonate while waiting for the ampicillin to arrive from the pharmacy. If the patient remains hemodynamically unstable and the nurse is unable to obtain or maintain peripheral venous access, then it is appropriate to speak with the physician regarding measures that would ensure more stable access, such as a central line or a PICC line.

106. Correct answer: B
Dobutamine has been linked with profound hypokalemia in some patients due to beta$_2$-adrenergic stimulation. Monitor the patient's urine output to determine renal function prior to implementing any potassium replacement. Consider alternative vasoactive drugs if blood pressure support continues to be required. Long-term dobutamine use may result in tolerance and decreased effectiveness after the medication is administered for several days.

107. Correct answer: C
When starting dopamine, it is important to ensure that the patient's hypovolemia has been treated appropriately. As part of the treatment for septic shock, the patient may receive as many as 3 to 10 fluid boluses until pulmonary edema is noted or the boluses fail to have an effect on blood pressure. Central venous access is the preferred route of administering dopamine, but the physician is responsible for obtaining parental consent. If central access is unavailable, peripheral access is acceptable. However, the site must be monitored closely for infiltration, and additional IV access points must be available. Phentolamine mesylate should be available in case infiltration does occur, but its administration is not the first action to be performed.

108. Correct answer: D
Dopamine should not be titrated any faster than every 5 minutes: Its onset of action is 5 minutes, and the duration of its action is 10 minutes. Titrating this medication more

frequently than every 5 minutes may result in greater hemodynamic instability and more difficulty in determining the effective dosage. The minimum systolic blood pressure limit for this patient is 78 mmHg. The calculation is as follows: age $\times$ 2 + 70 for patients older than 1 year.

109. Correct answer: A

In patients receiving high-dose epinephrine, glucose levels should be monitored closely for potential hyperglycemia. The risk for hyperglycemia is even greater if the patient is diabetic. Potassium levels—not calcium, chloride, or sodium—should also be monitored for potential hyperkalemia or hypokalemia.

110. Correct answer: A

Isuprel (Isoproterenol) is the better choice for vasoactive support for the asthmatic patient in decompensated shock. This catecholamine promotes smooth muscle relaxation, bronchodilation, and pulmonary vasodilation, thereby decreasing PVR and increasing heart rate and contractility. In contrast, dopamine increases peripheral vasoconstriction, which in turn increases blood pressure, but does not affect pulmonary blood flow. Vasopressin results in systemic vasoconstriction; it acts on the renal tubules to increase water reabsorption. Neo-Synephrine causes arteriolar vasoconstriction, resulting in greater PVR and more VQ shunting and there is also the possibility of the patient becoming hypoxemic.

111. Correct answer: D

Patient confusion, listlessness, and headache should be reported to the physician immediately due to the potential for water intoxication. You would also expect to see a sudden weight gain, anuria, and hyponatremia. Monitor urine output closely and serum electrolytes daily. Abdominal cramps and nausea are expected side effects and can be treated by drinking water.

112. Correct answer: A

Norepinephrine bitartrate (Levophed) infusions require blood pressure monitoring at least every 5 minutes. Direct arterial monitoring is preferred for more accurate evaluation. The solution should be clear without particulates and mixed in D_5W, D_5W with normal saline, or normal saline; and kept protected (i.e. covered) from direct light. Levophed may be infused with dopamine, but the nurse should monitor the patient's peripheral circulation closely due to the potential for severe vasoconstriction and extravasation. Patients should be weaned off of Levophed over at least 6 to 24 hours to prevent rebound hypotension.

113. Correct answer: B

The appropriate action would be to contact the physician and wean the patient off of phenylephrine hydrochloride (Neo-Synephrine) if her blood pressure remains stable. The drop in Emma's heart rate is likely due to the high dose effects of Neo-Synephrine, which increases SVR and PVR, thereby triggering a baroreceptor response that leads to vagal stimulation and, consequently, a decreased heart rate. Emma's minimum heart rate given her age should be greater than 75, and her minimum systolic blood pressure should be 74 mmHg. After the Neo-Synephrine dose is decreased, the heart rate should increase within 15 to 20 minutes as the effects of this medication wear off. Atropine is not indicated unless cessation of the Neo-Synephrine does not increase the heart rate. No data have been provided indicating that Emma requires additional oxygen support.

114. Correct answer: D
Education about digoxin is vital for parents to understand the importance of taking the medication as prescribed and of not doubling up on any dose when the previous dose was skipped. Placing Harry on a schedule will help his parents comply with the dosage regimen. If a liquid formulation is used, teach the parents to use the medicine dropper correctly to prevent either underdosing or overdosing. Parents should be able to accurately return demonstrate obtaining a pulse rate. The parents should be taught to report and withhold the digoxin for any heart rate less than 60. Digoxin may also cause nausea and vomiting. Parents should report any weight loss or decreased appetite and should be taught to watch for signs and symptoms of hyperkalemia.

115. Correct answer: D
Atropine administration may result in headaches, dizziness, and coma. You should also observe the patient for urinary retention, hypotension, and tachycardia due to blocking of parasympathetic receptor sites.

116. Correct answer: A
Lidocaine infusion may cause respiratory arrest. A respiratory rate of 7 indicates impending failure; immediate action is required to provide respiratory support via resuscitation bag and to prepare for intubation. The infusion should be stopped if respiratory failure occurs, if a widening QRS complex is noted, if the patient's heart rate drops below 60, and if the patient becomes hypotensive. The infusion must also be stopped if the patient has difficulty speaking or experiences numbness and tingling as they are also symptoms of lidocaine toxicity.

117. Correct answer: C
After five days, Maria may have gained enough weight so that her initial dosage is no longer adequate to maintain therapeutic drug levels. It will be important to teach the parents to monitor Maria's weight at home and notify the physician of any significant weight gain.

118. Correct answer: A
Life-threatening side effects of propranolol include laryngospasm and bronchospasm, in addition to bradycardia, bone marrow suppression, and hypotension. Complete heart block and dizziness are side effects of propafenone (Rythmol). Lidocaine may cause respiratory depression and cardiovascular collapse. Polymorphic VT and dyspnea are life-threatening side effects of sotalol (Betapace).

119. Correct answer: B
Esmolol is incompatible with furosemide. Furosemide administration will require alternative venous access or oral administration. Esmolol is compatible with cimetidine, penicillin, and midazolam.

120. Correct answer: C
Enlargement of the right atrium, right ventricle, and pulmonary artery and a heart that exhibits a "snowman" appearance on a chest radiograph indicate a total anomalous pulmonary venous return. The "snowman" appearance is due to widening of the superior mediastinum—a rare phenomenon caused by connecting blood vessels. Cardiomegaly and increased pulmonary vascular markings are also seen with this condition.

121. Correct answer: D

An allergy to fish places patients at an increased risk for an allergic reaction to protamine sulfate. Patients who have undergone other cardiac procedures or patients with diabetes who have used protamine insulin are also at risk for experiencing an allergic reaction to protamine sulfate. Protamine may also cause rebound bleeding as long as 18 hours postoperatively. Note that males who have undergone a vasectomy or who are infertile may have developed antibodies to protamine.

122. Correct answer: B

The modified Blalock-Taussig procedure attaches the subclavian and pulmonary arteries to redirect blood flow through the heart.

123. Correct answer: C

Severe cyanosis usually occurs when tricuspid atresia is present. Blood flow is unable to proceed through to the right ventricle and subsequently to the pulmonary circulation. Increased right-side pressures cause unoxygenated blood to shunt through the foramen ovale to the left side and then to the systemic circulation. Temporary management is to maintain a patent ductus arteriosus to shunt some blood to the pulmonary circulation and to oxygenate the patient. Surgical intervention is required for long-term treatment.

124. Correct answer: B

Indications for pacemaker insertion include symptomatic bradycardia, bradycardia with escape beats, overdrive pacing, bradycardia/arrest, acute MI with sinus dysfunction, Mobitz type II block, complete heart block, and development of a new bundle branch block.

125. Correct answer: A

Alpha-adrenergic effects of norepinephrine include peripheral arteriolar vasoconstriction. Increased SA node firing and increased force of myocardial contraction are effects of beta-adrenergic sympathetic stimulation.

126. Correct answer: A

Treatment for malignant hyperthermia consists of the administration of dantrolene sodium. It is also important to immediately discontinue all agents that might trigger this condition.

127. Correct answer: A

Signs and symptoms of right-sided congestive heart failure include respiratory distress and hepatomegaly. The respiratory distress is the result of blood's failure to flow to the lungs, which leads to hypoxemia. As blood backs up into the hepatic system, hepatomegaly and splenomegaly may result.

128. Correct answer: B

Quinidine and hypomagnesemia can lead to torsades de pointes (also known as polymorphic ventricular tachycardia)—a recurrent ventricular tachycardia that turns on its axis every six to eight beats, giving the EKG a twisting or "turning on point" look. Hypomagnesemia can occur when the patient receives total parenteral nutrition.

129. Correct answer: D

Rapid infusion of Lasix can cause tinnitus and hearing loss.

130. **Correct answer: A**
Calcium channel blockers act primarily on arteries to arterioles. Large lumen vessels in the arterial system are affected. The advantage of this action is that both systolic and diastolic pressures are reduced and the patient will not experience a drop in blood pressure. The blood pressure may be lowered slightly and cause a reflex baroreceptor response that speeds up the heart rate to maintain cardiac output.

131. **Correct answer: B**
Continuous-wave echocardiography shows the quantity of flow across an obstruction. This type of echocardiography is used to detect the direction of shunting, estimate cardiac output, and assess ventricular diastolic function. It provides a good estimate of pressure gradients.

132. **Correct answer: A**
M-mode echocardiography is used to identify motion of cardiac valves and to detect the presence of pericardial fluid. This type of echocardiography enables evaluation of anatomic relationships and the relative sizes of the valves.

133. **Correct answer: A**
Dong quai, gingko biloba, and ginseng can all increase bleeding times.

134. **Correct answer: B**
The high-contrast media used in cardiac catheterizations all have a high sodium content.

135. **Correct answer: B**
The PICU nurse should closely monitor the urine output and liver function tests of a patient receiving a loading dose of amiodarone. The high concentration of amiodarone may cause renal necrosis and impaired output, leading to vascular congestion and respiratory distress. Amiodarone has been linked to hepatocellular damage and impaired liver function. Its other side effects include anemia, neutropenia, pancytopenia, and thrombocytopenia. The thyroid levels of patients receiving this medication should also be monitored, as amiodarone may cause either hypothyroidism or hyperthyroidism. In addition, long-term use of amiodarone has been linked to bluish gray pigmentation in patients who are exposed to sunlight.

136. **Correct answer: C**
Discharge instructions for a patient prescribed amiodarone include avoiding grapefruit and grapefruit juice, as they will increase the level of amiodarone in the blood. In terms of outside activities, patients should restrict their participation in contact sports and use sunscreen and sun-protective clothing to protect their skin from exposure to sunlight. Amiodarone may impair liver function and lead to thrombocytopenia. Sunlight exposure may result in a bluish gray cast to the skin. If the patient normally uses theophylline to treat his or her asthma, the dosage may need to be decreased as amiodarone increases serum theophylline levels. Dark urine, respiratory distress, or edema should be reported immediately to the physician, as these are signs of renal and pulmonary impairment.

137. **Correct answer: A**
Verapamil is contraindicated in children younger than 1 year of age because it has been linked to cardiovascular collapse and death. Adenosine, procainamide, and esmolol may all be used in children younger than 1 year.

138. Correct answer: D

Isoptin (verapamil) is a calcium channel blocker used to slow conduction through the SA and AV nodes. If the patient's blood pressure falls suddenly due to vascular collapse and bradycardia, calcium chloride should be administered immediately. Normal saline would not be indicated in this scenario, given that the vascular collapse is due to an impaired heart rate, rather than volume depletion or vascular dilation. Regitine is used when infiltration of dopamine, epinephrine, or norepinephrine into the tissues occurs, to prevent sloughing.

139. Correct answer: A

Patients taking both diazoxide and furosemide should have their glucose levels monitored closely for possible hyperglycemia. Diazoxide inhibits pancreatic release of insulin and stimulates the liver to release glucose.

140. Correct answer: D

When administering nitroglycerin, it is important to have normal saline or another volume expander available at the bedside in case of vascular collapse. The potential for collapse results from the possibility of peripheral venous and arterial dilation (relative hypovolemia). Only nonpolyvinyl chloride tubing may be used for infusion: Nitroglycerin may absorb PVC if that type of tubing is used. Filtration is not required prior to infusion. Nitroglycerin is compatible only with D_5W, normal saline, lactated Ringer's solution, D_5NS, and half normal saline for infusion.

141. Correct answer: B

Alisa is presenting with possible transposition of the great vessels with VSD. Prostaglandin E_1 is used to open the ductus arteriosus to allow for blood mixing, thereby improving the flow of oxygenated blood to the body. In fact, without an open ductus arteriosus and the VSD, the newborn would not have any method of transporting oxygenated blood to the body. PGE_2 (prostaglandin E_2) is effective in improving renal blood flow via dilation. Dopamine and normal saline are not indicated. The structure of this patient's heart is impaired and inhibiting normal circulation. A saline bolus may further cause fluid overload, worsening heart failure and increasing the patient's distress.

142. Correct answer: A

Numerous foods should be avoided when taking warfarin. Those highest in vitamin K (the antagonist to warfarin) concentrations are broccoli, Brussels sprouts, cabbage, spinach, turnip greens, endive, scallions, and parsley. Other foods to be avoided include red leaf lettuce, watercress, oils (e.g., soybean, canola), and salads in general. All of these foods decrease the effectiveness of warfarin.

143. Correct answer: A

A pulmonary embolism is probably not the cause of Luis's condition. The high wedge pressure in association with a low CVP indicates a problem on the left side of his heart. A pulmonary embolism would have resulted in a high right atrial pressure and equal right atrial and wedge pressures. A clue to this patient's condition is the increase in his pulmonary capillary wedge pressure and pulmonary artery pressure. The pulmonary diastolic pressure roughly equals the wedge pressure, indicating that no increase in pulmonary venous resistance has occurred. Thus the most likely problem is something involving the left heart—diagnoses that include coronary artery disease, cardiomyopathy, aortic stenosis, mitral regurgitation or stenosis, and aortic insufficiency.

144. Correct answer: D
Pulmonary atresia is complete obstruction of the pulmonic valve, resulting in a hypoplastic right ventricle and tricuspid valve.

145. Correct answer: D
The least likely diagnosis is obstruction of the left anterior descending coronary artery. Steven is not exhibiting either chest pain or EKG changes. In addition, this patient has a normal PAOP, indicating normal left-sided cardiac function, but the pressures in the right heart are elevated. The RAP and PAP are elevated. Therefore, the problem involves the right heart. Conditions that would cause these results include RV dysfunction, pulmonary embolism, pulmonary stenosis, and RV hypertrophy.

146. Correct answer: B
A change in the position or level of the transducers would produce these data. Most units keep the transducer for the arterial pressure and central hemodynamics on the same manifold. Changes in the bed position or transducers are very common in a PICU.

This question can be quite tricky. The first thing to notice is that all of the pressures rose by 8 mmHg. Unless there was some major coincidence, this would not happen. The patient did not have any change in his blood pressure or cardiac index. It is possible that the mediastinal tubes may have stopped draining or dramatically slowed down postoperatively. The patient is currently not showing any signs of tamponade, however, nor do the hemodynamics support that diagnosis.

147. Correct answer: C
A heart rate of 160 may make it nearly impossible to obtain a stable wedge pressure reading. Tricuspid regurgitation should not have any effect on a wedge pressure measurement, because the wedge reflects pressure to the left atrium. Aortic stenosis also is not a problem, because obstruction of the aortic valve should show an increase in left atrial pressure if the patient had heart failure. Measurement of wedge pressure can be difficult in patients with severe mitral regurgitation, as these individuals may demonstrate a superimposed V wave on the wedge tracing.

148. Correct answer: D
The new-onset dysrhythmia most commonly seen in a patient with a diagnosis of pulmonary edema is atrial fibrillation. Atrial fibrillation is the result of the constant stretching and disruption of normal pathways in the atrium due to increased preload from the pulmonary congestion.

149. Correct answer: D
The nurse would be expected to monitor the patient's vital signs, condition of the wound, and LOC. However, this family is so eager to help with the patient's care that they would probably have someone at the bedside many hours during the day. Any change in mentation is very significant, and the family can help monitor the patient when the nurse is away from the room. This family will be ready to embrace learning and assume more caregiving tasks as time passes if they are positively reinforced for their efforts.

150. Correct answer: B
Matthew's blood pressure, PAS/PAD pressures, and RAP are low. The cardiac output and cardiac index are low, as are the heart rate and respiratory rate. Matthew's mentation is diminished. Collectively, these symptoms indicate hypovolemic shock.

151. **Correct answer: C**
Jeffrey is developing cardiogenic shock. When the left ventricle fails, fluid backs up into the pulmonary vasculature. In this case, the high wedge pressure indicates that the fluid is already backed up in the patient's left heart. The PAP and RAP are high, indicating pulmonary congestion. Cardiac output and cardiac index are low, and the BP is not being maintained.

152. **Correct answer: D**
Congestive heart failure results in a systemic venous engorgement, as blood does not flow forward and is allowed to pool in organs and peripheral circulation. Tissues become hypoxic and further diminish the body's functioning until complete failure and death occur.

153. **Correct answer: B**
Chlorothiazide reduces urinary calcium losses and does not result in profound potassium losses.

154. **Correct answer: B**
A common cause of restrictive cardiomyopathy is glycogen storage disease. Amyloidosis is another cause of restrictive cardiomyopathy. The myocardium (especially the left ventricle) becomes rigid from fibrosis, which results in inadequate left ventricular filling and increased atrial dilatation. Left ventricular diastolic dysfunction occurs, and the LVEDP becomes markedly increased. Systolic function remains normal in this type of cardiomyopathy. Fluid backs up into the lungs, and the patient looks as if he or she has congestive heart failure. There is no cure for restrictive cardiomyopathy. Symptoms are treated as they occur.

155. **Correct answer: C**
Arrhythmogenic cardiomyopathy (a relatively new classification for cardiomyopathy) is characterized by replacement of normal cells by fatty tissue. The right ventricle is primarily affected. Conduction cannot occur normally and the patient will have multiple ventricular arrhythmias and right ventricular failure. Young people are at risk for sudden death. The cause of this condition is unknown, but some research has shown a possible link to an autosomal dominant gene.

156. **Correct answer: B**
In hypertrophic cardiomyopathy, the myocardium thickens, but not symmetrically. There is more thickening of the ventricular septum than the ventricle. If you were to look at a heart with this condition, it might appear normal externally. When the septum is thicker, it creates a hyperdynamic state by increasing contractility, which in turn increases the ejection fraction. In rare conditions where the septum is asymmetrically thickened, the left ventricular outflow will be impaired, leading to decreased cardiac output.

157. **Correct answer: B**
Even though the exact causes are unknown, a large number of alcoholics develop dilated cardiomyopathy. Three possible reasons have been identified:
    1. Either the alcohol itself or its metabolites have a toxic effect.
    2. Alcohol sometimes contains additives, such as cobalt.
    3. The cause may be nutritional in origin, such as a thiamine deficiency.

New research suggests that there may be a viral link between dilated cardiomyopathy and chronic alcoholism.

Potentially, this type of cardiomyopathy might reverse itself if the patient ceases alcohol use. Other types of cardiomyopathy are not reversible.

158. **Correct answer: B**
Harold has dilated cardiomyopathy that is causing systolic dysfunction. A patient with this type of cardiomyopathy will exhibit S_3 and S_4 gallops, and the EKG may show atrial fibrillation, ventricular dysrhythmias, or a sinus tachycardia most of the time. The patient may also have a systolic murmur of the AV valves. Signs and symptoms associated with dilated cardiomyopathy include peripheral edema or ascites, hepatomegaly, and pale, cool extremities. Changes in mentation are also possible. Hypertrophic and restrictive cardiomyopathies are diastolic dysfunctions.

159. **Correct answer: B**
Although Kirk has a congenital heart disease, physical activity is still important for him to feel included and normal as well as developing normal coordination, achieve muscle development, and form friendships. Physical therapy can help Kirk develop improved muscle strength and coordination. Keeping him home or forcing him to stop physical activity can impede normal development. It is important that his mother understand that Kirk will typically limit his own activity based on his fatigue level. Dottie should not enroll her son in contact sports, however, as the activity may be too exhausting and could lead to injuries.

160. **Correct answer: A**
Transposition of the great vessels results in an increased pulmonary blood flow. Blood from the lungs is circulated through the left heart in a closed loop, and systemic blood flow circulates via the right side of the heart in a closed loop. Survivability depends on the presence of a patent ductus arteriosus or concurrent septal defects that allow mixing of blood in the heart.

161. **Correct answer: D**
Dobutamine improves cardiac output primarily by increasing cardiac contractility. Unlike dopamine, dobutamine does not increase heart rate and can be used in tachycardic patients.

162. **Correct answer: D**
Bart has increased exercise intolerance, edema, dyspnea, and increased PAP and wedge pressures. The RAP is normal. These are all signs of left ventricular failure.

163. **Correct answer: A**
Using ICHD nomenclature, the first "V" is the chamber paced.

164. **Correct answer: C**
Using ICHD nomenclature, the second "V" is the chamber sensed.

165. **Correct answer: C**
Graciana's problem involves the right ventricle. Her PAP and wedge pressures are normal. The RAP is high and there is some jugular distention, which indicates a problem with the right ventricle—it cannot pump effectively. The lungs do not seem to be the problem, because the pulmonary artery pressures are normal. Graciana's lethargy

may be unrelated and needs to be evaluated because it represents a significant change for this patient.

166. Correct answer: D

Carla was admitted for anaphylactic shock, but she now appears to be in distributive shock. She is 6 months pregnant, and the baby is probably pressing on her aorta and vena cava. A simple change of position might fix the problem. In anaphylactic shock, the PAP would be low in the initial stages because of vasodilation. In obstructive shock, the PAP and PAOP may be either normal or high. Symptoms usually resolve once the underlying problem is eliminated.

167. Correct answer: D

Brandon is in the hyperdynamic or "warm" stage of septic shock. The endotoxins are increasing his metabolism and acting as vasodilators. His temperature is elevated because of the increased metabolism and infection. The RAP, PAP, SVR, and PAOP are all decreased because of vasodilation. The cardiac output and cardiac index are high because they are compensating for the other imbalances. Hypotension occurs because of vasodilation. Urine output should be quite high.

Brandon needs immediate treatment with large quantities of fluids, vasopressors, antibiotics, and antiendotoxins.

168. Correct answer: B

The pulmonary artery pressures, RAP, and PAOP are all elevated and the values are virtually identical. Heart sounds are muffled, and the blood pressure is characterized by converging systolic and diastolic pressures. A pericardiocentesis for a pericardial tamponade must be performed immediately.

169. Correct answer: C

Daniel is probably suffering from biventricular failure. All of his pulmonary pressures are elevated. His heart cannot pump the fluid out, and his lungs are congested (dyspnea). Edema is a sign of pump failure. This patient will probably develop ascites and hepatomegaly.

170. Correct answer: C

The effects of epinephrine are shown here:

	HR	MAP	CVP	SVR	CO
C.	↑	↑	↑	↑	↑

171. Correct answer: C

The hemodynamic effects of milrinone are shown here:

	HR	MAP	CVP	SVR	CO
C.	0/↑	↓	0/↓	↓	↑

172. **Correct answer: B**
A left atrial catheter is usually placed via the right superior pulmonary vein into the left atrium.

173. **Correct answer: B**
The a wave from a left atrial catheter represents the pressure increase produced with atrial systole.

174. **Correct answer: A**
The x wave on a left atrial catheter tracing represents mitral valve closure with a decrease in atrial pressure.

175. **Correct answer: D**
In a left atrial catheter, absent a waves may occur with atrial fibrillation.

176. **Correct answer: A**
In a VSD, the pressure is higher in the left ventricle, which shunts blood to the right ventricle. This shunting can lead to right ventricular failure, with a subsequent decrease in cardiac output. The IABP decreases afterload and decreases the right-to-left shunt.

177. **Correct answer: C**
A relative contraindication for the use of an IABP would be thrombocytopenia. With a relative contraindication, the potential risk must be weighed against the potential benefit before deciding which treatment is appropriate. Additional relative contraindications to IABP therapy include coagulopathies, peripheral vascular disease, end-stage cardiomyopathies, and terminal diseases.

178. **Correct answer: B**
Diastolic augmentation follows the dicrotic notch of an assisted beat on the IABP. The dicrotic notch should take on a "V" shape between the unassisted systole and the augmented diastolic wave.

179. **Correct answer: B**
On the IABP, balloon deflation is optimal when the assisted end-diastolic pressure is less than the unassisted systolic pressure. Also, the assisted end-diastolic pressure should be less than the unassisted aortic end-diastolic pressure.

180. **Correct answer: A**
In an early IABP balloon inflation, the balloon inflates prior to closure of the aortic valve. When the balloon inflates too early, it will result in aortic regurgitation and reduced stroke volume. Additionally, myocardial oxygen demand and end-diastolic volumes will increase.

181. **Correct answer: D**
The loss of the left radial pulse during treatment with an IABP is due to upward migration of the balloon catheter. The catheter is probably occluding the left subclavian artery and requires immediate repositioning.

182. **Correct answer: C**
The most common complication of IABP therapy is lower limb ischemia. Other, less common complications of IABP therapy include bleeding, thrombocytopenia, anemia, catheter migration, infection, aortic dissection, and compartment syndrome.

183. Correct answer: A
An absolute contraindication to IABP therapy is an aortic dissection. In addition, irreversible brain damage, abdominal aortic aneurysm, and aortic insufficiency are all reasons that patients should not undergo IABP therapy.

184. Correct answer: D
In patients with pulmonary emboli, the PAOP is less than the LVEDP. Mitral valve disease, COPD, positive-pressure ventilation, and tachycardia will cause the PAOP to be greater than the LVEDP.

185. Correct answer: B
The PAD reflects the pressure in the area between the pulmonic and aortic valves. It is often a reliable indicator of left ventricular function.

186. Correct answer: C
Use of induction agents such as halothane, succinylcholine, and desflurane may initiate an episode of malignant hyperthermia. Stress and depolarizing muscle relaxants may also trigger MH. In malignant hyperthermia, excess calcium builds up in the microplasm. The patient then suffers from sustained skeletal muscular contractions, which ultimately leads to a hypermetabolic state.

187. Correct answer: B
Late signs of malignant hyperthermia include rhabdomyolysis, increased temperature, and bleeding from venipuncture sites.

188. Correct answer: D
Early signs of malignant hyperthermia include elevated serum creatinine phosphokinase (CPK), jaw rigidity, tachycardia, and respiratory and metabolic acidosis. Malignant hyperthermia can develop up to 24 hours postoperatively.

189. Correct answer: A
The most difficult part of the arterial switch is dealing with the coronary arteries. The arteries are very small and somewhat friable. Once the procedure is complete, normal blood flow should be established and the child will have the anatomy of a normal heart.

190. Correct answer: A
The heart is the first organ to become functional during embryonic development. It begins to beat from the sinus venosus once the endothelial tubes fuse to form the heart tube, around day 21 of development. The lungs become functional as soon as 23 to 24 weeks gestation, with vascularization and alveolar development occurring at delivery. The kidneys begin to form urine and perform glomerular filtration at 9 to 10 weeks gestation. The liver is a multifunctional organ whose actions support gastrointestinal, endocrinologic, and hematological functions that emerge at different intervals in fetal development. For example, the liver synthesizes and secretes bile as soon as 16 weeks gestation. From weeks 6 to 20 of gestation, the liver functions as the primary source of hematopoiesis until the fetal bone marrow matures and dominates production.

191. Correct answer: A
Marge's stress may increase due to her body image fears related to surgical scars, cyanosis, and feeding tubes. To decrease her stress, be sure to explain the procedure to Marge and introduce her to another patient who has undergone the same surgery. Conversing with a peer may give Marge an opportunity to speak more openly about

her fears. A family conference will assist Marge's parents in understanding the procedure and care plan, thereby decreasing both overall family stress and patient stress.

192. **Correct answer: C**
The only effective treatment for a severely stenosed aortic valve is replacement. About all that can be done is to treat the patient's symptoms with diuretics, inotropic support, vasodilators, ICDs, and sometimes interventional procedures. All of these treatments are only temporary because eventually, the valve will have to be replaced.

193. **Correct answer: A**
New-onset atrial fibrillation frequently develops as a sequela to pulmonary edema.

194. **Correct answer: B**
Aortic regurgitation increases LVEDP. This condition also increases preload in the left ventricle, leading to development of a diastolic blowing murmur and decreasing cardiac output.

195. **Correct answer: C**
Mitral valve regurgitation results in a decreased cardiac output, an increased LVEDP, decreased afterload, and an enlarged left atrium. Many patients also develop atrial fibrillation.

196. **Correct answer: D**
Primary tricuspid regurgitation may be caused by rheumatic fever.

197. **Correct answer: C**
According to the American Heart Association 2010 guidelines, one-third of the anterior posterior chest depth equates to approximately 1.5 inches in most infants and 2 inches in most older children. Compressions of less than the minimum one-third anterior–posterior chest depth will not provide sufficient compression of the heart to produce the needed blood flow to maintain circulation to the heart, lungs, and brain.

198. **Correct answer: D**
It is important that the family be notified that a complete, unrestricted autopsy be done on the child as soon as possible. According to the American Heart Association 2010 guidelines, a child who has died suddenly and unexpectedly from a cardiac arrest may have had an underlying condition called "channelopathy." This genetic calcium channel ion irregularity may predispose other family members to cardiac arrhythmias leading to sudden death.

199. **Correct answer: C**
According to the American Heart Association 2010 guidelines, healthcare providers should begin chest compressions immediately on infants and children if they cannot palpate a pulse within 10 seconds. Research has shown that both lay people and healthcare personnel are unable to accurately palpate pulses in arrested and compromised patients in less than 30 seconds. Therefore, compressions should be started in any patient who is unresponsive, fails to demonstrate effective breathing (i.e., agonal respirations), and has no palpable pulse.

200. **Correct answer: A**
Per the American Heart Association 2010 guidelines, if the patient is obese, the healthcare provider should calculate the drug dosage based on the ideal weight and using

the body length measured on a resuscitation tape. Subsequent administrations of medications can be titrated for effect and observation of toxicity. Drug dosages should never exceed the adult dosage. If the patient is within the ideal body weight range for his or her length, medications should be administered based on body length using the resuscitation tape.

CARDIOVASCULAR REFERENCES

Adler, A., Litmanovitz, I., Bauer, S., & Dolfin, T. (2004, September/October). Aspirin treatment for neonatal infectious endocarditis. *Pediatric Cardiology, 25*(5), 562–564.

Aehlert, B. (2002). *ECGs made easy* (2nd ed.). Philadelphia: Mosby.

Aehlert, B. (Ed.). (2005). *Comprehensive pediatric emergency care.* St. Louis, MO: Mosby.

Al Dhahri, K., Sandor, G., & Duncan, W. (2006). Intra-atrial thrombus in a neonate with coarctation of the aorta. *Cardiology in the Young, 16*(4), 392–394.

Alexander, C. P., Sood, B. G., Zilberman, M. Z., Becker, C., & Bedard, M. P. (2006). Congenital hepatic arteriovenous malformation: An unusual cause of neonatal persistent pulmonary hypertension. *Journal of Perinatology, 26*(5), 316–318.

Allocca, G., Slavich, G., Nucifora, G., Slavich, M., Frassani, R., Crapis, M., & Badano, L. (2007, August). Successful treatment of polymicrobial multivalve infective endocarditis: Multivalve infective endocarditis. *International Journal of Cardiovascular Imaging, 23*(4), 501.

American Association of Critical-Care Nurses (AACN). (2007). *AACN certification and core review for high acuity and critical care* (6th ed.). Philadelphia: Saunders.

American Association of Critical-Care Nurses (AACN). (2008). ST segment monitoring: AACN practice alert. Retrieved from http://www.aacn.org

American Association of Critical-Care Nurses (AACN). (2009). Pulmonary artery pressure monitoring: AACN practice alert. Retrieved from http://www.aacn.org

American Heart Association. (2010). *Congenital cardiovascular defects: Statistics.* Retrieved September 12, 2010, from http://www.americanheart.org/presenter.jhtml?identifier=4576

American Heart Association. (2010). *Guidelines 2010 for cardiopulmonary resuscitation and emergency cardiovascular care.* Retrieved from www.americanheart.org

American Heart Association. (2010). *Heart failure in children and adolescents.* Retrieved August 25, 2010, from http://www.americanheart.org/presenter.jhtml?identifier=3016405#

Anatomy. (2009, March). Studies from H. G. Lim et al. have provided new data on anatomy. *Cardiovascular Week,* 26–28.

Ariyan, C. E., & Sosa, J. A. (2004, April). Assessment and management of patients with abnormal calcium. *Critical Care Medicine, 32*(4 suppl), S146–S154.

Bakiler, A. R., & Arun-Ozer, E. (2008). An unusual case of acute rheumatic fever presenting with unilateral pulmonary edema. *Turkish Journal of Pediatrics, 50*(6), 589–591.

Barrett, M. J., Lacey, C. S., Sekara, A. E., Linden, E. A., & Gracely, E. J. (2004). Mastering cardiac murmurs: The power of repetition. *Chest, 126*(2), 470–475.

Barter, P. J., Nicholls, S., Rye, K. A., Anantharamaiah, G. M., Navab, M., & Fogelman, A. M. (2004). Antiinflammatory properties of HDL. *Circulation Research, 95*(8), 764–772.

Batlle, M. A., & Wilcox, W. D. (1993, February). Pulmonary edema in an infant following passive inhalation of free-base ("crack") cocaine. *Clinical Pediatrics, 32*(2), 105–106.

Baur, L. H. B. (2008, March). Three dimensional echocardiography: A valuable tool to assess left atrial function in non-compaction cardiomyopathy! *International Journal of Cardiovascular Imaging, 24*(3), 243.

Boneparth, A., & Flynn, J. T. (2009). Evaluation and treatment of hypertension in general *pediatric* practice. *Clinical Pediatrics, 48*(1), 44–49.

Bozza, F. A., Salluh, J. I., Japiassu, A. M., Soares, M., Assis, E. F., Gomes, R. N., . . . Bozza, P. T. (2007). Cytokine profiles as markers of disease severity in sepsis: A multiplex analysis. *Critical Care, 11,* R49.

Brucato, A., Jonzon, A., Friedman, D., Allan, L. D., Vignati, G., Gasparini, M., . . . Stein, J. I. (2003). Proposal for a new definition of congenital complete atrioventricular block. *Lupus, 12*(6), 427–435.

Bueltmann, M., Kong, X., Mertens, M., Yin, N., Yin, J., Liu, Z., . . . Kuebler, W. M. (2009). Inhaled milrinone attenuates experimental acute lung injury. *Intensive Care Medicine, 35*(1), 171–178.

Caforio, A. L. P, Daliento, L., Angelini, A., Bottaro, S., Vinci, A., Dequal, G., & Kenna, W. J. (2005). Autoimmune myocarditis and dilated cardiomyopathy: Focus on cardiac autoantibodies. *Lupus, 14*(9), 652–655.

Calkins, H., Reynolds, M. R., Spector, P., Sondhi, M., Xu, Y., Martin, A., . . . Sledge, I. (2009). Treatment of atrial fibrillation with antiarrhythmic drugs or radiofrequency ablation: Two systematic literature reviews and meta-analyses. *Circulation: Arrhythmia and Electrophysiology, 2*(4), 349–361.

Carabello, B., & Paulus, W. (2009). Aortic stenosis. *Lancet, 373*(9667), 956–966.

Carcillo, J. A. (2002). Clinical practice parameters for hemodynamic support of pediatric and neonatal patients in septic shock. *Critical Care Medicine, 30*(6), 1365–1378.

Carmona, I. T., Dios, P. D., & Scully, C. (2007, December). Efficacy of antibiotic prophylactic regimens for the prevention of bacterial endocarditis of oral origin. *Journal of Dental Research, 86*(12), 1142.

Catchpole, K. R., Giddings, A. E., de Leval, M. R., Peek, G. J., Godden, P. J., Utley, M., . . . Dale, T. (2006). Identification of systems failures in successful paediatric cardiac surgery. *Ergonomics, 49*(5–6), 567–588.

Chambers, M. A., & Jones, S. (Eds.). (2007). *Surgical nursing of children*. Philadelphia: Elsevier.

Chaudhari, M., & Brodile, M. (2008). Hypertrophic cardiomyopathy and transportation of great arteries associated with maternal diabetes and presumed gestational diabetes. *Acta Paediatrica, 97*(12), 3.

Chaudhari, M., Hamilton, L., & Hasan, A. (2006). Correction of coronary arterial anomalies at surgical repair of common arterial trunk with ischemic left ventricular dysfunction. *Cardiology in the Young, 16*(2), 179–181.

Chernecky, C., & Berger, B. (2004). *Laboratory tests and diagnostic procedures* (4th ed.). Philadelphia: Saunders.

Chowdary, Y. C., & Patel, J. P. (2001). Recurrent pulmonary edema: An uncommon presenting feature of childhood obstructive sleep apnea hypoventilation syndrome in an otherwise healthy child. *Clinical Pediatrics, 40*(5), 287.

Conover, M. B. (2003). *Understanding electrocardiography* (8th ed.). St. Louis, MO: Mosby.

Costedoat-Chalumeau, N., Georgin-Lavialle, S., Amoura, A., & Piette, J. C. (2005). Anti-SSA/Ro and anti-SSB/La antibody-mediated congenital heart block. *Lupus, 14*(9), 660–664.

Crandall, M. A., Bradley, D. J., Packer, D. L., & Asirvatham, S. J. (2009). Contemporary management of atrial fibrillation: Update on anticoagulation and invasive management strategies. *Mayo Clinic Proceedings, 84*(7), 643–662.

Curfam, G. D., Morrissey, S., & Drazen, J. M. (2008). Cardiac transplantation in infants. *New England Journal of Medicine, 359*(7), 749.

Dabir, T., Mccrossan, B., Sweeney, L., Magee, A., & Sands, A. J. (2008). Down syndrome, achondroplasia and tetralogy of Fallot. *Neonatology, 94*(1), 68–70.

Darovic, G. O. (2002). *Hemodynamic monitoring: Invasive and noninvasive clinical application* (3rd ed.). Philadelphia: Saunders.

den Uil, C. A., Lagrand, W. K., Valk, S. D., Spronk, P. E., & Simoons, M. L. (2009). Management of cardiogenic shock: Focus on tissue perfusion. *Current Problems in Cardiology, 34*(8), 330–349.

Deymann, A. J., & Goertz, K. K. (2003). Myocardial infarction and transient ventricular dysfunction in an adolescent with sickle cell disease. *Pediatrics, 11*(2), E183.

Dickerson, H., Cooper, D. S., Checchia, P. A., & Nelson, D. P. (2008). Endocrinal complications associated with the treatment of patients with congenital cardiac disease: Consensus definitions from the Multi-Societal Database Committee for Pediatric and Congenital Heart Disease. *Cardiology in the Young, 18*(2), 256–264.

Dong, L., Zhang, F., Shu, X., Zhou, D., Guan, L., Pan, C., & Chen, H. (2009). Left ventricular torsional deformation in patients undergoing transcatheter closure of secundum atrial septal defect. *International Journal of Cardiovascular Imaging, 25*(5), 479–486.

Drake Melander, S. (Ed.). (2004). *Case studies in critical care nursing: A guide for application and review* (3rd ed.). Philadelphia: Saunders.

Emergency Nurses Association, & Newberry, L. (2003). *Sheehy's emergency nursing: Principles and practice* (5th ed.). St. Louis, MO: Mosby/Elsevier.

Francis, M. L. (2009). Atrial septal defects: Not always so simple. *British Journal of Cardiac Nursing, 4*(2), 68–74.

Gandhi, S. K., Powers, J. C., Nomeir, A. M., Fowle, K., Kitzman, D. W., Rankin, K. M., & Little, W. C. (2001, January 4). The pathogenesis of acute pulmonary edema associated with hypertension. Cardiology Section, Wake Forest University School of Medicine, Winston-Salem, NC 27157-1045. *New England Journal of Medicine, 344*(1), 17–22.

Garin, E. H., & Araya, C. E. (2009). Treatment of systemic hypertension in children and adolescents. *Current Opinion in Pediatrics, 21*(5), 600–604.

Gervasi, L., & Basu, S. (2009). Atrial septal defect devices used in the cardiac catheterization laboratory. *Progress in Cardiovascular Nursing, 24*(3), 86–89.

Giuliano, J. S., Sekar, P., Dent, C. L., Border, W. L. Hirsch, R., Manning, P. B., & Wheeler, D. S. (2008). Unilateral pulmonary edema and acute rheumatic fever. *European Journal of Pediatrics, 167*(4), 465.

Gora-Harper, M. (1998). *The injectable drug reference*. Princeton, NJ: Bioscientific Resources.

Hakuno, D., Kimura, N., Yoshioka, M., & Fukuda, K. (2009). Molecular mechanisms underlying the onset of degenerative aortic valve disease. *Journal of Molecular Medicine, 87*(1), 17–24.

Hanson, S. J., Punzalan, R. C., Greenup, R. A., Liu, H., Sato, T. T., & Havens, P. L. (2010). Incidence and risk factors for venous thromboembolism in critically ill children after trauma. *Journal of Trauma, 68*(1), 52–56.

Hardin, S. R., & Kaplow, R. (Ed.). (2010). *Cardiac surgery essentials for critical care nursing*. Sudbury, MA: Jones and Bartlett.

Hay, W. W. Jr., Levin, M. J., Sondheimer, J. M., & Deterding, R. R. (Eds.). (2007). *Current diagnosis and treatment in pediatrics* (18th ed.). New York: McGraw-Hill.

Hetzel, P. G., Glanzmann, R., Günthard, J., Bruder, E., Godi, E., & Buhrer, C. (2007). Failed detection of complex congenital heart disease (including double outlet right ventricle and total anomalous pulmonary venous return) by neonatal pulse oximetry screening. *European Journal of Pediatrics, 166*(6), 625–626.

Hill, E. E., Vanderschueren, S., Verhaegen, J., Herijgers, P., Claus, P., Herregods, M. C., & Peetermans, W. E. (2007, October). Risk factors for infective endocarditis and outcome of patients with *Staphylococcus aureus* bacteremia. *Mayo Clinic Proceedings, 82*(10), 1165

Hinton, R. B., Martin, L. J., Rame-Gowda, S., Tabangin, M. E., Cripe, L. H., & Benson, D. W. (2009). Hypoplastic left heart syndrome links to chromosomes 10q and 6q and is genetically related to bicuspid aortic valve. *Journal of the American College of Cardiology, 53*(12), 1065–1071.

Huhta, J. (2004). Neonatal hemodynamics in patients with hypoplastic left heart syndrome. *Cardiology in the Young: Controversies Relating to the Hypoplastic Left Heart, 14*(S1), 22–26.

Jackson, P. C., & Morgan, J. M. (2008). Perioperative thromboprophylaxis in children: Development of a guideline for management. *Paediatric Anaesthesia, 18*(6), 478–487.

Jeger, R. V., Radovanovic, D., Hunziker, P. R., Pfisterer, M. E., Stauffer, J. C., Erne, P., & Urban, P. (2008). Ten-year trends in the incidence and treatment of cardiogenic shock. *Annals of Internal Medicine, 149*(9), 618–626.

Jones, K. L. (2006). Smith's recognizable patterns of human malformation (6th ed.). Philadelphia: Elsevier.

Jones & Bartlett Learning (2011). *2011 nurse's drug handbook* (10th ed.). Sudbury, MA: Jones & Bartlett Learning.

Kaestner, M., Handke, R., Photiadis, J., Sigler, M., & Schneider, M. B. (2008). Implantation of stents as an alternative to reoperation in neonates and infants with acute complications after surgical creation of a systemic-to-pulmonary arterial shunt. *Cardiology in the Young, 18*(2), 177–184.

Kaminer, S. J., Pickoff, A. S., Dunnigan, A., Sterba, R., & Wolff, G. S. (1990). Cardiomyopathy and the use of implanted cardio-defibrillators in children. *Pacing and Clinical Electrophysiology: PACE, 13*(5), 593–597.

Karlsen, K. A., & Tani, L. Y. (2008). *S.T.A.B.L.E.: Cardiac module handbook: Recognition and stabilization of neonates with severe congenital heart disease*. Park City, UT: S.T.A.B.L.E. Program.

Karpawich, P. P. (2007). Pediatric cardiac resynchronization pacing therapy. *Current Opinion in Cardiology, 22*(2), 72–76.

Karpawich, P. P., Pettersen, M. D., Gupta, P., & Shah, N. (2008). Infants and children with tachycardia: Natural history and drug administration. *Current Pharmaceutical Design, 14*(8), 743–752.

Kawasaki, T., Akakabe, Y., Yamano, M., Miki, S., Kamitani, T., Kuribayashi, T., & Sugihara, H. (2008, January/February). R-wave amplitude response to myocardial ischemia in hypertrophic cardiomyopathy. *Journal of Electrocardiology, 41*(1), 68.

Kelly, N. F. A., Walters, D. L., Hourigan, L. A., Burstow, D. J., & Scalia, G. M. (2010). The relative atrial index (RAI): A novel, simple, reliable, and robust transthoracic echocardiographic indicator of atrial defects. *Journal of the American Society of Echocardiography, 23*(3), 275–281.

Kleinman, M., de Caen, A., Chameides, L., Atkins, D., Berg, R. A., Berg, M. D., . . . Zideman, D. (2010). Part 10: Pediatric basic and advanced life support: 2010 International consensus on cardiopulmonary resuscitation and emergency cardiovascular care science with treatment recommendations. *Circulation*. Retrieved October, 18, 2010, from http://www.circ.aha journals.org/cgi/content/full/122/16_suppl_2/S466

Koo, S., Yung, T. C., Lun, K. S., Chau, A. K., & Cheung, Y. F. (2008). Cardiovascular symptoms and signs in evaluating cardiac murmurs in children. *Pediatrics International, 50*(2), 145–149.

Koschel, M. J. (2006, August). Management of the cyanide-poisoned patient. *Journal of Emergency Nursing, 32*(4 suppl), S19–S28.

Krahn, G. (2007). Continuous central venous saturations during pericardial tamponade case report. *Pediatric Critical Care Medicine, 8*(3), 18.2.153.

Kumar, A., Kumar, A., Paladugu, B., Mensing, J., & Parrillo, J. E. (2007). Transforming growth factor-beta1 blocks in vitro cardiac myocyte depression induced by tumor necrosis factor-alpha, interleukin-1beta, and human septic shock serum. *Critical Care Medicine, 35*, 358–364.

Kutsal, A., Yavuz, T., & Ulusan, V. (2006). Right atrial and tricuspid hypoplasia. *Journal of Cardiovascular Surgery, 47*(3), 353–354.

Larmay, H. J., & Strasburger, J. F. (2004). Differential diagnosis and management of the fetus and newborn with an irregular or abnormal heart rate. *Pediatrics Clinics of North America, 51*, 1033–1050.

Lennestål, R., Otterblad Olausson, P., & Källén, B. (2009). Maternal use of antihypertensive drugs in early pregnancy and delivery outcome, notably the presence of congenital heart defects in the infants. *European Journal of Clinical Pharmacology, 65*(6), 615–625.

Mackie, A. S., Jutras, L. C., Dancea, A. B., Rohlicek, C. V., Platt, R., & Beland, M. (2009). Can cardiologists distinguish innocent from pathologic murmurs in neonates? *Journal of Pediatrics, 154*(1), 50–54.

Macksey, L. F. (2009). *Pediatric anesthetic and emergency drug guide*. Sudbury, MA: Jones and Bartlett.

Marks, K. A., Zucker, N., Kapelushnik, J., Karplus, M., & Levitas, A. (2002, January). Infective endocarditis successfully treated in extremely low birth weight infants with recombinant tissue plasminogen activator. *Pediatrics, 109*(1), 153.

Martin, B. (2010). Family presence during resuscitation and invasive procedures: AACN practice alert. Retrieved from http://www.aacn.org

McCalmont, V., & Ohler, L. (2008). Cardiac transplantation: Candidate identification, evaluation, and management. *Critical Care Nursing Quarterly, 31*(3), 216–231.

Meissner, U., Scharf, J., Dotsch, J., & Schroth, M. (2008). Very early extubation after open-heart surgery in children does not influence cardiac function. *Pediatric Cardiology, 29*(2), 317–320.

Melegh, Z., Patel, Y., & Ramani, P. (2008). Solitary pulmonary infantile hemangioma in an infant with atrial septal defect. *Pediatric and Developmental Pathology, 11*(6), 465–468.

Menon, T., Nandhakumar, B., Jaganathan, V., Shanmugasundaram, S., Malathy, B., & Nisha, B. (2008, January–March). Bacterial endocarditis due to Group C streptococcus. *Journal of Postgraduate Medicine, 54*(1), 64.

Meyer, S., Gortner, L., McGuire, W., Baghai, A., & Gottischling, S. (2008). Vasopressin in catecholamine-refractory shock in children. *Anaesthesia, 63*(3), 228.

Mittnachy, A. J., Wax, D. B., Srivastava, S., Nguyen, K., & Joashi, U. (2008). Development and implementation of a pediatric cardiac anesthesia/intensive care database. *Seminars in Cardiothoracic and Vascular Anesthesia, 12*(1), 12–17.

Morgan, T. (2007). Turner syndrome: Diagnosis and management. *American Family Physician, 76*(3), 405–410.

Obesity, Fitness & Wellness Week Staff. (2010, September). Tetralogy of Fallot: New tetralogy of Fallot findings from McGill University, Health Center described. *Obesity, Fitness & Wellness Week Newsletter,* 1740.

Obesity, Fitness & Wellness Week Staff. (2010, September). Tetralogy of Fallot: Research from General Hospital provides new data about tetralogy of Fallot. *Obesity, Fitness & Wellness Week Newsletter,* 2482.

Padalino, M., Castellani, C., Toffoli, S., Della Barbera, M., Milanesi, O., Thiene, G., . . . Angelini, A. (2008). Pathological changes and myocardial remodelling related to the mode of shunting following surgical palliation for hypoplastic left heart syndrome. *Cardiology in the Young, 18*(4), 415–422.

Paul Collison, S., & Singh Dagar, K. (2007). The role of the intra-aortic balloon pump in supporting children with acute cardiac failure. *Postgraduate Medical Journal, 83*(979), 308–311.

Peddy, S. B., Hazinski, M. F., Laussen, P. C., Thiagarajan, R. R., Hoffman, G. M. Nadkarni, V., & Tabbutt, S. (2007). Cardiopulmonary resuscitation: Special considerations for infants and children with cardiac disease. *Cardiology in the Young, 17*(2), 116–126.

Peel, D. A. (2007). Endocarditis due to a nutritionally variant *Streptococcus*: A lesson in recognition and isolation. *British Journal of Biomedical Science, 64*(4), 175.

Prescribing reference. (2009, Summer). NPPR: Nurse practitioner's prescribing reference, 16(2).

Pulmonary atresia: New pulmonary atresia research from Children's Hospital, Department of Cardiology outlined. (2010, September). Pediatrics Week, 252.

Romp, R. L., & Lau, Y. R. (2010). Congenital heart disease. In R. E. Rakel & E. T. Bope (Eds.), *Conn's current therapy 2010* (pp. 337–342). Philadelphia: Saunders Elsevier.

Siles, A., & Lapierre, C. (2008). Infracardiac total anomalous pulmonary venous return (TAPVR). *Pediatric Radiology, 38*(12), 1354.

Slota, M. C. (Ed.). (2006). *Core curriculum for pediatric critical care nursing* (2nd ed.). St. Louis, MO: Saunders.

Soongswang, J., Sangtawesin, C., Durongpisitkul, K., Laohaprasitiporn, D., Nana, A. Punlee, K., & Kangkagate, C. (2005). The effect of coenzyme Q10 on idiopathic chronic dilated cardiomyopathy in children. *Pediatric Cardiology, 26*(4), 361–366.

Spratto, G. R., & Woods, A. L. (2001). *PDR: Nurse's drug handbook.* Montvale, NJ: Delmar & Medical Economics.

Stumper, O. (2010). Hypoplastic left heart syndrome. *Heart, 96*(3), 231–236.

Taeusch, H. W., Ballard, R. A., & Gleason, C. A. (2005). *Avery's diseases of the newborn* (8th ed.). Philadelphia: Elsevier.

Trivits Verger, J., & Lebet, R. M. (Eds.). (2008). *AACN procedure manual for pediatric acute and critical care.* St. Louis, MO: Saunders.

Tweddell, J. S., Hoffman, G. M., Mussatto, K. A., Fedderly, R. T., Berger, S., Jaquiss, R. D., . . . Litwin, S. B. (2002). Improved survival of patients undergoing palliation of hypoplastic left heart syndrome: Lessons learned from 115 consecutive patients. *Circulation, 106*(12 suppl 1), I82–I89.

Tweddell, J. S., Ghanayem, N. S., Mussatto, K. A., Mitchell, M. E., Lamers, L. J., Musa, N. L., . . . Hoffman, G. M. (2007). Mixed venous oxygen saturation monitoring after stage 1 palliation for hypoplastic left heart syndrome. *Annals of Thoracic Surgery, 84,* 1301–1311.

University of California. (2008, July). Atrioventricular canal defects: Reports outline atrioventricular canal defects research from University of California. *Cardiovascular Week,* 33.

Van Hare, G. F., & Javitz, H. (2004). Prospective assessment after pediatric cardiac ablation: Demographics, medial profiles, and initial outcomes. *Pediatric Electrophysiology Society, Journal of Cardiovascular Electrophysiology, 15*(7), 759–770.

Vasudevan, A., & Mahesh, N. (2009). Acute respiratory distress syndrome in a child with cerebral palsy. *Internet Journal of Anesthesiology, 20*(2). 3.

Watson, S., & Gorski, K. A. (2011). *Invasive cardiology: A manual for cath lab personnel.* Sudbury, MA: Jones & Bartlett Learning.

Wessels, M. W., De Graaf, B. M., Cohen-Overbeek, T .E., Spitaels, S. E., de Groot-de Laat, L. E., Ten Cate, F. J., . . . Willems, P. J. (2008, January). A new syndrome with noncompaction cardiomyopathy, bradycardia, pulmonary stenosis, atrial septal defect and heterotaxy with suggestive linkage to chromosome 6p. *Human Genetics, 122*(6), 595.

Yildirim, S., Tokel, K., Saygili, B., & Varan, B. (2008). The incidence and risk factors of arrhythmias in the early period after cardiac surgery in pediatric patients. *Turkish Journal of Pediatrics, 50*(6), 549–553.

Young, T. E., & Magnum, B. (2009). *Neofax 2009.* Montvale, NJ: Thomson Reuters.

SECTION 4

Pulmonary

1. **Your patient was admitted to the PICU and is septic. You have just drawn an ABG sample from an arterial line and handed the sample to the respiratory therapist. The respiratory therapist asks if the patient has a fever. The possibility of fever will have what effect on the sample you collected?**
   A. The PO_2 will be falsely elevated
   B. The pH will rise
   C. Fever has no effect
   D. The HCO_3 will be elevated

2. **You ask an orientee to carry a newly drawn ABG specimen to the lab. She does not place the sample on ice and walks away. What effect will the lack of icing have on the sample?**
   A. None
   B. It will invalidate the sample
   C. The pH will rise
   D. The PaO_2 will rise

3. **You are asked to draw an arterial blood gas sample. You prepare a glass syringe with heparin. What effect will too much heparin have on the sample?**
   A. It will increase the $PaCO_2$
   B. No effect
   C. It will decrease the bicarbonate
   D. It will totally prevent clotting

4. **You are attempting to draw an arterial blood gas sample from an arterial line. The syringe requires a lot of force to move the cylinder. What effect will this high friction on the syringe have on the blood gas results?**
   A. It will put the artery into spasm
   B. It will increase the $PaCO_2$
   C. It will decrease the PaO_2
   D. No effect

5. **Which of the following drugs is classified as a methylxanthine?**
   A. Morphine
   B. Theophylline
   C. Prednisone
   D. Atropine

6. **Jerold has been hypoxic since his admission three days ago for a tension pneumothorax. Which potential imbalance would be expected with this prolonged hypoxic state?**
   A. Hypochloremia
   B. Respiratory alkalosis
   C. Decreased bicarbonate levels
   D. Hypokalemia

7. **A student nurse asks you to explain the concept of hypoxemia. Hypoxemia is best defined as**
   A. A decrease in oxygen at the cellular level
   B. A decrease in oxygen at the alveolar level
   C. A decrease in oxygen levels in venous blood
   D. A decrease in oxygen levels in arterial blood

8. **Anatomic dead space is defined as**
   A. A conducting airway
   B. Wasted ventilation
   C. End expiratory volume
   D. Minute ventilation

9. **The cells that are responsible for forming a barrier for alveoli are**
   A. Histocytes
   B. Type II alveolar epithelial cells
   C. Macrophages
   D. Type I alveolar epithelial cells

10. **Chronic hypoxia usually results in which of the following electrolyte imbalances?**
   A. Decreased chloride
   B. Decreased potassium
   C. Decreased calcium
   D. Decreased bicarbonate

11. **Familial emphysema is a condition that results in a deficiency of**
   A. Adenosine monophosphate
   B. The ability to produce mucus
   C. Alveoli
   D. Serum alpha-antitrypsin

12. **Victor was finally released from the hospital after a difficult course of treatment for sepsis. He plans to visit his family in Colorado Springs. Part of the patient teaching for Victor and his parents should include information on the effects of high altitude on his ability to oxygenate effectively. Which of the following changes would be expected with his blood gas results?**
   A. The PaO_2 will increase
   B. No effect
   C. The O_2 saturation will decrease
   D. The pH will decrease

13. Mary Margaret is a 16 year old admitted to your PICU with status asthmaticus. She has been taking Accolate, Allegra and using a Proventil HFA rescue inhaler at home. Today she was skateboarding with her friends and could not catch her breath. Her bronchospasms worsened, and she was transported to the ED. In the ED, Mary Margaret received albuterol, oxygen, and epinephrine without significant improvement. During the initial assessment in the PICU, you note that she is using accessory muscles for respiration and is tachycardic and tachypneic. On auscultation, inspiratory and expiratory wheezing with a prolonged expiratory phase is heard throughout the lung fields. Mary Margaret is placed on 2 L/min via NC and ABGs are drawn. Blood gas results are as follows: pH 7.53, PaO_2 104 mmHg, $PaCO_2$ 27 mmHg, and HCO_3 23 mEq/L. These blood gas results indicate

A. Compensated metabolic alkalosis
B. Uncompensated respiratory acidosis
C. Compensated metabolic acidosis
D. Uncompensated respiratory alkalosis

14. Which of the following conditions would be the most probable cause of the acid–base imbalance of uncompensated respiratory alkalosis?

A. Kidney failure
B. A side effect of theophylline
C. Hyperventilation
D. Hypoventilation

15. The hospitalist for the PICU orders Inderal (propranolol) for your patient who is an asthmatic. As a nurse, you know that propranolol is contraindicated for asthmatics because

A. It will lead to severe respiratory acidosis
B. It will exacerbate the tachycardia
C. Pneumonia may result
D. Bronchospasm may worsen

16. Falsely low readings on a pulse oximeter may be due to

A. Vasodilation
B. Vascular dyes
C. Phototherapy
D. Fever

17. Your 13 year old patient needs to be placed on mechanical ventilation. The anesthesiologist uses pancuronium bromide (Pavulon) to paralyze the respiratory muscles. Which of the following drugs will counteract the effects of Pavulon?

A. Atropine
B. Neostigmine
C. Narcan
D. Regitine

18. The best treatment to improve air flow in status asthmaticus is the use of

A. PEEP
B. Heliox
C. Norepinephrine
D. Nebulizer treatments

19. **Type II alveolar cells produce**
    A. Surfactant
    B. Phagocytes
    C. Macrocytes
    D. CO_2

20. **Your patient has had 2 cm H2O PEEP added on his ventilator. The use of PEEP may cause an increase in**
    A. SVR
    B. PVR
    C. PAOP
    D. CO

21. **Increased PEEP may cause**
    A. Barotrauma
    B. Increased cardiac output
    C. Hemothorax
    D. A decrease in left atrial pressure

22. **Patients can develop pulmonary air leaks while on mechanical ventilation. A risk factor for the development of an air leak would be**
    A. PEEP set too low
    B. Asynchrony
    C. Use of SIMV
    D. A malfunctioning ETT

23. **If you hear faint breath sounds on the left side of the chest and normal sounds on the right side of the chest immediately after your patient has been intubated, most likely**
    A. The ETT has an air leak
    B. The physician has intubated the esophagus
    C. The ETT is at the carina
    D. The right mainstem bronchus has been intubated

24. **On a ventilator, a high-pressure-limit alarm may sound if**
    A. The ventilator tubing contains excess water
    B. A leak occurs in a chest tube
    C. A pneumothorax occurs
    D. The tubing is disconnected

25. **Persistent pulmonary hypertension of the newborn (PPHN) is caused by**
    A. Shunting through the ventricles
    B. Right-to-left shunting through fetal channels
    C. Increased SVR
    D. Low PVR and pulmonary artery pressures

26. The most common precipitating factor for developing PPHN is

A. Hypoxia/asphyxia
B. Cardiomegaly
C. Bacterial sepsis
D. Pulmonary parenchymal disease

27. Which of the following pulmonary dilators is used for the treatment of pulmonary hypertension?

A. Dobutamine
B. Dopamine
C. Inhaled nitric oxide
D. Epinephrine

28. An action of nitric oxide is

A. Vascular smooth-muscle relaxation
B. Augmentation of prostaglandin synthesis
C. Release of macrophages
D. Increased pulmonary vascular resistance

29. Congenital lobar emphysema predominantly affects which lung field?

A. The right upper lobe
B. The right middle lobe
C. The left upper lobe
D. The left lower lobe

30. An intrinsic factor that may contribute to the pathogenesis of congenital lobar emphysema is

A. An adenoma
B. Pulmonary artery dilation
C. Lymph node compression
D. Hyperplasia

31. The infant you are caring for will require oxygen therapy at home, so it is important that the parents are taught

A. To secure oxygen tanks in a vertical position
B. To have the child wear synthetic clothing to reduce the risk of static electricity
C. To use alcohol-based swabs to reduce oral dryness
D. To use only a nasal cannula, and not a mask

32. Which of the following statements is true regarding the administration of CPAP?

A. CPAP cannot be delivered via an endotracheal tube.
B. CPAP allows for a decrease in functional residual capacity.
C. CPAP provides decreased pressure to the posterior pharynx.
D. CPAP may be administered via nasal prongs.

33. An adverse effect of excessive CPAP is

A. A continuous need to increase oxygen over time
B. A rise in intrathoracic pressure
C. Intraventricular hemorrhage
D. A sudden change in cerebral blood flow

34. One means of decreasing pCO_2 when using a pressure ventilator is to

A. Increase FiO_2
B. Add PEEP
C. Increase the ventilator rate
D. Decrease the tidal volume

35. A disadvantage of using a pressure ventilator is

A. Laryngeal deviation
B. Possible overdistention
C. Changes in pressure occur on a timed cycle
D. PEEP cannot be adjusted

36. Which of the following statements is true regarding pressure ventilators?

A. Pressure ventilators are widely used in PICUs
B. Pressure ventilators deliver a constant tidal volume with each breath
C. Pressure ventilators are pressure-limited, have constant flow, and are time cycled
D. Peak inspiratory pressure varies throughout inspiration

37. In a volume-limited ventilator, an increase in ventilation may be achieved by

A. Decreasing the ventilator rate
B. Increasing the delivered tidal volume
C. Decreasing the PEEP
D. Increase the FiO_2

38. A drug given to lessen the effects of respiratory syncytial virus is

A. Curosurf
B. Palivizumab
C. Attenovir
D. Gentamycin

39. Mary is 3 months old and is receiving lipids. When lipids are given, sometimes the pleural fluid may appear milky in color and be confused with

A. Infectious exudate
B. A pleural effusion
C. A cardiac effusion
D. Chylothorax

40. The risk of pulmonary hemorrhage in an infant is increased if the infant is receiving

A. Adenosine
B. Digoxin
C. Surfactant
D. Intralipids

41. Joey is 6 years old and requires mechanical ventilation. If positive inspiratory pressure (PIP) is increased on a mechanical ventilator, what effect should this change have on the patient's blood gases?

A. It will increase the $PaCO_2$ and decrease the PaO_2
B. It will decrease the $PaCO_2$ and decrease the PaO_2
C. It will decrease the $PaCO_2$ and increase the PaO_2
D. It will decrease the pH and decrease the $PaCO_2$

42. When utilizing transcutaneous PO_2 measurements, some conditions may make the results unreliable. Underestimation of oxygenation may occur

A. If the patient is febrile
B. If the alignment is improper
C. If the patient's skin is hypoperfused
D. If an air bubble forms between the electrode and the patient's skin

43. Which of the following statements is true about high-frequency jet ventilators?

A. Exhalation is an active function
B. High-frequency jet ventilators deliver high-flow, short duration pulses
C. Exhalation is active and forced
D. No conventional breaths can be delivered during HFJV

44. An advantage of high-frequency ventilators over conventional ventilators is

A. Mean airway pressures do not have to be monitored
B. HF ventilators can transport CO_2 out of the lungs while using lower pressures
C. HF ventilators should not cause barotrauma because of the lower pressures used
D. HF ventilators have an advantage only over pressure ventilators

45. Which of the following conditions is most likely to lead to inaccurate oxygen saturation values on a pulse oximeter?

A. Probe placement on an earlobe
B. Hyperthermia
C. Decreased peripheral perfusion
D. Cyanotic heart disease

46. Martha is 2 months old with Pierre Robin sequence and has been admitted to your PICU prior to undergoing a surgical procedure. As a PICU nurse, you know

A. Martha must be fed in the prone position
B. Martha has a thoracic cyst
C. Martha will require at least five successive operations
D. The infant's condition is often fatal

47. Your patient is 1 week old and has undergone a diaphragmatic hernia repair. While preparing the infant for discharge, it is necessary to teach the parents about the possibility of long-term

A. Gastroesophageal reflux
B. Recurrence of ascites
C. Spontaneous pneumothoraces
D. Necrotizing enterocolitis

48. **Your patient is suffering from cardiogenic shock and requires ECMO therapy. Which of the following statements about ECMO is true?**
   A. ECMO is used for treatment of pulmonary hypoplasia
   B. ECMO has replaced nitric oxide as the therapy of choice for PPHN
   C. ECMO should not be used in cases of intravascular hemorrhage
   D. ECMO may be used in cases of immunosuppression

49. **Which of the following high-frequency ventilation modalities is exhalation active?**
   A. High-frequency, flow-interrupted ventilation
   B. High-frequency oscillator ventilation
   C. High-frequency modal ventilation
   D. High-frequency jet ventilation

50. **Veronica was placed on high-frequency jet ventilation (HFJV) for severe respiratory acidosis unresponsive to surfactant replacement and conventional ventilation. During your assessment, you note that her chest is not vibrating and there are secretions in the ETT. Which of the following statements is true regarding suctioning a patient on HFJV?**
   A. Suctioning may be done only with the ventilator on standby
   B. Suctioning may be done when ventilation is in use
   C. Suctioning is not possible due to the size of the ETT
   D. Suction must be applied while inserting and withdrawing the catheter

51. **High-frequency ventilators have a "sigh" setting. This setting is used to**
   A. Allow time for proper suctioning
   B. Decrease microatelectasis and recruit alveoli
   C. Assess lung sounds apart from ventilator sounds
   D. Deliver respirations to fully exchange gases within the lungs

Questions 52–67 require interpretation of arterial blood gas results. On occasion, exam writers will attempt to provide additional, unnecessary information in the stem of a question. The goal is simply to identify the acid–base abnormality.

52. **Analyze the following arterial blood gas results from a toddler on 2 L O_2 via a nasal cannula**
   pH 7.48
   CO_2 31
   HCO_3 22
   A. Normal
   B. Compensated respiratory acidosis
   C. Uncompensated respiratory alkalosis
   D. Uncompensated metabolic alkalosis

53. **Analyze the following arterial blood gas values**
   pH 7.37
   CO_2 29
   HCO_3 18

A. Compensated metabolic acidosis
B. Compensated respiratory acidosis
C. Uncompensated metabolic acidosis
D. Uncompensated respiratory acidosis

54. Analyze the following capillary blood gas results from a patient in room air

pH 7.40
CO_2 40
HCO_3 24

A. Compensated respiratory acidosis
B. Compensated respiratory alkalosis
C. Normal
D. Compensated metabolic acidosis

55. Analyze the following arterial blood gas results from a toddler with a ventricular septal defect

pH 7.55
CO_2 24
HCO_3 31

A. Uncompensated (mixed) respiratory/metabolic alkalosis
B. Compensated respiratory acidosis
C. Compensated metabolic alkalosis
D. Uncompensated respiratory alkalosis

56. Analyze the following arterial blood gas values

pH 7.36
CO_2 69
HCO_3 37

A. Uncompensated metabolic alkalosis
B. Compensated respiratory acidosis
C. Compensated metabolic acidosis
D. Uncompensated respiratory acidosis

57. Analyze the following arterial blood gas results from an infant with tetralogy of Fallot

pH 7.16
CO_2 42
HCO_3 13

A. Normal
B. Compensated respiratory acidosis
C. Uncompensated respiratory acidosis
D. Uncompensated metabolic acidosis

58. Interpret the following capillary blood gas values

pH 7.23
CO_2 61
HCO_3 23

A. Compensated respiratory acidosis
B. Uncompensated metabolic acidosis
C. Uncompensated respiratory acidosis
D. Normal

59. **Analyze the following arterial blood gas values**
    pH 7.52
    CO_2 40
    HCO_3 35
    A. Uncompensated metabolic alkalosis
    B. Compensated metabolic acidosis
    C. Uncompensated respiratory alkalosis
    D. Uncompensated mixed respiratory/metabolic alkalosis

60. **Analyze the following arterial blood gas values**
    pH 7.41
    CO_2 37
    HCO_3 24
    A. Compensated respiratory acidosis
    B. Normal
    C. Compensated metabolic acidosis
    D. Compensated metabolic alkalosis

61. **Analyze the following arterial blood gas values**
    pH 7.09
    CO_2 68
    HCO_3 15
    A. Uncompensated respiratory acidosis
    B. Uncompensated metabolic alkalosis
    C. Compensated metabolic acidosis
    D. Uncompensated (mixed) respiratory/metabolic acidosis

62. **Analyze the following capillary blood gas values**
    pH 7.38
    CO_2 25
    HCO_3 16
    A. Compensated respiratory alkalosis
    B. Compensated metabolic acidosis
    C. Uncompensated metabolic acidosis
    D. Uncompensated respiratory acidosis

63. **Analyze the following blood gas values**
    pH 7.49
    CO_2 30
    HCO_3 22
    A. Uncompensated respiratory alkalosis
    B. Compensated respiratory acidosis
    C. Compensated metabolic alkalosis
    D. Uncompensated metabolic acidosis

64. Analyze the following arterial blood gas values

pH 7.44
CO_2 30
HCO_3 20

A. Uncompensated metabolic alkalosis
B. Uncompensated respiratory alkalosis
C. Compensated respiratory alkalosis
D. Compensated metabolic alkalosis

65. Analyze the following arterial blood gas values

pH 7.31
CO_2 65
HCO_3 26

A. Uncompensated metabolic alkalosis
B. Uncompensated respiratory acidosis
C. Compensated metabolic acidosis
D. Compensated respiratory acidosis

66. Analyze the following arterial blood gas values

pH 7.38
CO_2 38
HCO_3 22

A. Normal
B. Compensated respiratory acidosis
C. Compensated metabolic acidosis
D. Compensated respiratory alkalosis

67. Analyze the following arterial blood gas results from a term infant on room air

pH 7.15
CO_2 57
HCO_3 21

A. Uncompensated metabolic alkalosis
B. Uncompensated (mixed) respiratory/metabolic acidosis
C. Compensated metabolic acidosis
D. Uncompensated respiratory acidosis

68. Naomi is a 15 year old who was prescribed steroids by her obstetrician. Antenatal corticosteroids affect lung maturation and help prevent respiratory distress syndrome. Steroids work by

A. Decreasing the size of the alveoli
B. Accelerating the rate of glycogen depletion
C. Reducing the number of lamellar bodies inside the cells
D. Thickening the intra-alveolar septa

69. **Luigi is in respiratory distress and is having retractions. Retractions may best be described as**
    A. A neurological sign indicating no pleural pressure
    B. The chest wall caving inward with a small decrease in pleural pressure
    C. The chest wall caving inward with a large increase in pleural pressure
    D. The chest wall caving inward with a moderate decrease in pleural pressure

70. **When caring for an infant with an expiratory grunt, the infant**
    A. Needs to be intubated immediately
    B. Requires monitoring of vital signs every hour
    C. Is exhaling against a closed glottis
    D. Is exhibiting a neurological sign due to hypoxia

71. **Which of the following actions should be done routinely when caring for an infant with a pulse oximeter?**
    A. Check the disposable sensor q 24 hours
    B. Use a disposable cuff
    C. Apply the pulse oximeter only to a toe
    D. Eliminate all arterial blood gas draws to prevent unnecessary pain for the infant

72. **Samuel is 2 weeks old. He has been receiving antibiotics for a respiratory infection for the past four days. When you change his diaper, you note some small, bright red, raised areas on his buttocks. In the buccal area in his mouth, you note white plaques and you suspect that Samuel is suffering from**
    A. Thrush
    B. An abscess
    C. Herpes virus
    D. Strep throat

73. **Which of the following considerations should the PICU nurse take into account prior to the administration of vancomycin?**
    A. Vancomycin is nephrotoxic
    B. Vancomycin must be administered intramuscularly
    C. Vancomycin should always be given with an aminoglycoside
    D. Vancomycin is specific for *Staphylococcus aureus*

74. **You are part of the patient safety team for your PICU and are responsible for evaluating compliance with hospital-acquired infection procedures. To prevent ventilator-associated pneumonia (VAP) in the PICU, the Centers for Disease Control and Prevention (CDC) recommends that respiratory equipment that comes in direct contact with patient mucosal membranes be**
    A. Cleaned with an alcohol-based solution prior to autoclaving
    B. Washed with sterile normal saline at 90 °F for 5 minutes prior to use
    C. Steam sterilized or autoclaved by the facility regardless if the item is multiuse or single-use
    D. Wet-heat pasteurized at temperatures > 158 °F for 30 minutes and packaged sterile for next use

75. Precautions used when handling respiratory equipment or providing respiratory patient care include

A. Using an alcohol-based antiseptic agent, if your hands are visibly soiled prior to, during, and after patient care

B. Using an alcohol-based antiseptic solution only if you have worn gloves during contact with the patient

C. Using an antimicrobial soap and water prior to and after providing patient care

D. Only decontaminating your hands after providing care if gloves are worn

76. Tiffany has contracted a wound infection secondary to removal of her appendix four days ago. She was started on intravenous gentamycin. Gentamycin is useful in the treatment of

A. Otitis media

B. Gram-positive rods

C. *Pseudomonas aeruginosa*

D. *Bacillus*

77. Fluid therapy in ARDS is directed toward

A. Keeping a high CO state

B. Maintaining a low protein content

C. Maintaining hyponatremia

D. Maintaining a low circulating fluid volume

78. A diagnosis of asthma may be made by

A. A PEFR of 100–125

B. An FEF of 80%

C. A decreased FEV_1

D. Wheezing

79. Your patient required placement of a chest tube after aspiration of a pleural effusion. When assessing a patient with a chest tube drainage system, which of the following statements would be correct?

A. Check for subcutaneous emphysema around the insertion site by auscultation

B. If using a Pleur-Evac with autotransfusion connection, make certain all clamps are open

C. The average chest tube size for an adult is 20 Fr

D. If using a chest tube drainage system with a one-way value and suction, water is required to maintain a seal

80. The nurse just coming on shift to care for your patient brought several ampules of normal saline to the bedside in preparation for suctioning your patient. Research has shown that use of normal saline does not thin secretions and may cause which of the following adverse effects?

A. Decreased mean arterial pressure

B. Decreased intrathoracic pressure

C. Anxiety

D. Bronchodilation

81. **In the PICU, patients are mechanically ventilated by a variety of ventilator modes. Which of the following ventilator modes allows the patient to breathe spontaneously?**
    A. HFV
    B. SIMV
    C. CMV
    D. Oscillator

82. **A patient recently admitted to the PICU requires immediate intubation. The physician orders succinylcholine. Which of the following conditions is not a side effect of succinylcholine?**
    A. Hypotension
    B. Malignant hypothermia
    C. Hypokalemia
    D. Smooth-muscle contraction

83. **Vecuronium (Norcuron) is eliminated primarily via the**
    A. Hepatic/biliary system
    B. Spleen
    C. Renal glomerulus
    D. Large bowel

84. **Patients with uncontrolled asthma may receive steroids and neuromuscular blocking agents in an attempt to mitigate their symptoms. These patients are at increased risk for**
    A. Hypertension
    B. Prolonged muscle weakness
    C. Renal failure
    D. Hepatic failure

85. **The FiO_2 for a nasal cannula set at a flow rate of 6 L/min is**
    A. 21%
    B. 24%
    C. 30%
    D. 40%

86. **Your patient has been on a nasal cannula and now requires a nonrebreathing mask to maintain his oxygenation saturation at acceptable levels. A non-rebreathing mask can deliver what percentage of oxygen when the O_2 flow rate is set at 10–15 L/min?**
    A. 24–40%
    B. 30–40%
    C. 60–80%
    D. 50–60%

87. **Pulse oximetry readings are considered unreliable when the oxygen saturation falls below**
    A. 55%
    B. 60%
    C. 80%
    D. 70%

88. **One cause of decreased SVO_2 in a pediatric patient would be**
    A. An increased metabolic rate
    B. Sedation
    C. A decreased metabolic rate
    D. Increased cardiac output

89. **Many of the ventilator circuits used in a PICU utilize a closed catheter suction system. What is one disadvantage of closed catheter suctioning in a mechanically ventilated patient?**
    A. The patient does not receive oxygen during the procedure
    B. The extra weight of the inline tubing
    C. The cost is higher with a single-use catheter
    D. This type of suctioning is cost-effective only if used sporadically

90. **Your patient requires a stoma stent. What is the function of a stoma stent?**
    A. To prevent aspiration
    B. To avoid translaryngeal intubation
    C. To provide the ability for the patient to speak
    D. To keep the stoma tract open

91. **The ED nurse caring for your patient reported that your patient had been previously intubated by paramedics with an LMA. The patient is now conscious and is on a nasal cannula at 2 L/min. Which of the following statements is true regarding the use of LMAs?**
    A. Nurses routinely insert these airways
    B. There is a low risk of aspiration
    C. The LMA is a temporary airway
    D. The vocal cords must be visualized

92. **Which of the following statements about silicone or plastic tracheostomy tubes is true?**
    A. Silicone holds up to repeated cleaning
    B. Wire-reinforced tubes cannot be used during MRI imaging
    C. A one-way speaking valve is easy to use
    D. The tubes offer a lower cost to the facility

93. **Ashley is a 12 year old patient with severe bronchitis. She has been treated with a nonrebreather mask for five days. Today, she is exhibiting increased distress with chest discomfort, restlessness, a dry hacking cough with dyspnea, and numbness in her extremities. Pulmonary function tests (PFTs) indicate a decreased vital capacity (VC), decreased compliance, and decreased functional residual capacity (FRC). As the nurse caring for this patient, you should**

A. Administer Lasix 40 mg IV
B. Prepare for intubation with 100% FiO_2
C. Take the patient for a CT scan and prepare to give tPA
D. Check the pulse oximeter correlation with an arterial blood gas and decrease the FiO_2

94. Bryce is an 8 year old patient with ARDS. He has been on mechanical ventilation for four days. During your assessment, you note a temperature of 100.6 °F, a heart rate of 126, and a respiratory rate of 28. Bryce also has an increased cough and decreased breath sounds on the right side without tracheal deviation. You suspect his symptoms are the result of
A. Pulmonary edema
B. A pneumothorax
C. Sepsis
D. Atelectasis

95. As patients age from birth through young adulthood, chest wall compliance decreases. One reason for this change is
A. Increased arterial oxygen tension
B. Decreased total lung capacity
C. Costal cartilage degeneration
D. Decreased residual volume

96. The oxyhemoglobin dissociation curve may be shifted to the right by
A. Alkalosis, hyperthermia, and hypercapnia
B. Acidosis, hypocarbia, and hypothermia
C. Acidosis, hypercarbia, and hyperthermia
D. Alkalosis, hypothermia, and hypercapnia

97. The nursing student assigned to you for the day asks you to explain the oxyhemoglobin dissociation curve. You reply that the oxyhemoglobin dissociation curve is
A. A relation between dissolved oxygen and the affinity for oxygen by the hemoglobin molecule
B. A graphic representation of carbon dioxide content versus oxygen content in arterial blood
C. A measure of methemoglobin
D. A way to calculate gas transport across the alveoli

98. If the oxyhemoglobin dissociation curve shifts to the right, one factor that will promote this shift is
A. A decrease in 2,3-DPG
B. A decrease in temperature
C. A decrease in pH
D. A decrease in CO_2

99. If the oxyhemoglobin dissociation curve shifts to the left, which of the following conditions could precipitate this change?
A. Increased temperature and increased pH
B. Increased $PaCO_2$
C. Increased 2,3-DPG
D. Decreased temperature

100. Your patient will require long-term ventilatory support via a tracheostomy. One disadvantage of a tracheostomy tube is

A. Subcutaneous emphysema
B. Increased airway resistance
C. A less stable airway
D. The possibility of right mainstem intubation

101. A complication/contraindication of a nasal endotracheal intubation could be

A. It cannot be used for a patient with a cervical injury
B. It provides easy access to the right mainstem bronchus
C. The patient cannot drink
D. It may cause otitis media

102. Your patient has just been intubated with an ETT. Documentation of the procedure usually would not include

A. The time the intubator took to complete the task
B. The size of the tube
C. The depth of the tube
D. If a CXR was taken

103. Your patient required endotracheal intubation. Which of the following statements is true regarding the use of capnography to verify endotracheal tube placement?

A. Placement of the device can be difficult to learn initially
B. It is not necessary to auscultate lung sounds when capnography is used
C. $ETCO_2$ is a moderately reliable indicator of correct tube placement
D. Capnography is not a substitute for pulse oximetry

104. A patient with acute respiratory failure will benefit from the use of which of the following ventilator strategies?

A. Limiting plateau pressure
B. Hyperventilation
C. Lower CO_2 levels
D. Maintain PEEP < 5 cm H_2O

105. Mask continuous positive airway pressure (CPAP) should be used with caution if a pediatric patient has

A. A low functional residual capacity (FRC)
B. A basilar skull fracture
C. Sinusitis
D. Pneumonia

106. What is the purpose of grunting?

A. Grunting increases lung compliance
B. Grunting pushes more air through an ETT
C. Grunting decreases the need for abdominal muscle use
D. Grunting helps maintain functional residual capacity

107. Croup is a respiratory infection that primarily affects children

A. Age 3 months to 9 months
B. Age 6 months to 3 years
C. Age 12 months to 5 years
D. Age 18 months to 36 months

108. A child exhibits moderate retractions, normal air entry, stridor when agitated, no cyanosis, and is restless. Using the Westley Croup Score, this child would be classified as having

A. Mild croup
B. Mild moderate croup
C. Moderate croup
D. Severe croup

109. Which of the following medications is given orally to inhibit a rapid rise in pulmonary artery pressure secondary to hypoxia?

A. Calcium channel blockers
B. Nitric oxide
C. Sildenafil
D. Prostacycun

110. Which of the following medications is both an analgesic and an amnestic?

A. Barbiturates
B. Propofol
C. Atropine
D. Ketamine

111. A measurement of total oxygen consumption is

A. SvO_2
B. $EtCO_2$
C. $PtCO_2$
D. SjO_2

112. In the lungs, communicating channels through holes in the alveolar wall allowing gas movement between alveoli are called

A. A preacinar artery
B. Alveolar pores of Kohn
C. A cycindric canae of Smolder
D. The palmar artery

113. Which of the following statements about infant and child airways is false?

A. The chest wall is composed of more cartilage than bone
B. Because of rib pliability, the ribs may fail to support the lungs
C. A pneumothorax is easy to auscultate because breath sounds are easily transmitted
D. Internal injury may be present without extreme signs

114. An accessory pathway connecting a small airway to an airspace normally supplied by another pathway is called

A. A cartilaginous bronchus
B. A membranous bronchiole
C. A canal of Lambert
D. The portal of Menifer

115. Gas exchange in the lungs requires movement of gas between the atmosphere, alveoli, and pulmonary vasculature. This movement of gases occurs via
A. Passive diffusion
B. Osmotic pressure
C. Airway resistance
D. Hydrostatic pressure

116. The driving pressure of air divided by air flow rate determined by airway diameter is known as
A. A V-Q mismatch
B. A compliance curve
C. Airway resistance
D. A driving force curve

117. The volume of gas remaining in the lungs at the end of one normal expiration is called
A. Residual volume
B. Capacitance
C. Total lung capacity
D. Functional residual capacity

118. The volume of gas left in the lung following a maximal respiratory effort is known as the
A. Vital capacity
B. Total lung capacity
C. Residual volume
D. Dead airspace

119. An intubated patient who is stable with some residual factors that will affect readiness to wean from the ventilator is said to be in the
A. Acute stage of weaning
B. Prewean stage
C. Weaning stage
D. Chronic weaning stage

120. Mort's father was driving his car through an intersection when the vehicle was T-boned by another car. Mort suffered a fractured pelvis and left femur and was stabilized in the ED. Mort was then transferred to your unit to await surgical fixation of the fractures. When auscultating lung sounds, you hear what you believe to be bowel sounds in his chest. Mort also states he has moderate shoulder pain on the left side and he is mildly tachypneic. Mort will probably be diagnosed with
A. A fractured scapula
B. A hemothorax
C. Diaphragmatic rupture
D. Bowel rupture

121. **Which of the following statements about cyanosis is true?**
   A. Cyanosis is directly related to increased $PaCO_2$
   B. Fingertip clubbing is an indication of chronic hypoxia
   C. Cyanosis may be observed when 1 to 3 grams of Hgb is desaturated
   D. Cyanosis may be easily observed in cases of anemia and polycythemia

122. **Brianna fell down a flight of stairs, breaking her ribs and suffering internal injuries. Which of the following conditions mandates the use of pain control?**
   A. Flail chest
   B. ARDS
   C. Splenectomy
   D. Hemothorax

123. **Your patient has a confirmed flail chest. Which alteration in acid–base balance would you expect with this condition?**
   A. Metabolic alkalosis
   B. Metabolic acidosis
   C. Respiratory acidosis
   D. Respiratory alkalosis

124. **Your patient had a mixed venous sample drawn from his pulmonary artery catheter with a PaO_2 result of 38 mmHg. This result would indicate**
   A. Acute respiratory acidosis
   B. Hypoxemia
   C. A normal value
   D. Hypoxia

125. **Douglas had 1250 mL of pleural effusion removed via thoracentesis and immediately began coughing and became dyspneic. You believe he has developed**
   A. Reexpansion pulmonary edema
   B. A pneumothorax
   C. A cardiac tamponade
   D. A hemothorax

126. **Joseph's endotracheal tube cuff has been requiring increasing pressures all shift to maintain a good air seal. The cuff now requires 64 mmHg for a tight seal. What is the probable cause for the increasing pressure?**
   A. Tracheal stenosis
   B. A cuff leak
   C. Tracheal atresia
   D. A wider endotracheal tube is necessary

127. **Endotracheal cuff pressures should not exceed**
   A. PAOP
   B. Tracheal capillary filling pressure
   C. RAP
   D. Pulmonary artery diastolic pressure

128. The respiratory therapist tells you he is covering another unit and cannot perform postural drainage on your patient. He says your patient needs the left upper lobes drained if possible. The correct position to help this patient is

A. Flat on his left side
B. Flat with his hips elevated
C. Supine
D. Semireclining

129. The respiratory therapist has just given Dolly an aerosol treatment. Dolly is 8 months pregnant. Which of the following conditions is contraindicated for this treatment?

A. Pleural effusions
B. Head injury
C. Asthma
D. Stridor

130. Joey was directly admitted to your PICU by his physician after Joey aspirated an unknown substance at home. One of the factors to be considered when assessing a patient for possible aspiration and chemical/aspiration pneumonitis is

A. The possibility of using syrup of ipecac
B. The pH of the aspirate
C. The type of infiltrates on CXR
D. The ABG results

131. Grace is 9 years old and has a hemothorax. What is the proper location of a chest tube for evacuation of a hemothorax?

A. Second intercostal space, midclavicular line
B. Second intercostal space, midaxillary line
C. Fifth intercostal space, midaxillary line
D. Fifth intercostal space, midclavicular line

132. The hypoxemic type of respiratory failure is defined as

A. Increased dead airspace
B. ARDS
C. $PaO_2 < 60$ mmHg while a person is at rest, at sea level, on room air
D. COPD

133. Betty has been diagnosed with right ventricular hypertrophy. A term for a patient who has been diagnosed with right ventricular hypertrophy caused by pulmonary hypertension, secondarily caused by lung disease, is known as

A. Hyperplasia
B. Thrombotic syndrome
C. Cor pulmonale
D. ARDS

134. PEEP is useful in acute respiratory distress syndrome (ARDS) because

A. PEEP decreases cardiac output
B. PEEP decreases venous return so lungs drain more effectively
C. PEEP prevents barotrauma
D. PEEP can open collapsed alveoli

135. You suspect your patient is developing a pulmonary embolism. Signs and symptoms of a pulmonary embolus can include

A. Sinus bradycardia or a normal EKG
B. Pleuritic chest pain, decreased cardiac output
C. ABGs showing respiratory acidosis, increased respiratory rate
D. Decreased PAS pressure

136. A patient who is being mechanically ventilated with continuous end-tidal CO_2 (pet CO_2) monitoring, develops a pulmonary embolism. An expected change in the patient's parameters would include

A. Increased PaO_2
B. Decreased CVP
C. Decreased pet CO_2
D. Increased $PaCO_2$

137. Which of the following statements is true when a patient has a pulmonary embolism?

A. Respiratory acidosis will occur
B. Heparin is used to dissolve clots
C. Normal D-dimer results can rule out a pulmonary embolism
D. Metabolic alkalosis will develop

138. Multiple organ dysfunction (MODS) may be directly caused by

A. Venous thrombosis
B. Shunting
C. Oral estrogen therapy
D. Pulmonary embolism

139. Pulmonary embolism is actually considered a complication of deep venous thrombosis. To assess for deep venous thrombosis, which of the following signs should be assessed?

A. Moses' sign
B. Davis' sign
C. Corrigan's sign
D. Hamman's sign

140. Nathan had a pulmonary artery catheter placed to closely monitor his fluid status. The physician ordered PAOP pressures q 8 hours. You obtain the initial readings on your shift. The next afternoon, when you attempt to take another wedge pressure, you notice decreased resistance to the syringe. Which of the following complications may have occurred?

A. Syringe malfunction
B. Embolization
C. Balloon rupture
D. This is an expected finding

141. Lauren was admitted to the PICU following a fall from a tree. She complains of stabbing substernal pain each time she changes her position. She has been diagnosed with a pneumomediastinum. A common significant finding is

A. Cullen's sign
B. Grey-Turner's sign
C. Hamman's sign
D. Handes' sign

142. An indication for the use of PEEP would be
A. To reduce FiO_2
B. To assess mean arterial pressure
C. To increase surfactant
D. To reduce mediastinal bleeding post CABG

143. Where does the hypoxemic drive to breathe originate?
A. The cerebellum
B. The aortic and carotid arteries
C. The hypothalamus
D. The medulla

144. The functional residual capacity is defined as
A. The amount of air in the lungs after normal expiration
B. The amount of gas that can be forcefully exhaled after maximum inspiration
C. The amount of gas normally exhaled after a maximum inhalation
D. The amount of gas left in the lungs after a maximum exhalation

145. Severe carbon monoxide poisoning occurs when carboxyhemoglobin levels are higher than
A. 10–15%
B. 20–40%
C. 40–50%
D. 50–60%

146. Carbon monoxide has an affinity for hemoglobin thought to be 200–300 times greater than oxygen's affinity for hemoglobin. Elimination of carbon monoxide from the body is via the
A. Kidneys
B. Liver
C. Spleen
D. Lungs

147. Tyler and his family lost their home to a fire this morning. Tyler was burned on the chest, head, and neck while trying to put out the fire. He is dyspneic and has soot on his face, and his eyebrows and nares are singed. The priority of treatment is for Tyler is
A. To maintain cardiac output
B. To maintain airway patency
C. To treat burned areas
D. To obtain ABGs and a carboxyhemoglobin level

148. The nurse reporting to you on a new patient states that the patient has developed subcutaneous emphysema. Subcutaneous emphysema usually occurs in the area of the

A. Head
B. Neck
C. Abdomen
D. Thorax

149. Pulse oximetry has not been shown to be affected by

A. Dark skin
B. Elevated bilirubin
C. Dark nail polish
D. Presence of hemoglobin

150. Pulse oximetry should never be used

A. To determine oxygen saturation values
B. During a cardiac arrest
C. As a determinant for predicting hemoglobin affinity for oxygen
D. To determine a patient's activity tolerance

151. An SpO_2 value of 95% correlates with which of the following PaO_2 values?

A. 75
B. 80
C. 90
D. 95

152. To prevent complications with chest tube drainage systems, the suction level should not be set higher than

A. -20 cm H_2O
B. -30 cm H_2O
C. -40 cm H_2O
D. -50 cm H_2O

153. Which of the following statements is true regarding chest tube drainage systems?

A. Drainage of frank blood in amounts $>$ 100 mL/hour is not significant
B. Drainage tubing should be placed horizontally on the bed and down to the collection chamber
C. All drainage tubing should be dependent to the insertion site
D. Chest tube drainage from a mediastinal tube should always bubble in the water seal chamber

154. Patients often experience decreases in lung compliance. Which of the following conditions will increase lung compliance?

A. Pulmonary edema
B. Pleural effusions
C. Obesity
D. Emphysema

155. Which of the following statements about laryngeal mask airways is true?
A. The LMA may be inserted by any nurse
B. The LMA may cause hoarseness after its removal
C. The patient must have an absent gag reflex
D. The LMA eliminates the risk of aspiration

156. Which of the following drugs would be considered a mucolytic agent?
A. Atropine
B. Terbutaline
C. Acetyl-cysteine
D. Albuterol

157. Side effects of acetyl-cysteine include
A. Red urine
B. Headache
C. Hypertension
D. Bronchospasm

158. One of the most effective ways to relieve bronchospasm is to administer
A. Adrenalin
B. An antihistamine
C. Prednisone
D. A β_2-receptor agonist

159. To determine if your patient has a genetic predisposition toward malignant hyperthermia, which of the following drugs might be used for sensitivity testing?
A. Halothane
B. Caffeine
C. Accolate
D. Singulair

160. During a cardiac arrest, your patient aspirated gastric contents. Which of the following statements is true regarding this type of aspiration?
A. If the pH of the material is <2.5, necrosis will be minimal
B. The patient will always develop ARDS
C. Onset of symptoms is gradual
D. There is little danger of atelectasis

161. Placement of a central line via a subclavian vein may cause
A. Cardiac tamponade
B. An open pneumothorax
C. A tension pneumothorax
D. Limb pain

162. **As the resident attempts to place a central line, air is accidentally introduced into the line when the IV tubing becomes disconnected. The best position in which to place this patient to minimize a venous air embolism is**
   A. Reverse Trendelenburg
   B. On his right side
   C. Trendelenburg with left decubitus tilt
   D. On his left side

163. **The definitive study to confirm the presence of thrombolic emboli is**
   A. Pulmonary ventilation–perfusion scan
   B. Mixed venous oxygen saturation
   C. Pulmonary angiography
   D. PAWP

164. **Risk factors for thrombolic emboli include**
   A. A patient who is one week post partum
   B. Carcinoma
   C. Long bone fractures
   D. Heparin administration

165. **A venous air embolism may be caused by**
   A. Hemodialysis
   B. Arterial blood gas draws
   C. Radial arterial catheters
   D. Peritoneal dialysis

166. **A shift to the left on the oxyhemoglobin dissociation curve is caused by**
   A. Decreased pH, decreased $PaCO_2$, increased temperature
   B. Increased pH, decreased temperature, decreased $PaCO_2$
   C. Increased 2,3-DPG, decreased pH, decreased $PaCO_2$
   D. Decreased pH, increased $PaCO_2$, increased temperature

167. **You are assisting with the insertion of an orally placed endotracheal tube for an apneic 6 year old child. Which endotracheal tube size (internal diameter) and insertion depth would you anticipate?**
   A. Number 6 uncuffed ETT at 15 cm
   B. Number 5.5 cuffed ETT at 20 cm
   C. Number 5 cuffed ETT at 15 cm
   D. Number 4.5 uncuffed ETT at 18 cm

168. **Blood gases you would expect to see in a patient with thrombotic emboli are**
   A. pH 7.42, PaO_2 88, $PaCO_2$ 28, HCO_3 22
   B. pH 7.45, PaO_2 59, $PaCO_2$ 30, HCO_3 24
   C. pH 7.32, PaO_2 86, $PaCO_2$ 29, HCO_3 26
   D. pH 7.32, PaO_2 90, $PaCO_2$ 30, HCO_3 24

169. **Alexis was admitted for multiple fractures and contusions following a motor vehicle accident this evening. She complains of dyspnea, and petechiae are noted. Alexis probably has**

A. A pulmonary embolus
B. Thrombocytopenia
C. A venous air emboli
D. A fat embolus

170. The best position for a patient with ARDS is
A. Prone
B. On the right side
C. On the left side
D. Supine

171. Fluid therapy for a patient with ARDS is directed toward
A. Keeping a high CO state
B. Maintaining a low protein content
C. Maintaining hyponatremia
D. Maintaining a low circulating fluid volume

172. When managing a patient with persistent pulmonary hypertension, the pH should be maintained between ________, while the $PaCO_2$ should be between __________.
A. 7.35 and 7.45; 40 and 50
B. 7.45 and 7.6; 20 and 30
C. 7.30 and 7.40; 50 and 70
D. 7.28 and 7.35; 50 and 60

173. Pulmonary interstitial emphysema (PIE) may be treated with
A. Cefotaxime
B. Clonidine
C. Dexamethasone
D. Gentamycin

174. Darla is 14 years old and just delivered a male infant at 39 weeks gestation via cesarean section. The infant was a complete placenta previa. Soon after birth, he developed respiratory distress requiring supplemental oxygen and mechanical ventilation. After two weeks in the NICU, the infant was discharged. Two days later, the infant was readmitted to the PICU. His chest X-ray now shows decreased lung volumes and a diffuse "ground glass pattern" with air bronchograms. Which of the following conditions is the most likely cause of his respiratory distress syndrome (RDS)?
A. Persistent pulmonary hypertension of the newborn (PPHN)
B. Deficient surfactant
C. Fluid retention in the lungs
D. Aspiration

175. Pulmonary hypertension is generally defined as a mean pulmonary artery pressure of
A. $\geq$ 10 mmHg
B. $\geq$ 15 mmHg
C. $\geq$ 25 mmHg
D. $\geq$ 35 mmHg

176. Which of the following is a cause of primary hypertension?

A. BPD

B. Histological changes in the vasculature

C. Tetralogy of Fallot

D. Chronic thrombotic disease

177. Ella was a passenger in a car accident and has been diagnosed with pulmonary hypertension. Which of the following drug therapies is most appropriate for her at this time?

A. Nitric oxide

B. Flolan (epoprostenol sodium)

C. Endothelin-1

D. Thromboxane A

178. You are receiving a report on Daren, a 4 year old with pulmonary hypertension related to a VSD. Which of the following symptoms is consistent with presentation of pulmonary hypertension?

A. A prominent S_4

B. Decreased respiratory rate

C. Dyspnea with exertion

D. Left-side heart failure

179. Sally is suffering from primary pulmonary hypertension. Which of the following classes of medications would be used to treat this condition?

A. Beta blockers

B. Calcium channel blockers

C. MAO inhibitors

D. Catecholamines

180. Which of the following conditions may cause cardiac collapse in a child if left untreated?

A. Hyperthermia

B. Infection

C. Constipation

D. Influenza

181. If left untreated, pulmonary hypertension may result in which of the following sequelae?

A. Increased left atrium pressures

B. Irreversible thinning of the medial smooth muscles in the arterioles

C. Reversible thickening of the lateral smooth muscle in the arterioles

D. Increased right ventricular pressures

182. What is the purpose of screening for collagen vascular disease and coagulation disorders in a patient with suspected pulmonary hypertension?

A. Hypoxemia triggers a decrease in collagen creation

B. Hypoxia results in decreased elastin production

C. Decreased blood flow results in blood pooling

D. Hypoxemia destroys collagen

183. Your patient has malignant hyperthermia. Which of the following arterial blood gas results would be expected from a patient with this condition?

A. pH 7.35, pCO_2 40, pO_2 80
B. pH 7.28, pCO_2 49, pO_2 60
C. pH 7.40, pCO_2 38, pO_2 90
D. pH 7.42, pCO_2 41, pO_2 70

184. Your post-op heart patient is being discussed at the biweekly meeting between nurses and physicians for the PICU. You believe your patient is ready to wean from mechanical ventilation. Because this patient has been on prolonged ventilatory support, which of the following parameters would probably result in continuation of mechanical ventilation?

A. Elevated serum creatinine
B. An ejection fraction of 50%
C. A history of a long bone fracture
D. An SPO_2 of 96%

185. Pertussis in infants younger than 1 month old who received erythromycin may mean the infants are at increased risk for

A. Infantile hypertrophic pyloric stenosis
B. Toxoplasmosis
C. Rubella
D. Pulmonary hypertension

186. Which of the following statements about respiratory diphtheria is true?

A. Protection against respiratory diphtheria is predominantly provided by immunoglobulin G antibodies
B. Respiratory diphtheria occurs only during the third trimester of pregnancy
C. The mortality rate of respiratory diphtheria is approximately 90% if left untreated
D. Maternal antitoxin is not transferred to the fetus

SECTION 4

Pulmonary Answers

1. **Correct answer: B**
   Fever will cause the pH to rise. Most ABG machines are calibrated to 37 °C. If the patient has a fever, the oxyhemoglobin curve will be shifted to the right. More oxygen will be given off to the tissues, so the machine has to be calibrated to account for the temperature.

2. **Correct answer: B**
   Not placing the ABG sample on ice will invalidate the sample by causing the $PaCO_2$ to rise approximately 3–10 mmHg per hour. The PaO_2 and the pH will decrease. Even with the advent of new technology, in some facilities samples have to be manually transported to a central testing site.

3. **Correct answer: C**
   Too much heparin in a glass syringe will have dilutional effects and will decrease the bicarbonate and the $PaCO_2$.

4. **Correct answer: C**
   Using a vacutainer or a high-friction syringe will create a vacuum. When that occurs, dissolved gases come out of solution, which decreases PaO_2 and $PaCO_2$. The increased effort to move the cylinder may cause the artery to spasm and impede obtaining the sample, but will not directly affect the test results.

5. **Correct answer: B**
   Methylxanthines are an important class of drugs. In addition to theophylline, caffeine and theobromine are methylxanthines. Methylxanthines can be found in coffee, tea, and cocoa. Low doses of drugs in this classification can stimulate cortical arousal and in higher doses cause insomnia. These drugs can cause tachycardias and increase production of gastric acid and digestive enzymes. Methylxanthines also inhibit histamine release.

6. **Correct answer: A**
   Jerold is probably hypochloremic. Chronic hypoxia leads to chronic respiratory acidosis. The kidneys then retain bicarbonate in the form of sodium bicarbonate. The bicarbonate is exchanged for sodium chloride. Ammonia is an acid, so excess amounts must be removed from the body by releasing ammonium chloride. In chronic hypoxia, there is an increase in bicarbonate levels and a decrease in chloride levels. Other causes of hypochloremia include NG suction, vomiting, and diarrhea.

7. **Correct answer: D**
   Hypoxemia is defined as a decreased oxygen level in the arterial blood or a PaO_2 of < 80 mmHg. Hypoxia is a decreased oxygen level at the cellular level.

8. **Correct answer: A**
   Anatomic dead space is defined as a conducting airway. Conducting airways (e.g., trachea, bronchi) are ventilated, but perfusion (gas exchange) does not take place there. Wasted ventilation is the amount of ventilation that does not participate in gas exchange.

9. **Correct answer: D**
   Type I epithelial cells are responsible for forming a barrier for alveoli. These cells line the outside of the alveoli and are easily inflamed by inhaled toxins or heated air. In addition, type I cells maintain the blood–gas interface. Type II cells produce surfactant.

10. **Correct answer: A**
    Chronic hypoxia usually results in decreased chloride levels. The kidneys try to correct the imbalance by retaining bicarbonate. Chronic hypoxia results in increased CO_2, leading to chronic respiratory acidosis. The bicarbonate is exchanged for the chloride to maintain a balance.

11. **Correct answer: D**
    Familial emphysema is a condition that results in a deficiency in serum alpha-antitrypsin. This disease is extremely rare: Its incidence is estimated to be only 1–3%. It is believed that serum alpha-antitrypsin destroys lung tissue through enzymatic action. Usually Caucasians of European descent express this disease, which is caused by an autosomal recessive trait. Symptoms usually appear when the patient is a teenager; this age of onset facilitates the diagnosis because most emphysema occurs in older patients.

12. **Correct answer: C**
    At higher altitudes, there is decreasing atmospheric pressure to force oxygen into the lungs. To compensate for this lower pressure, the person must breathe faster. The percentage of oxygen remains the same, but the partial pressure of the oxygen decreases. Arterial PaO_2 and O_2 saturation decrease. The rapid breathing results in hyperventilation, raising the pH and lowering the $PaCO_2$ level.

13. **Correct answer: D**
    The pH is elevated, indicating alkalosis. The HCO_3 is normal and the $PaCO_2$ is decreased, which indicates an uncompensated respiratory alkalosis.

14. **Correct answer: C**
    Hyperventilating will cause respiratory alkalosis because the patient is unable to get enough oxygen due to bronchial constriction. Hypoventilation causes a buildup of CO_2, leading to respiratory acidosis.

15. **Correct answer: D**
    Propranolol is contraindicated for asthmatics because it may cause bronchospasm. Propranolol works by blocking the beta-adrenergic effects of the sympathetic nervous system (like bronchodilation). Some antihypertensive drugs are cardioselective, such as atenolol. Newer agents, such as nebivolol, provide for cardioselective beta blockade with vasodilation.

16. **Correct answer: C**
    Falsely low readings on a pulse oximeter may be due to phototherapy. If the patient is hypothermic or has decreased peripheral perfusion, the results will be inaccurate. Phototherapy, the position of the probe, and patient motion can also cause inaccurate readings on a pulse oximeter.

17. **Correct answer: B**
    Neostigmine will counteract the effects of Pavulon. Neostigmine is an enzyme that prevents the breakdown of acetylcholine into its enzyme, thereby improving impulse transmission. Sometimes neostigmine causes bradycardia and increases bronchial secretions. Atropine may be used with neostigmine to mitigate these effects. Narcan is an opioid antagonist.

18. **Correct answer: B**
    Air flow in a patient with status asthmaticus may be improved by the use of heliox. Heliox is a helium–oxygen mixture that can facilitate the delivery of inhaled medications, thereby decreasing the work of breathing. The PEEP must be carefully regulated so as not to cause barotrauma or a dynamic hyperinflation. Adjusting this pressure might improve air flow. Norepinephrine is a vasoconstrictor. Nebulizers may also work, but if the patient is compromised their effectiveness will be minimal at best.

19. **Correct answer: A**
    Type II alveolar cells produce surfactant. Surfactant is a lipoprotein and functions by increasing the surface tension of alveoli and allows alveoli to expand and contract. Some residual pressure should remain in the alveoli at the end of respiration to keep the alveoli open (physiologic PEEP). If surfactant production is impaired, the alveoli's ability to exchange O_2 is compromised. Type I cells line the outside of the alveoli.

20. **Correct answer: B**
    Because PEEP raises intrathoracic pressure and PVR, blood backs up, which can cause hepatic congestion. The increased intrathoracic pressure may also compress blood vessels, cause or exacerbate hypovolemia, and cause low cardiac output.

21. **Correct answer: A**
    Increased PEEP may cause barotrauma. Any pressure in the thorax decreases preload, cardiac output, and blood pressure. Forward blood flow is impeded by increased pressure in the pulmonary vasculature. A pulmonary air leak could occur from the increased pressure caused by PEEP.

22. **Correct answer: B**
    Asynchrony is a risk factor for the development of an air leak. Many PICUs use conventional mechanical ventilators that deliver intermittent positive-pressure inflations and positive end-expiratory pressure at a preset rate, which may be out of synch with the patient's respiratory efforts. The resulting barotrauma may increase bronchopulmonary dysplasia (BPD).

23. **Correct answer: D**
    If you hear faint breath sounds on the left side of the chest and normal sounds on the right side immediately after the patient has been intubated, most likely the tube has been placed in the right mainstem bronchus. The right mainstem bronchus is somewhat wider and has less of an angle off the mainstem bronchus, so it is much more readily intubated.

24. **Correct answer: C**
    On a ventilator, a high-pressure-limit alarm may sound if a pneumothorax has occurred. The increases and changes in thoracic pressure in the presence of a pneumothorax will set off a high-pressure alarm to alert staff. In addition, alarms for saturation and possibly heart rate may sound on the cardiorespiratory monitor. A low-limit alarm may sound if tubing is disconnected and a leak in the chest tube occurs.

25. **Correct answer: B**
PPHN is the result of right-to-left shunting through the fetal shunts at the atrial and ductal levels. The PVR and pulmonary artery pressures are also elevated. The high PVR and pulmonary hypertension restrict pulmonary blood flow, which in turn promotes the development of hypoxemia, acidemia, and lactic acidosis. Most newborns who have PPHN are diagnosed within the first 24 hours of life.

26. **Correct answer: A**
The most common precipitating factors for developing PPHN are hypoxia and asphyxia. Hypoxia and asphyxia are correlated with remodeling small pulmonary arteries and abnormal muscularization. In particular, asphyxia may lead to persistent pulmonary vasospasm. Pulmonary parenchymal diseases (pneumonia, meconium aspiration, RDS, and aspiration syndromes) may also cause pulmonary vasospasm. In rare cases, bacterial sepsis may lead to PPHN.

27. **Correct answer: C**
Inhaled nitric oxide (iNO) is a selective pulmonary vasodilator that is used to treat pulmonary hypertension. iNO reduces the risk of death and the need for extracorporeal membrane oxygenation (ECMO). Do not administer iNO to patients who are dependent on a right-to-left shunt.

28. **Correct answer: A**
One action of nitric oxide is vascular smooth-muscle relaxation, which occurs when NO molecules are released from the endothelium. NO inhibits platelet aggregation and adherence and is thought to alter vascular permeability. It may also participate in nonspecific immunity because it is generated when macrophages are activated.

29. **Correct answer: C**
In congenital lobar emphysema, the left upper lobe is affected 41% of the time, the right middle lobe 34% of the time, and the right upper lobe 21% of the time. In rare cases, both lungs are affected. Congenital lobar emphysema may take one of two forms: hypoalveolar (affecting less than the expected number of alveoli) and polyalveolar (affecting more than the expected number of alveoli).

30. **Correct answer: A**
An intrinsic factor that may contribute to the pathogenesis of congenital lobar emphysema is an adenoma. Pulmonary artery dilation and lymph node compression are extrinsic factors influencing the development of congenital lobar emphysema. Other intrinsic factors include infection, tuberculosis, retained secretions, absence of cartilage, stenosis, and hypoplasia.

31. **Correct answer: A**
Education for the parents should emphasize that oxygen tanks should be stored in the upright position. Synthetic materials often cause static electricity. Only lemon-glycerin swabs (not alcohol-based swabs) should be used. In this case, we do not know whether the infant will be given O_2 via a mask or a cannula.

32. **Correct answer: D**
Continuous positive airway pressure may be delivered by nasal prongs, nasopharyngeal tubes, or endotracheal tubes. CPAP provides increased pressure to the posterior pharynx and increases transpulmonary pressure. It can prevent alveolar collapse and helps prevent obstructive apnea.

33. Correct answer: B

Excessive CPAP may increase intrathoracic pressure to the point of compressing the right atrium and vena cava. The preload will be decreased and cardiac output will be reduced.

34. Correct answer: C

If a patient is retaining CO_2, it is possible to help wash it out by increasing the respiratory rate (the ventilator rate, in this case) or by increasing the tidal volume.

35. Correct answer: B

One potential disadvantage of using a pressure ventilator is overdistention. Lung compliance can change fairly quickly. Compliance can be likened to the elasticity of the lung. If it is less compliant, it can be described as stiffer. If it is more compliant, it can be said to be easier to inflate and deflate. If a pressure ventilator is used and the lung becomes more compliant, the alveoli and lung may become overdistended. If the lung is less compliant, less tidal volume will be delivered because the ventilator only delivers to a preset volume.

36. Correct answer: C

Infants can only generate very small inspiratory efforts. Pressure ventilators provide a constant flow of gas through an endotracheal tube. Breaths are provided at fixed intervals, and a peak inspiratory pressure (PIP) is maintained throughout inspiration.

37. Correct answer: B

In a volume-limited ventilator, it is possible to increase ventilation by increasing either the delivered tidal volume or the ventilator rate. Oxygenation can be increased by increasing the PEEP, FiO_2, or tidal volume.

38. Correct answer: B

Two medications are recommended for babies at high risk for RSV to protect them against the serious complications associated with this illness. During the peak RSV season, either respiratory syncytial virus immune globulin intravenous (RSV-IGIV) or palivizumab (an antibody against RSV) is usually given monthly. These medications are not vaccines and do not prevent infection with the virus. Nevertheless, they do lessen the severity of the resultant illness and may help shorten the hospital stay. There are no medications available to treat the virus itself. Care of a child with RSV involves treating the effects of the virus on the respiratory system. Because a virus causes the illness, antibiotics are not useful.

39. Correct answer: D

Mary is 3 months old and is receiving lipids. Sometimes the pleural fluid may appear milky in color and be confused with chylothorax. Chylothorax is an accumulation of lymphatic fluid that may be either congenital or acquired. If it is acquired, it may occur secondary to a perforated or obstructed thoracic duct. It also may be a surgical complication from repair of a congenital heart defect, diaphragmatic hernia, or tracheoesophageal fistula. If the chylothorax is congenital, it may impede ventilatory efforts in a newborn.

40. Correct answer: C

The risk of pulmonary hemorrhage is increased approximately 5% if the infant is receiving surfactant. Suction can cause bleeding if the respiratory endothelium is damaged. Pulmonary hemorrhage is rarely isolated and often accompanies other conditions such as RDS, aspiration of gastric contents or maternal blood, asphyxia, or DIC.

41. **Correct answer: C**
If positive inspiratory pressure (PIP) is increased on a mechanical ventilator, the result will be a decrease in $PaCO_2$ and an increase in PaO_2.

42. **Correct answer: C**
When utilizing transcutaneous PO_2 measurements, underestimation of oxygenation may occur when the skin is hypoperfused or the calibration is improperly performed. Overestimation of oxygenation may occur if an air bubble or leak between the electrode and the skin occurs.

43. **Correct answer: B**
High-frequency jet ventilators (HFJV) deliver high-flow, short-duration pulses of pressurized gas directly into the upper airway through a specially made endotracheal lumen. These pulses are delivered to the upper airway and are superimposed on gas flow from a conventional ventilator that provides positive end-expiratory pressure (PEEP). In addition, conventional breaths may be delivered in conjunction with the jet ventilation. The systems operate at rates of 150–600 breaths per minute and exhalation is passive.

44. **Correct answer: B**
High-frequency ventilators have the advantage of transporting CO_2 out of the lungs with lower pressure and smaller volume fluctuations than are required during conventional mechanical ventilation. Originally it was thought that adequate gas exchange could be achieved at relatively low mean airway pressures, but now it is known that recruiting lung volume is essential not only for optimizing oxygenation but also for minimizing lung injury.

45. **Correct answer: C**
Adequate perfusion must exist if the probe on a pulse oximeter is to register an accurate evaluation of hemoglobin saturation. If the infant is hypothermic or has decreased peripheral perfusion, the results will be inaccurate. Phototherapy, position of the probe, and patient motion may also cause inaccurate readings on a pulse oximeter.

46. **Correct answer: A**
Pierre Robin sequence is a condition present at birth in which an infant has a very small lower jaw, a tongue that tends to fall back and downward, and a soft cleft palate. An affected infant may choke, so feeding in the prone position may be necessary. Also, the infant should not be placed on his or her back. The mandible may grow and the problem resolve when the infant reaches 6 to 12 months of age.

47. **Correct answer: A**
When a patient has undergone a diaphragmatic hernia repair, it is necessary to teach the parents about the possibility of long-term gastroesophageal reflux issues. In addition, it is important to emphasize that the patient could also suffer other potential side effects such as growth restrictions, recurrent diaphragmatic hernias, and delayed neurological development.

48. **Correct answer: C**
ECMO should not be used for intravascular hemorrhage because systemic heparinization is required. ECMO also increases the risk for intravascular hemorrhage in premature infants, especially those born at less than 35 weeks gestation.

49. Correct answer: B

During high-frequency oscillator ventilation, the exhalation phase is active, with the oscillator controlling inspiration and expiration. Frequency or rate of breaths per minute is expressed in units of hertz (Hz).

50. Correct answer: D

To prevent alveolar rupture, suction should be applied during both insertion and withdrawal of the suction catheter when using high-frequency jet ventilation. If suction is not applied while inserting the catheter, the circuit may become overpressurized due to the occlusion, and the alveoli may rupture. Suctioning may be done when the ventilator is in use or on stand-by. Suctioning while in stand-by mode will prevent airway damage from opposing pressures generated by the ventilator and suction catheter.

51. Correct answer: B

On a high-frequency ventilator, the "sigh" setting is a backup rate that provides a set number of ventilations per minute with the goal of recruiting additional alveoli and minimizing microatelectasis.

52. Correct answer: C

This result is uncompensated respiratory alkalosis. The pH is greater than 7.45, so the value is an uncompensated alkalosis. To determine whether the alkalosis is respiratory or metabolic, find the value that represents alkalosis—in this case, $CO_2 < 35$ mmHg.

53. Correct answer: A

This result is compensated metabolic acidosis. The pH is between 7.35 and 7.45, so the value is compensated, but because it is closer to 7.35, the value is considered acidotic. To determine whether the acidosis is respiratory or metabolic, find the value that represents acidosis—in this case, $HCO_3 < 22$ mEq/L.

54. Correct answer: C

The pH is between 7.35 and 7.45, the CO_2 is between 35 and 45 mmHg, and the HCO_3 is between 22 and 26 mEq/L. All the results are within normal ranges, so this ABG is considered normal.

55. Correct answer: A

This is an uncompensated (mixed) respiratory/metabolic alkalosis. The pH is greater than 7.45, so the value is uncompensated. To determine whether the acidosis is respiratory or metabolic, find the value that represents alkalosis—in this case, $HCO_3 > 26$ mEq/L and $CO_2 < 35$ mmHg. Thus the cause of the alkalosis is both respiratory and metabolic in nature.

56. Correct answer: B

This ABG result is a compensated respiratory acidosis. The pH is between 7.35 and 7.45, so the value is compensated, but because it is closer to 7.35, the value is considered acidotic. To determine whether the acidosis is respiratory or metabolic, find the value that represents acidosis—in this case, $CO_2 > 45$ mmHg.

57. Correct answer: D

The result of this blood gas analysis is an uncompensated metabolic acidosis. The pH is less than 7.35, so the value is uncompensated acidosis. To determine whether the acidosis is respiratory or metabolic, find the value that represents acidosis—in this case, $HCO_3 < 22$ mEq/L.

58. **Correct answer: C**
This capillary blood gas is an uncompensated respiratory acidosis. The pH is < 7.35, so the value indicates an uncompensated acidosis. Next, determine which respiratory or metabolic value represents acidosis—in this case, $CO_2 > 45$ mmHg.

59. **Correct answer: A**
This result is an uncompensated metabolic alkalosis. The pH is greater than 7.45, so the value is uncompensated. To determine whether the alkalosis is respiratory or metabolic, find the value that represents alkalosis—in this case, $HCO_3 > 26$ mEq/L.

60. **Correct answer: B**
The pH is between 7.35 and 7.45, the CO_2 is between 35 and 45 mmHg, and the HCO_3 is between 22 and 26 mEq/L. All the results are within normal ranges, so this ABG is considered normal.

61. **Correct answer: D**
This is an uncompensated (mixed) respiratory/metabolic acidosis. The pH is less than 7.35, so the value is uncompensated acidosis. To determine whether the acidosis is respiratory or metabolic, find the value that represents acidosis—in this case, $HCO_3 < 22$ mEq/L and $CO_2 > 45$ mmHg. Thus the cause of the acidosis is both respiratory and metabolic in nature.

62. **Correct answer: B**
This capillary blood gas indicates a compensated metabolic acidosis. The pH is between 7.35 and 7.45, so the gas is compensated, but the value is closer to acidosis, indicating compensated acidosis. Next, determine which respiratory or metabolic value is acidotic—in this case, $HCO_3 < 22$ mEq/L.

63. **Correct answer: A**
This result signifies an uncompensated respiratory alkalosis. The pH is greater than 7.45, so the value is uncompensated alkalosis. To determine whether the alkalosis is respiratory or metabolic, find the value that represents alkalosis—in this case, $CO_2 < 35$ mmHg.

64. **Correct answer: C**
This result demonstrates a compensated respiratory alkalosis. The pH is between 7.35 and 7.45, so the value is compensated, but because it is closer to 7.45, the value is considered alkalotic. To determine whether the alkalosis is respiratory or metabolic, find the value that represents alkalosis—in this case, $CO_2 < 35$ mmHg.

65. **Correct answer: B**
This result is an uncompensated respiratory acidosis. The pH is less than 7.35, so the value is uncompensated. To determine whether the acidosis is respiratory or metabolic, find the value that represents acidosis—in this case, $CO_2 > 45$ mmHg.

66. **Correct answer: A**
The pH (between 7.35 and 7.45), the CO_2 (between 35 and 45 mmHg), and the HCO_3 (between 22 and 26 mEq/L) are within normal ranges, so the ABG is considered normal.

67. **Correct answer: B**
This result is an uncompensated (mixed) respiratory/metabolic acidosis. The pH is less than 7.35, so the value is uncompensated acidosis. To determine whether the acidosis

is respiratory or metabolic, find the value that represents acidosis—in this case, HCO_3 < 22 mEq/L and $CO_2 > 45$ mmHg. Thus the cause of the acidosis is both respiratory and metabolic in nature.

68. **Correct answer: B**
Antenatal corticosteroids affect lung maturation and help prevent respiratory distress syndrome. Steroids work by accelerating the rate of glycogen depletion and glycerophospholipid biosynthesis. This process results in thinning of the intra-alveolar septa and increases the size of the alveoli.

69. **Correct answer: D**
Retractions occur when parenchymal disease is present and the chest wall produces a greater negative pressure. The chest wall is very compliant and caves inward with a moderate decrease in pleural pressure. Retractions are best seen at the xiphoid and intercostal markings of the chest.

70. **Correct answer: C**
An infant with an expiratory grunt is performing a Valsalva maneuver in which the infant exhales against a closed glottis, producing a sound similar to a moan. With this behavior, transpulmonary pressure is increased, which decreases or prevents atelectasis. Oxygenation and alveolar ventilation are improved. Intubation should not be tried unless the infant's condition is rapidly deteriorating, because the ETT prevents the Valsalva maneuver and the alveoli will collapse.

71. **Correct answer: B**
When caring for an infant with a pulse oximeter, it is important to use a disposable cuff. A reusable cuff will wear down and allow ambient light to get in and invalidate the readings. The disposable sensor should be checked at least every 8 hours. The pulse oximeter is useful for trending, but arterial blood gases must be drawn to correlate with the pulse oximeter.

72. **Correct answer: A**
Small, raised, bright red areas around the diaper line and white plaques in the buccal area, on the cheeks, on the tongue, or on the gums usually indicate thrush. Samuel has been on antibiotic therapy, so he is probably experiencing overgrowth of bacteria.

73. **Correct answer: A**
Prior to the administration of vancomycin, the PICU nurse should know that vancomycin is nephrotoxic, especially if used in combination with aminoglycosides. Vancomycin is used in the treatment of methicillin-resistant strains of pathogens (e.g., *Staphylococcus epidermidis*) and must be administered by slow intravenous drip.

74. **Correct answer: D**
The 2003 guidelines from the Centers for Disease Control and Prevention (CDC) recommend that any equipment that comes in direct contact with patient mucosal membranes undergo wet-heat pasteurization at a temperature greater than 158 °F for at least 30 minutes and be packaged in sterile wrapping for the next use. An autoclave may also be used for reusable equipment. Any single-use equipment is recommended for resterilization per FDA guidelines by a third-party agency prior to use with another patient. If equipment must be washed after sterilization, the CDC recommends the use of sterile water, not normal saline. Many PICU units use the services of the respiratory

therapy department to maintain and sterilize all respiratory equipment. As a patient advocate, the bedside nurse should be aware of this issue and ensure that equipment is properly sterilized prior to use on his or her patient.

75. **Correct answer: C**
Antimicrobial soap and water may be used to decontaminate the provider's hands prior to, during, and after patient care, regardless of glove use, visible soiling, or no apparent soiling. Hands should always be decontaminated using soap and water, waterless soap, or alcohol-based antiseptic agent prior to and after patient care to prevent the spread of organisms from patient to patient or from surfaces. Alcohol-based antiseptic agents should be used only if no visible soiling is observed.

76. **Correct answer: C**
Gentamycin is effective against gram-negative rods and penicillin-resistant staphylococci, *Escherichia coli* strains, and *Pseudomonas aeruginosa.* It may cause ototoxicity and nephrotoxicity. The nurse needs to follow serum levels (peak and trough). Gentamycin must never be given as IV push—only as a drip over at least 30–60 minutes. If the patient has oliguria or anuria, the dose must be decreased or discontinued.

77. **Correct answer: D**
Fluid therapy in ARDS is directed toward maintaining a low circulating fluid volume. The fluid volume is kept low to maintain PAOP (PCWP) at minimal levels. If too much fluid is present, leakage may occur through damaged capillaries so that fluid moves into the interstitial space.

78. **Correct answer: C**
A diagnosis of asthma may be made based on a decreased FEV_1. The forced expiratory volume (FEV) is how much air is exhaled during the first second of effort. This amount should be $\geq$ 75% of the predicted normal value. In asthmatics, this value is decreased because of obstruction. The forced vital capacity (FVC) is the total amount of gas exhaled as forcefully and rapidly as possible after taking a maximal inspiration. This value should be greater than 80%.

79. **Correct answer: B**
If using a Pleur-Evac with autotransfusion connection, make certain all clamps are open. When using any autotransfusion drainage system, make sure to connect the system per the manufacturer's recommendations. Most connections will be color coded for easy connecting. Clamps must remain open to allow for blood collection and prevent increases in intrathoracic pressures. Subcutaneous air should be checked by palpation and borders marked for further monitoring. If a one-way valve system and suction are used, water is not required to maintain a seal because the valve serves this function.

80. **Correct answer: C**
Research into normal saline use in tracheal suctioning has proven that normal saline is associated with anxiety, increased risk for hospital-acquired pneumonia, and bronchoconstriction. Current recommendations focus on dry suctioning, frequent oral care, balanced hydration, and position changes to prevent complications associated with intubation and mechanical ventilation.

81. **Correct answer: B**
Synchronized intermittent mandatory ventilation provides a set frequency of breaths and either volume or pressure. The patient is permitted to breathe spontaneously at his

or her own volume between mandatory ventilations. If the spontaneous breath occurs at the same time as a mandatory breath, the ventilator will synchronize with the patient, thereby preventing "stacked" breaths. The other modes of ventilation listed as options (CMV, HFV and oscillation) require full control of setting by an operator and not the patient's responses.

82. **Correct answer: D**
Succinylcholine combines with acetylcholine to cause smooth-muscle relaxation, not contraction. Prolonged use may change the blocking action and result in potassium-regulated alterations in electrical activity. Other side effects of succinylcholine include malignant hyperthermia, either hypertension or hypotension, hyperkalemia, anaphylaxis, and increased intraocular pressure.

83. **Correct answer: A**
Norcuron is eliminated via the hepatic/biliary system. Use this agent with caution in patients with known or suspected hepatic or biliary compromise, such as cirrhosis or hepatitis. Norcuron may take twice as long to clear a patient's system.

84. **Correct answer: B**
Uncontrolled asthma symptoms during an attack may lead to prolonged and extensive muscle use in an attempt to maintain independent respirations. Prolonged effort may result in respiratory failure due to respiratory muscle fatigue. Administration of a neuromuscular blocking agent further inhibits the smooth-muscle retractions. Long-term steroid use has been linked to muscle wasting. Ventilatory weaning may be prolonged as respiratory muscles must recover from both the disease process and the pharmacologic intervention.

85. **Correct answer: D**
The FiO_2 for a nasal cannula set at a flow rate of 6 L/min is 40%. The nasal cannula is generally considered a low-flow oxygen device unless it is connected to a high-flow system. If the flow exceeds 4 L/m, the oxygen should be humidified to prevent drying of the mucosal membranes.

86. **Correct answer: C**
A nonrebreathing mask can deliver 60–80% of oxygen when the O_2 flow rate is 10–15 L/min. If both exhalation ports have one-way valves, then nearly 100% oxygen may be delivered. To prevent suffocation in patients when the oxygen is disconnected, nonrebreathing masks now come equipped with only a single one-way valve to prevent or limit inhalation of room air. This results in decreasing the highest concentration of actual inspired oxygen to 60–80%.

87. **Correct answer: D**
Pulse oximetry readings are considered unreliable when oxygen saturation falls to a level less than 70%. Pulse oximetry accuracy is influenced by patient motion, low perfusion, venous pulsation, light, poor probe positioning, edema, anemia, and carbon monoxide levels. It is important to compare pulse oximetry values against arterial blood gas results to validate values reported as less than 70%.

88. **Correct answer: A**
One cause of decreased SVO_2 would be an increased metabolic rate. An increased metabolic rate would increase the O_2 uptake by tissues, resulting in a lower value

measured by venous blood gases. The other answers result in a lower tissue oxygen requirement, so that a larger concentration of oxygen remains in the bloodstream.

89. **Correct answer: B**

Lack of available oxygen and lower cost-effectiveness are characteristics of open catheter suctioning. The inline system can be used multiple times and is more cost-effective.

When a closed system is used, an extra weight is present that can increase tension on the catheter or tubing. In turn, this tension may cause the ETT to move. Many manufacturers make the inline tubing for both ETTs and tracheostomy tubes. Nurses must make certain they are using the correct tube for suctioning.

Another problem with the inline catheters relates to the extra tubing that hangs out when the catheter is not in use. Patients may easily reach this tubing and extubate themselves or push the catheter down the airway, where it will obstruct air flow.

90. **Correct answer: D**

The function of a stoma stent is to keep the stoma tract open. The stents can be manufactured to have either a straight or curved configuration to accommodate the differing nature of patients' air passages. The stent rests against the anterior wall of the trachea, where it allows for freer passage of air. The patient can then breathe spontaneously around the tube.

91. **Correct answer: C**

The laryngeal mask airway was intended for use as a temporary airway. It requires minimal training to insert, but cannot be placed by RNs as a matter of course. The patient must be unconscious and/or without a gag reflex. The low-pressure seal around the mask means that it cannot be used on patients with high peak ventilator pressures. The LMA is also associated a significant risk of aspiration.

Advantages with use of this airway are that it is simply blindly inserted into the hypopharynx, does not require visualization of the vocal cords, and does not traumatize the trachea. Patients will not have hoarseness or lose their voice altogether. At best, patients will complain of a mild sore throat.

92. **Correct answer: B**

Silicone or plastic tracheostomy tubes contain wires. The magnet in the MRI will attract the wires in the tube. The silicone or plastic tubes cannot tolerate repeated cleanings. Use of a one-way speaking valve is contraindicated when using a foam cuff because the cuff may lie at an angle to the valve due to its orientation in the airway. The cost of using silicone or plastic tubes is actually higher to facilities because the tubes are difficult to keep clean and are labor intensive.

93. **Correct answer: D**

Ashley is exhibiting signs and symptoms of oxygen toxicity after five days of oxygen therapy at $>50\%$ FiO_2. Non-rebreather masks provide a minimum of 60% FiO_2 at 6 L/min. An arterial blood gas analysis would show an increased $PaO_2 > 100$ mmHg, ruling out respiratory failure ($PaO_2 < 60$) that would require intubation. The dry, hacking cough rules out pulmonary edema and the need for Lasix. The numbness in the patient's extremities is caused by oxygen radicals in her blood, not a neurologic impairment that would indicate the need for a CT scan with possible tPA administration.

94. **Correct answer: D**
Four days of high FiO_2 has produced a nitrogen washout, resulting in atelectasis. Nitrogen's high partial pressure is necessary to maintain alveolar inflation. It is important to titrate FiO_2 to maintain oxygen saturation within a prescribed range when oxygen therapy is utilized. Pulmonary edema would result in coarse breath sounds. With a unilateral pneumothorax, the patient would demonstrate tracheal deviation. Sepsis would not necessarily present with diminished breath sounds, but would be accompanied by additional findings of increased purulent secretions, coarse breath sounds, and altered laboratory diagnostic results.

95. **Correct answer: C**
From birth, chest wall compliance decreases. Much of this decrease is due to calcification of the costal cartilage, but the elasticity decreases as well. Vertebrae develop osteoporosis and a degree of kyphosis can occur. Weight gain is common and posture is affected. In today's society, children are more commonly suffering from obesity and frequently develop back problems. The chest wall compliance decreases, as does vital capacity. Residual volume increases, PaO_2 decreases, and $PaCO_2$ increases.

96. **Correct answer: C**
Acidosis, hypercarbia and hyperthermia will all lead to a rightward shift in the oxyhemoglobin dissociation curve. Hemoglobin in this instance has a decreased affinity for oxygen and enhances tissue uptake of oxygen.

97. **Correct answer: A**
The oxyhemoglobin dissociation curve reflects the patient's physiological circumstances. It is a relation between dissolved oxygen and the affinity for oxygen by the hemoglobin molecule.

98. **Correct answer: C**
A shift to the right in the oxyhemoglobin dissociation curve means hemoglobin has less affinity for oxygen. If the pH decreases and the patient becomes more acidotic, the tissues will need more oxygen. 2,3-Diphosphoglyceride is needed to help force O_2 off the hemoglobin molecule. Thus, if the level of 2,3-DPG is decreased, the hemoglobin will hang onto the O_2. If the temperature is increased, the tissues need more O_2. If the PCO_2 is elevated, the tissues need more oxygen.

99. **Correct answer: D**
If the oxyhemoglobin dissociation curve shifts to the left, hemoglobin holds onto the oxygen. This may be caused by decreased temperature, CO_2 and levels of 2,3-DPG. Tissues would not need as much O_2.

100. **Correct answer: A**
A disadvantage associated with the use of a tracheostomy tube is the potential for development of subcutaneous emphysema. The tracheal tube provides a more stable airway, can be placed in an ICU setting, and decreases airway resistance. The tube is not near the right mainstem bronchus, so it will not facilitate intubation of the bronchus. A large number of potential complications are associated with the use of a tracheostomy tube. Some of these complications include tracheal stenosis, tracheal malacia, aspiration, infection, hemorrhage, subcutaneous emphysema, and pneumothorax.

101. Correct answer: D

Because of the direct connection via the Eustachian tube, infection in the ear is possible. If a cervical injury has been stabilized, it is certainly possible for a skilled intubator to place the tube. Additional complications associated with placement of nasal endotracheal tubes include nasal bleeding, sinusitis, accidental esophageal intubation, vocal cord injuries, necrosis, cuff leak or failure, and obstruction.

102. Correct answer: A

Generally, the time it took for the intubator to complete the task is not documented. However, if an unusual occurrence or a complication occurred during this process, it should be properly documented. The depth of the tube is important to chart because it gives a reference point for any questions about tube migration. The size of the tube may be too small or large, so it would have to be adjusted to the next appropriate size. A CXR is done to confirm tube placement, and the time when the X-ray is taken should be documented. Any medications given during the procedure should be documented as to reason for administration, patient response, and follow-up such as vital sign measurements or untoward reactions.

103. Correct answer: D

Capnography is not a substitute for pulse oximetry. A pulse oximeter measures the availability of sites on the hemoglobin molecule for oxygen transport versus the percentage of sites actually occupied. The $ETCO_2$ measures whether gas exchange is taking place at the cellular level. If CO_2 is being given off, it will react with chemically treated paper in the detector. If the esophagus has been intubated, the $ETCO_2$ can give a false-positive reading if the patient has consumed a carbonated beverage within the past few hours.

104. Correct answer: A

This is a very advanced question. The topic is discussed here more for your awareness, rather than test content. The plateau or alveolar pressure should be limited to 30 cm H_2O, maximum. If a higher pressure is maintained, microvascular permeability is increased. The high pressure may also cause a stress fracture of capillary endothelium, epithelium, and basement membranes, leading the lung to completely rupture. If this happens, blood, fluids, proteins, and exudates will leak into the air spaces and the tissue. The reverse is also true—air may leak into the tissues. If the pressure can be maintained at 30 cm H_2O, the CO_2 level may rise and increase the intracranial pressure, eventually resulting in a respiratory acidosis will result. By slowly reducing tidal volume, the kidneys will be able to compensate for the respiratory acidosis.

105. Correct answer: B

CPAP should be used with caution in patients with basilar skull fractures. Research has shown that pneumocephalus may occur if a basilar skull fracture exists. CPAP increases the functional residual capacity by helping to reexpand the alveoli. Patients who have acute cardiogenic pulmonary edema may also benefit from the use of CPAP.

106. Correct answer: D

Grunting helps the patient maintain functional residual capacity.

107. Correct answer: B
Croup is a respiratory infection that primarily affects children between ages 6 months and 3 years.

108. Correct answer: C
According to the Westley Croup Score, moderate croup is diagnosed when a child exhibits moderate retractions, normal air entry, stridor when agitated, no cyanosis, and restlessness.

109. Correct answer: C
Sildenafil is given orally to inhibit a rapid rise in pulmonary artery pressure secondary to hypoxia.

110. Correct answer: D
Ketamine is an analgesic and an amnestic.

111. Correct answer: A
SvO_2 is a measurement of total oxygen consumption.

112. Correct answer: B
In the lungs, communicating channels through holes in the alveolar wall allowing gas movement between alveoli are called alveolar pores of Kohn.

113. Correct answer: C
A pneumothorax is difficult to auscultate because breath sounds are easily transmitted.

114. Correct answer: C
A canal of Lambert is an accessory pathway that connects a small airway to an airspace normally supplied by another pathway.

115. Correct answer: A
Gas exchange in the lungs requires passive diffusion of gas between the atmosphere, alveoli, and pulmonary vasculature.

116. Correct answer: C
Airway resistance is the driving pressure of air divided the by air flow rate as determined by the airway diameter.

117. Correct answer: D
Functional residual capacity is the volume of gas remaining in the lungs at the end of one normal expiration.

118. Correct answer: C
Residual volume is the volume of gas left in the lungs following a maximal respiratory effort.

119. Correct answer: B
This patient is in the prewean stage. During this stage, interventions and patient care are focused on restoring the patient to baseline status or improving the baseline status. Ventilator settings may be changed frequently to increase patient interaction, change modes, decrease FiO_2, or decrease PEEP. The prewean stage in a patient who has been ventilated for a short period of time is often quite brief and may last only hours. In a patient who has been ventilated for a longer period, this stage can last up to several months because even minute changes may dramatically alter the patient's condition.

120. **Correct answer: C**
Mort's abdominal contents have probably entered the thoracic cavity secondary to a diaphragmatic tear. If air also enters the thoracic cavity, it will increase the intrathoracic pressure and help to transmit sound. It is usually the left side of the diaphragm that ruptures—and Mort was injured on the left. It is postulated that perhaps the liver, because it is large, protects the right side of the diaphragm. A fractured pelvis increases the probability of a ruptured diaphragm by 50%.

121. **Correct answer: B**
Fingertip clubbing is an indication of chronic hypoxia.

122. **Correct answer: A**
Pain control is absolutely necessary with a flail chest. A flail chest results when two or more adjacent ribs are broken in two or more places. The chest wall is unstable. Usually during inspiration, the chest wall moves outward with an increase in negative intrathoracic pressure. In flail chest, the opposite movement of the chest wall is seen, a phenomenon known as "paradoxical" movement. Eventually, it will result in atelectasis and alveolar collapse, with possible development of ARDS. To adequately stabilize the fracture, sometimes neuromuscular blockade is used. The patient must be given pain medication and sedation. Also, pain is the priority because the work of breathing (WOB) needs to be reduced. To understand why pain control is necessary, just think about the last time you had a pain in your side and consider how difficult it was to take a full breath.

123. **Correct answer: C**
Flail chest is a very painful condition that limits respiratory effort either because of the pain or because of the effects of the analgesia and sedation that may be required. CO_2 will increase, PaO_2 will decrease, and the pH will be less than 7.35. The patient will develop respiratory acidosis.

124. **Correct answer: C**
The normal value is 35–40 mmHg, so perfusion is adequate. The mixed venous sample is a way of assessing ventilation and circulation. If the mixed venous PaO_2 is low, it means that the tissues extract a normal amount of oxygen and return deoxygenated blood to the heart. The sample is drawn from the distal port of the pulmonary artery catheter.

125. **Correct answer: A**
Removal of large amounts of pleural fluid increases the negative intrapleural pressure. Edema occurs when the lung does not reexpand. The patient develops a severe cough and dyspnea. If these symptoms occur during thoracentesis, the procedure should be stopped.

126. **Correct answer: D**
Pressures that exceed 60 mmHg usually mean that only one side of the tube is sealed. The trachea is somewhat oval, whereas the tube and cuff are circular. If a cuff leak occurs, the pressure would be lower and the patient might be able to speak or make noise with the tube in place.

127. **Correct answer: B**
The endotracheal cuff pressure should not exceed the tracheal capillary filling pressure. Blood flow to the trachea requires a tracheal filling pressure of approximately 15–25

mmHg. If the cuff pressure exceeds this amount, complications such as a tracheoesophageal fistula may occur. The overinflated cuff may also cause ischemia and possibly necrosis.

128. Correct answer: D
A semireclining or upright position will promote upper lobe drainage. Fluid or secretions will collect if the patient lies flat.

129. Correct answer: B
If the patient has a head injury, the intracranial pressure will be increased. It is also best to avoid postural drainage in a woman in the last two to three months of her pregnancy. The baby will shift toward the lungs and may cause respiratory distress. When giving aerosol treatments, it is also a good idea to wait an hour after a patient eats to avoid nausea, vomiting, and possible aspiration.

130. Correct answer: B
The pH of the aspirate is very important. If the aspirate is acidic, pulmonary edema will be created almost immediately, due to the collapse and breakdown of the alveoli, capillaries, and their interface. Atelectasis, intra-alveolar hemorrhage, and some interstitial edema may lead to hypoxia. Alkalotic aspirate destroys surfactant, which in turn causes alveolar collapse, leading to hypoxia. Other factors to identify include the type of material aspirated and the amount. Syrup of ipecac is used as a treatment for ingested poisons. ABG analysis would be considered more of a diagnostic tool.

131. Correct answer: C
To evacuate fluids, the tube is placed low in the thoracic cavity, and gravity is used to help clear the fluid. The chest tube should be placed at the fifth intercostal space, midaxillary line. If a hemothorax is not completely removed, an infection may potentially occur, leading to empyema. When assessing a patient, it is a good idea to ask (if possible) about the origin of any small scars on the thoracic area.

132. Correct answer: B
The hypoxemic type of respiratory failure is defined as ARDS. In this type of respiratory failure, the $PaCO_2$ may be decreased or normal. A ventilation–perfusion mismatch (pneumonia, atelectasis) may occur due to an intrapulmonary shunt. Alternatively, increased alveolar dead space may lead to shock, or pulmonary embolism.

133. Correct answer: C
Cor pulmonale also results from right ventricular failure or dilation secondary to pulmonary hypertension caused by lung disease. The important distinction here is that this condition is not caused by a problem with the left ventricle. Instead, acute cor pulmonale is usually the result of a massive pulmonary embolism that raises the PVR and places increased preload and strain on the right heart.

134. Correct answer: D
PEEP is useful in treating acute respiratory distress syndrome) because it can open collapsed alveoli. Barotrauma and decreased cardiac output and venous return are potential complications of PEEP. The pressure must be regulated so that it does not cause barotrauma, yet keeps alveoli from collapsing during expiration.

135. Correct answer: B

An acute pulmonary embolism can be associated with right heart failure. The PAS and PVR will be elevated. The patient may be having chest pain, dyspnea, tachycardia, hypotension, shock, and possibly coma.

136. Correct answer: C

The patient will have a sudden decrease in the pet CO_2 due to loss of blood flow in the pulmonary vasculature. The decrease in blood flow increases the amount of dead space, with a resultant decrease in the pet CO_2.

137. Correct answer: C

If the D-dimer is elevated, it may be caused by multiple other conditions. A normal D-dimer rules out a pulmonary embolism. Hyperventilation will occur subsequent to hypoxemia, so respiratory alkalosis will occur. Heparin does not dissolve existing clots.

138. Correct answer: D

If a pulmonary embolism decreases oxygen availability, the work of breathing increases, as does the respiratory rate. The thoracic respiratory muscles and the diaphragm will increase their oxygen demand. Respiratory muscle fatigue may result. Oxygen may be diverted to these muscles and deplete the oxygen and nutrient supplies necessary for other vital organs. These organs may become ischemic and develop multiple organ dysfunction. Venous thrombosis, shunting, and oral estrogen therapy may all contribute to the formation of a pulmonary embolus.

139. Correct answer: A

Traditionally, healthcare providers were taught to assess Homan's sign: dorsiflexion of the ankle while bending the knee. If that elicited pain, the patient had a problem with circulation and possibly DVT. Moses' sign is elicited by pressing the calf toward the tibia. It may also elicit pain. These results are not exclusive to DVT, but may complement the other diagnostic findings.

140. Correct answer: C

Sometimes balloons are old and weakened, in which case they may rupture easily. The balloons are made of rubber and will disintegrate in the presence of circulating lipoproteins. If the balloon does rupture, it will not wedge in the vessel, so you can attempt to aspirate blood through the inflation port. If you cannot aspirate the blood, the balloon is probably ruptured. Immediately place a piece of tape on the port with a notation that the balloon is ruptured. This step ensures that the next person will not attempt to use the port and inject air into the pulmonary circulation. Sometimes the balloon shatters into small parts, which become emboli. Another precaution is to determine if the patient has a preexisting rubber allergy.

141. Correct answer: C

A very common and significant finding in a patient with a pneumomediastinum is Hamman's sign. Hamman's sign is a "crunching" sound or a slight clicking sound with each heart sound auscultated over the apex of the heart.

142. Correct answer: A

One indication for the use of PEEP is to reduce the need for FiO_2. PEEP helps keep alveoli open, thereby raising PaO_2, so it will decrease need for FiO_2.

143. Correct answer: B

The hypoxemic drive to breathe originates in the aortic and carotid arteries. Chemoreceptors are found in the bifurcation of the internal and external carotid arteries, carotid bodies, and aortic bodies (in the carotid arch). When the supply of oxygen decreases, stimulation of the aortic and/or carotid bodies occurs, which in turn stimulates cortical activity. This activity produces adrenal gland secretions (epinephrine, norepinephrine), tachycardia, tachypnea, increased respiratory rate, and increased blood pressure.

144. Correct answer: A

The functional residual capacity is defined as the amount of air remaining in the lungs after normal expiration. The formula for functional residual capacity is FRC = ERV (expired residual volume) + the RV (residual volume). The normal FRC in healthy lungs is in the range of 2000–3000 mL.

145. Correct answer: D

If carbon monoxide levels are above 60%, the patient will be comatose and probably die. Smokers often have CO levels of 5–10%. Normal levels in nonsmokers are less than 2%.

146. Correct answer: D

Elimination of carbon monoxide from the body is via the lungs. In cases of severe carbon monoxide poisoning, hyperbaric therapy must be utilized to force the CO molecule off the hemoglobin. The CO is then eliminated by the lungs.

147. Correct answer: B

Airway patency is always a priority. Tyler probably inhaled superheated air and toxins. Most of the products found in a home will give off carbon monoxide when burned. These toxins, plus the CO, may cause edema of the air passages.

148. Correct answer: D

Subcutaneous emphysema usually occurs in the thorax as a result of a pulmonary air leak. This air leak may occur secondary to the patient receiving positive-pressure ventilation or from alveolar rupture caused by a pneumothorax. The air travels along under the skin and may be easily palpated—it feels like a crackling sensation. Patients who have chest tubes often have at least a small amount of subcutaneous emphysema at the tube insertion site. Sometimes the patient will feel pain when palpation is performed because the air tears the tissue. The free air must be reabsorbed, which may take several days.

149. Correct answer: B

Bilirubin is not within the color spectrum that will interfere with pulse oximetry results. Dark nail polish—especially black, brown, blue, and green colors—will interfere with light transmission and cause an artificially lowered SpO_2. Patients who have bruising under the nails may have SpO_2 values that are artificially decreased.

150. Correct answer: B

During resuscitation, blood pressure and blood flow may vary. The pharmacologic effects of medications such as vasoactive drugs used during resuscitation will compromise SpO_2 values.

151. Correct answer: B

Pulse oximetry values do not directly correlate with PaO_2. You must use ABGs to determine PaO_2, the amount of oxygen available to the tissues. SpO_2 measures the number of hemoglobin binding sites that are occupied compared to the number of hemoglobin binding sites available. The following table shows the probable correlation.

Values of Pulse Oximetry	Probable PaO_2
97	100
95	80
94	70
90	60
85	50
75	40
57	30
32	20
10	10

152. Correct answer: C

To prevent complications with chest tube drainage systems, the suction level should not be higher than −40 cm H_2O. Maintaining suction at a higher pressure may cause reexpansion pulmonary edema, pleural air leaks, and lung tissue entrapment. The lung may not be able to expand properly.

153. Correct answer: B

Chest tube drainage tubing should be placed horizontally on the bed and down to the collection chamber. If a mediastinal chest tube is in place, bubbling in the water seal chamber may indicate a communication between the mediastinal space and the pleural space. The physician should be notified immediately. Note that some sporadic bubbling will occur when suction is first turned on, simply because fluid has to displace air in the collection chamber. Chest tube tubing that is dependent or coiled will allow for the accumulation of drainage, and this obstruction may eventually increase pressure in the lung.

154. Correct answer: D

Emphysema will actually increase lung compliance. In contrast, pulmonary edema, pleural effusions, and obesity decrease lung compliance. Other factors that decrease compliance include atelectasis, fibrotic changes, abdominal distention, pain (causes splinting), and flail chest (pain and loss of structure).

155. Correct answer: C

Prior to insertion of an LMA, the patient must have an absent gag reflex. Nurses cannot insert an LMA unless they have specialized training. The LMA does not usually cause hoarseness because it does not pass through the vocal cords. There is a high risk of aspiration with LMA usage.

156. Correct answer: C
Acetyl-cysteine contains a sulfide group that effectively splits disulfide bonds in mucin molecules, which reduces the viscosity of the mucus. Atropine is an anticholinergic. Terbutaline and albuterol are β_2 agonists.

157. Correct answer: D
Side effects of acetyl-cysteine include bronchospasm. Thinning the mucus may promote excessive coughing with resultant bronchospasm. Additional side effects include rhinorrhea, stomatitus, nausea, and vomiting.

158. Correct answer: D
The β_2-receptor agonists lower cellular calcium levels and relax bronchial smooth muscle. The selective β_2-receptor agonists do not produce cardiac stimulation. The cardiac stimulation can result in tachycardia and reduced cardiac output.

159. Correct answer: B
In malignant hyperthermia, the use of anesthetic agents such as halothane causes muscles to contract and the patient to become hypothermic. Caffeine is used diagnostically because it can contract muscles at higher doses without the danger of depolarizing cell membranes. The antidote for malignant hyperthermia is dantrolene.

160. Correct answer: C
Symptoms from aspirated gastric contents have a gradual onset. The patient may develop ARDS, but not always. If the pH is > 2.5, very little necrosis will occur. If the pH is < 2.5, there is probability of pulmonary edema, necrosis, bleeding, and atelectasis.

161. Correct answer: B
Placement of a central line via a subclavian vein may cause an open pneumothorax. By definition, an open pneumothorax exists because air enters the pleural cavity from the atmosphere. The hole made into the subclavian vein allows air to pass from the atmosphere to the pleural cavity.

162. Correct answer: C
The best position in which to place this patient to minimize the risk of venous air embolism is Trendelenburg with left decubitus tilt. This position will minimize the risk of any air migrating through the heart and into the lungs.

163. Correct answer: C
The definitive study to confirm the presence of thrombolic emboli is pulmonary angiography. This study involves catheterization of the right ventricle and then dye is injected into the pulmonary artery. The pulmonary vasculature is readily visualized, and the embolus is easily found because the dye trail comes to a sudden end at the location of the embolus.

164. Correct answer: B
Risk factors for thrombolic emboli include carcinoma. Neoplasms, obesity, trauma, dysrhythmias, congestive heart failure (CHF), and prolonged immobility are also risk factors.

165. Correct answer: A
A venous air embolism may be caused by hemodialysis. Other potential causes of venous air emboli include central and pulmonary artery catheters, endoscopy, and automatic pressure-driven injectors.

166. Correct answer: B
A shift to the left of the oxyhemoglobin dissociation curve is caused by an increased pH, decreased temperature, and/or decreased $PaCO_2$.

167. Correct answer: C
A 6 year old child should have a number 5 cuffed ETT inserted to a depth of 15 cm. To estimate the appropriate ETT size, the formula is age divided by 4, plus 4, for an uncuffed ETT, and age divided by 4, plus 3.5, for a cuffed ETT. For this patient, the calculation is as follows: $6/4 + 3.5 = 5$. The insertion depth for an orally placed endotracheal tube is estimated by the formula age divided by 2, plus 12 cm. For this patient, the calculation is as follows: $6/2 + 12 = 15$ cm. For nasally placed endotracheal tubes, the insertion depth is calculated as age divided by 2, plus 15 cm.

168. Correct answer: B
Of the options presented here, the blood gas results you would expect to see in a patient with thrombotic emboli are pH 7.45, PaO_2 59, $PaCO_2$ 30, and HCO_3 24.

169. Correct answer: D
Fractures, usually of the long bones, often release free fatty acids that cause fatty emboli. With this disorder, fat globules float around and obstruct the pulmonary vasculature.

170. Correct answer: A
Prone positioning is the best position to promote drainage and oxygenation for a patient with ARDS. Prone positioning is often the most difficult position to achieve without proper lifting and safety devices.

171. Correct answer: D
In patients with ARDS, the fluid volume is kept low to keep the PAOP (PCWP) at minimal levels. If too much fluid is present, leakage may occur through damaged capillaries into the interstitial space.

172. Correct answer: B
When managing a patient with persistent pulmonary hypertension, the pH should be maintained between 7.45 and 7.6, while the $PaCO_2$ should remain between 20 and 30 mmHg.

173. Correct answer: C
Pulmonary interstitial emphysema (PIE) may be treated with dexamethasone to decrease tissue inflammation. Complications of dexamethasone administration place the infant at greater risk of infection, hypertension, hyperlipidemia, and hyperglycemia.

174. Correct answer: B
The most likely cause of respiratory distress syndrome (RDS) in a neonate is deficient surfactant due to prematurity. This question highlights the rare case where the baby is born near term. Replacement surfactant allows for greater alveolar expansion and oxygenation.

175. Correct answer: C
Pulmonary hypertension is generally defined as a mean pulmonary artery pressure of ≥ 25 mmHg. Pulmonary hypertension in smaller children and infants is defined as a

mean pulmonary artery pressure > 25% of the systemic pressure. The increase in pressure may be related to increased blood flow or obstruction of blood flow through the lungs.

176. **Correct answer: B**
Histological changes in the vasculature cause primary hypertension. Chronic lung disease such as BPD, chronic thrombotic disease, and congenital heart disease such as TOF all have been identified as leading to secondary hypertension.

177. **Correct answer: A**
Although nitric oxide and Flolan are powerful vasodilators, nitric oxide is the preferred option. Flolan is a platelet anti-aggregate. Given this patient's history of being in an accident, its use may increase the risk of internal and external bleeding. Endothelin-1 and thromboxane A are vasoconstrictors that are contraindicated in pulmonary hypertension.

178. **Correct answer: C**
Patients with pulmonary hypertension present with dyspnea during exertion, right-sided heart failure, increased respiratory and heart rates, and a prominent S_2. Additional signs of pulmonary hypertension include fatigue and lethargy, enlarged liver, and pulmonary congestion. Cyanosis is a late sign of pulmonary hypertension.

179. **Correct answer: B**
Calcium channel blockers are used to treat primary pulmonary hypertension. Patients treated with nitric oxide will improve more rapidly when treated with calcium channel blockers due to abnormalities in the membrane function.

180. **Correct answer: C**
If a patient becomes constipated or strains to stool, he or she may initiate a Valsalva maneuver and become bradycardic, resulting in cardiac collapse. Fever, infections, and increased myocardial demands will lead to increased respiratory distress and shunting. It is also important to maintain an immunization schedule to prevent additional infections and immunologic compromise.

181. **Correct answer: D**
Without initial, aggressive treatment of pulmonary hypertension, the medial smooth muscles in arterioles will become irreversibly thickened. This outcome is due to development of high right-sided ventricular pressures and heart failure.

182. **Correct answer: C**
Pulmonary hypertension results in hypoxia and hypoxemia, leading to vasoconstriction. As vasoconstriction continues, the vessel walls begin to undergo remodeling, marked by an increase in elastin and collagen. Prolonged vasoconstriction leads to increased shunting and blood pooling. Serum testing for abnormalities further increases the risks and progression of irreversible epithelial changes.

183. **Correct answer: B**
Malignant hyperthermia is a hypermetabolic state that results in metabolic and respiratory acidosis.

184. Correct answer: A

An elevated serum creatinine would be a concern and probably prolong the patient's time on mechanical ventilation. Sometimes, patients will develop acute renal failure following a cardiac procedure. Close monitoring of the serum creatinine is necessary to ensure the patient is not in danger of developing renal problems.

185. Correct answer: A

Infants younger than 1 month who receive erythromycin are at increased risk of infantile hypertrophic pyloric stenosis. For this reason, and because azithromycin is associated with fewer adverse effects than erythromycin, azithromycin is the preferred antimicrobial for prophylaxis of newborns exposed to pertussis. A macrolide antibiotic (erythromycin, azithromycin, or clarithromycin) is preferred for postexposure prophylaxis and treatment of pertussis. Antimicrobials generally do not affect the severity or course of this illness after paroxysmal cough has begun, but they can eliminate the pathogen, *Bordetella pertussis,* and stop transmission to newborns. A macrolide should be given to women with pertussis that is acquired late in pregnancy, to their household contacts, and to their infants. Early recognition of pertussis is necessary to ensure the effectiveness of this approach.

186. Correct answer: A

Protection against respiratory diphtheria is provided predominantly by the immunoglobulin G antibody. During pregnancy, the maternal antitoxin is transferred to the fetus. Transplacental maternal antitoxin provides newborns with protection against diphtheria if the mother is immune. Respiratory diphtheria can occur during any trimester of pregnancy, at term, or in the postpartum period. The mortality rate of obstetric respiratory diphtheria is estimated at 50% when no antitoxin is administered.

PULMONARY REFERENCES

Abman, S. (2007). Recent advances in the pathogenesis and treatment of persistent pulmonary hypertension of the newborn. *Neonatology, 91*(4), 283–290.

Abman, S. (2008). The dysmorphic pulmonary circulation in bronchopulmonary dysplasia: A growing story. *American Journal of Respiratory and Critical Care Medicine, 178*(2), 114–115.

Aehlert, B. (Ed.). (2005). *Comprehensive pediatric emergency care.* St. Louis, MO: Mosby.

Agbaht, K., et al. (2007). Management of ventilator-associated pneumonia in a multidisciplinary intensive care unit: Does trauma make a difference? *Intensive Care Medicine, 33*(8), 1387–1395.

Ahrens, T., & Sona, C. (2003). Capnography application in acute and critical care. *AACN Clinical Issues, 14,* 123–132.

American Heart Association. (2010). Guidelines 2010 for cardiopulmonary resuscitation and emergency cardiovascular care. Retrieved from www.americanheart.org

Antonelli, M., Azoulay, E., et al. (2010). Year in review in intensive care medicine 2009. Part III: Mechanical ventilation, acute lung injury and respiratory distress syndrome, pediatrics, ethics and miscellanea. *Intensive Care Medicine, 36*(4), 567–584.

Askin, D. F., & Diehl-Jones, W. (2009). Pathogenesis and prevention of chronic lung disease in the neonate. *Critical Care Nursing Clinics of North America, 21*(1), 11–25.

Bachman, T., Marks, N., & Rimensberger, P. (2008). Factors affecting adoption of new neonatal and pediatric respiratory technologies. *Intensive Care Medicine, 34*(1), 174–178.

Baird, J. S., Killinger, J. S., Kalkbrenner, K. J., Bye, M. R., & Schleien, C. L. (2010). Massive pulmonary embolism in children. *Journal of Pediatrics, 156*(1), 148–151.

Baltacioğlu, F., Çimşit, N., Bostanci, K., Yüksel, M., & Kodalli, N. (2010). Transarterial microcatheter glue embolization of the bronchial artery for life-threatening hemoptysis: Technical and clinical results. *European Journal of Radiology, 73*(2), 380–384.

Baraldi, E., & Filippone, M. (2007). Chronic lung disease after premature birth. *New England Journal of Medicine, 357,* 1946–1955

Bashore, T. M., Granger, C. B., Hranitzky, P., & Patel, M. R. (2010). Heart disease. In S. J. McPhee & M. A. Papadakis (Eds.), *Lange 2010 current medical diagnosis and treatment* (49th ed., pp. 358–366). New York: McGraw-Hill Medical.

Begheti, M., & Galiè, N. (2009). Eisenmenger syndrome: A clinical perspective in a new therapeutic era of pulmonary arterial hypertension. *Journal of the American College of Cardiology, 53*(9), 733–740.

Bhandari, V., Choo-Wing, R., Lee, C., et al. (2008). Developmental regulation of NO-mediated VEGF-induced effects in the lung. *American Journal of Respiratory Cell and Molecular Biology, 39*(4), 420–430.

Bialk, J. L. (2004). Ethical guidelines for assisting patients with end-of-life decision making. *Medsurg Nursing, 13*(2), 87–90.

Bigatello, L. M., Davidson, K. R., & Stelfox, H. T. (2005). Respiratory mechanics and ventilatory waveforms in the patient with acute lung injury. *Respiratory Care, 50,* 235–245.

Biss, T. T., Brandão, L. R., Kahr, W. H., Chan, A. K., & Williams, S. (2008). Clinical features and outcome of pulmonary embolism in children. *British Journal of Haematology, 142*(5), 808–818.

Bissinger, R., Carlson, C., Michel, Y., Dooley, C., Hulsey, T., & Jenkins, D. (2008). Secondary surfactant administration in neonates with respiratory decompensation. *Journal of Perinatology, 28*(3), 192–198.

Bohlin, K., Jonsson, B., Gustafsson, A., & Blennow, M. (2008). Continuous positive airway pressure and surfactant. *Neonatology, 93*(4), 309–315.

Boussemart, T., Nsota, J., Martin-Coignard, D., & Champion, G. (2009). Nephrogenic diabetes insipidus: Treat with caution. *Pediatric Nephrology, 24*(9), 1761–1763.

Burns, S. M. (Ed.). (2007). *American Association of Critical-Care Nurses (AACN): AACN protocols for practice: Healing environments* (2nd ed.). Sudbury, MA: Jones and Bartlett.

Carroll, C. L., & Zucker, A. R. (2008). Barotrauma not related to the type of positive pressure ventilation during severe asthma exacerbations in children. *Journal of Asthma, 45*(5), 421–424.

Caruana, J. A., Anain, P. M., & Pham, D. T. (2009). The pulmonary embolism risk score system reduces the incidence and mortality of pulmonary embolism after gastric bypass. *Surgery, 146*(4), 678–685.

Centers for Disease Control and Prevention. (2002). Guideline for hand hygiene in health-care settings: Recommendations of the Healthcare Infection Control Practices Advisory Committee and the HICPAC/SHEA/APIC/IDSA Hand Hygiene Task Force. *Morbidity and Mortality Weekly Report, 51*(RR16), 1–44.

Centers for Disease Control and Prevention. (2004). Guidelines for preventing health-care associated pneumonia: 2003 recommendations of the CDC and the Healthcare Infection Control Practices Advisory Committee. *Morbidity and Mortality Weekly Report, 53*(RR03), 1–36.

Centers for Disease Control and Prevention. (2010). Respiratory syncytial virus activity—United States, July 2008–December 2009. *Morbidity and Mortality Weekly Report, 59*(8), 230–233.

Centers for Disease Control and Prevention. (2010). Vaccines & immunizations. Vaccines and preventable diseases: Pertussis (whooping cough) vaccination. Retrieved September 1, 2010, from http://www.cdc.gov/vaccines/vpd-vac/pertussis/default.htm

Chambers, M. A., & Jones, S. (Eds.). (2007). *Surgical nursing of children*. Philadelphia, PA: Elsevier.

Chaudhry, K., & Sinert, R. (2010). Evidence-based emergency medicine/systematic review abstract. Is nebulized hypertonic saline solution an effective treatment for bronchiolitis in infants? *Annals of Emergency Medicine, 55*(1), 120–122.

Cheng, S., Naidoo, Y., da Cruz, M., & Dexter, M. (2009). Quality of life in postoperative vestibular schwannoma patients. *Laryngoscope, 119*(11), 2252–2257.

Chernecky, C., & Berger, B. (2004). *Laboratory tests and diagnostic procedures* (4th ed.). Philadelphia, PA: Saunders.

Cherry, J. D. (2008). Clinical practice: Croup. *New England Journal of Medicine, 358*(4), 384–391.

Chotirmall, S. H., Branagan, P., Gunaratnam, C., & McElvaney, N. G. (2008). Aspergillus/allergic bronchopulmonary aspergillosis in an Irish cystic fibrosis population: A diagnostically challenging entity. *Respiratory Care, 53*(8), 1035–1041.

Chun, J.-Y., & Belli, A.-M. (2010). Immediate and long-term outcomes of bronchial and non-bronchial systemic artery embolisation for the management of haemoptysis. *European Radiology, 20*(3), 558–565.

Church, D. G., Matthay, M. A., Liu, K., Milet, M., & Flori, H. . (2009). Blood product transfusions and clinical outcomes in pediatric patients with acute lung injury. *Pediatric Critical Care Medicine, 10*(3), 297–302.

Cosentini, R., Aliberti, S., Bignamini, A., Piffer, F., & Brambilla, A. M. (2009). Mortality in acute cardiogenic pulmonary edema treated with continuous positive airway pressure. *Intensive Care Medicine, 35*(2), 299–305.

Dabir, T., Mccrossan, B., Sweeney, L., et al. (2008). Down syndrome, achondroplasia and tetralogy of Fallot. *Neonatology, 94*(1), 68–70.

Dellamonica, J., Louis, B., Lyazidi, A., et al. (2008). Intrapulmonary percussive ventilation superimposed on conventional ventilation: Bench study of humidity and ventilator behaviour. *Intensive Care Medicine, 34*(11), 2035–2043.

Dimopoulos, K., Inuzuka, R., Goletto, S., Giannakoulas, G., Swan, L., Wort, S. J., & Gatzoulis, M. A. (2010). Improved survival among patients with Eisenmenger syndrome receiving advanced therapy for pulmonary arterial hypertension. *Circulation, 121*(1), 20–25.

Dincipi, N., & Esposito, S. (2009). Antigen-based assays for the identification of influenza virus and respiratory syncytial virus: Why and how to use them in pediatric practice. *Clinics in Laboratory Medicine, 29*(4), 649–660.

Dossey, B. M., Keegan, L., & Guzzetta, C. (2003). *Holistic nursing: A handbook for practice* (3rd ed.). Sudbury, MA: Jones and Bartlett.

Downard, C. D. (2008). Congenital diaphragmatic hernia: An ongoing clinical challenge. *Current Opinion in Pediatrics, 20*(3), 300–304.

Drake Melander, S. (Ed.). (2004). *Case studies in critical care nursing: A guide for application and review* (3rd ed.). Philadelphia, PA: Saunders.

Dueker, C. W. (2004). Immersion in fresh water and survival. *Chest, 126*(6), 2027–2028.

Durbin, C. G. (2005). Applied respiratory physiology: Uses of ventilator waveforms and mechanics in the management of critically ill patients. *Respiratory Care, 50,* 287–293.

Duster, M. C., & Derlet, M. N. (2009). High altitude illness in children. *Pediatric Annals, 38*(4), 218–223.

Emergency Nurses Association & Newberry, L. (2003). *Sheehy's emergency nursing: Principles and practice* (5th ed.). St. Louis, MO: Mosby/Elsevier.

Eppert, H. D. (2010). Disease prevention update: Tetanus toxoid, reduced diphtheria toxoid, and acellular pertussis—who, what, when, why, and how? *JEN: Journal of Emergency Nursing, 36*(2), 122–124.

Farhath, S., He, Z., Nakhla, T., Saslow, J., Soundar, S., Camacho J., & Aghai, Z. H. (2008). Pepsin, a marker of gastric contents, is increased in tracheal aspirates from preterm infants who develop bronchopulmonary dysplasia. *Pediatrics, 121*(2), e253–e259.

Fidkowski, C. W., Fuzaylov, G., Sheridan, R. L., & Coté, C. J. (2009). Inhalation burn injury in children. *Paediatric Anaesthesia, 19*(suppl 1), 147–154.

Fitzgerald Macksey, L. (2009). *Pediatric anesthetic and emergency drug guide.* Sudbury, MA: Jones and Bartlett.

Flume, P. A. (2009). Pulmonary complications of cystic fibrosis. *Respiratory Care, 54*(5), 618–627.

Foglia, E., Meier, M. D., & Elward, A. (2007, July). Ventilator-associated pneumonia in neonatal and pediatric intensive care unit patients. *Clinical Microbiology Reviews, 20*(3), 409–425.

Frankel, S. K., & Schwarz, M. (2009). Update in idiopathic pulmonary fibrosis. *Current Opinion in Pulmonary Medicine, 15*(5), 463–469.

Fung, Y. L., & Silliman, C. C. (2009). The role of neurophils in the pathogenesis of transfusion-related acute lung injury. *Transfusion Medicine Reviews, 23*(4), 266–283.

Galante, D. (2009). Intraoperative management of pulmonary arterial hypertension in infants and children. *Current Opinion in Anaesthesiology, 22*(3), 378–382.

Getahun, D., Strickland, D., Zeiger, R. S., Fassett, M. J., Chen, W., Rhoads, G. G., & Jacobsen, S. J. (2010). Effect of chorioamnionitis on early childhood asthma. *Archives of Pediatrics & Adolescent Medicine, 164*(2), 187–192.

Gien, J., Seedorf, G., Balasubramaniam, V., et al. (2007). Intrauterine pulmonary hypertension impairs angiogenesis in vitro: Role of vascular endothelial growth factor–nitric oxide signaling. *American Journal of Respiratory and Critical Care Medicine, 176*(11), 1146–1153.

Goissen, C., Ghyselen, L., Tourneux, P., et al. (2008). Persistent pulmonary hypertension of the newborn with transposition of the great arteries: Successful treatment with bosentan. *European Journal of Pediatrics, 167*(4), 437–440.

Gora-Harper, M. (1998). *The injectable drug reference.* Princeton, NJ: Bioscientific Resources.

Grewal, S., Ali, S., McConnell, D. W., Vandermeer, B., & Klassen, T. P. (2009). A randomized trial of nebulized 3% hypertonic saline with epinephrine in the treatment of acute bronchiolitis in the emergency department. *Archives of Pediatrics and Adolescent Medicine, 163*(11), 1007–1012.

Guyton, A. C., & Hall, J. E. (2005). *Textbook of medical physiology* (11th ed.). Philadelphia, PA: Saunders.

Hardin, S. R., & Kaplow, R. (Eds.). (2004). *Synergy for clinical excellence: The AACN Synergy Model for Patient Care.* Sudbury, MA: Jones and Bartlett.

Hay, W. W. Jr., Levin, M. J., Sondheimer, J. M., & Deterding, R. R. (Eds.). (2007). *Current diagnosis and treatment in pediatrics* (18th ed.). New York: McGraw-Hill.

Hermansen, C., & Lorah, K. (2007). Respiratory distress in the newborn. *American Family Physician, 76*(7), 987–994.

Hickey, J. V. (2008). *The clinical practice of neurological and neurosurgical nursing* (6th ed.). Philadelphia, PA: Lippincott Williams & Wilkins.

Hoshino, T., Kato, S., Oka, N., et al. (2007). Pulmonary inflammation and emphysema: Role of the cytokines IL-18 and IL-13. *American Journal of Respiratory and Critical Care Medicine, 176*(1), 49–62.

Huddleston, C. B. (2010). Lung transplantation for pulmonary hypertension in children. *Pediatric Critical Care Medicine, 11*(2 suppl), S53–S56.

Hummler, H. D., Engelmann, A., Pohlandt, F., & Franz, A. R. (2006). Volume-controlled intermittent mandatory ventilation in preterm infants with hypoxemic episodes. *Intensive Care Medicine, 32,* 577–584.

Hwang, J. H., Misumi, S., Sahin, H., Brown, K. K., Newell, J. D., & Lynch, D. A. (2009). Computed tomographic features of idiopathic fibrosing interstitial pneumonia: Comparison with pulmonary fibrosis related to collagen vascular disease. *Journal of Computer Assisted Tomography, 33*(3), 410–415.

Inal, M. T. (2007). Laryngospasm-induced pulmonary edema. *Internet Journal of Anesthesiology, 15*(1), 5.

Iyer, V., Joshi, A., & Ryu, J. (2009). Spontaneous pneumomediastinum: Analysis of 62 consecutive adult patients. *Mayo Clinic Proceedings, 84*(5), 417–421.

Johnson, J. M. (2009). Management of acute cardiogenic pulmonary edema: A literature review. *Advanced Emergency Nursing Journal, 31*(1), 36–43.

Jones, K. L. (2006). *Smith's recognizable patterns of human malformation* (6th ed.). Philadelphia, PA: Elsevier.

Jones & Bartlett Learning (2011). *2011 nurse's drug handbook* (10th ed.). Sudbury, MA: Jones & Bartlett Learning.

Kamath, B. D., Fashaw, L., & Kinsella, J. P. (2010). Adrenal insufficiency in newborns with congenital diaphragmatic hernia. *Journal of Pediatrics, 156*(3), 495–497.

Kealey, G. P. (2009). Carbon monoxide toxicity. *Journal of Burn Care and Research, 30*(1), 146–147.

Koehoorn, M., Karr, C. J., Demers, P. A., Lencar, C., Tamburic, L., & Brauer, M. (2008). Descriptive epidemiological features of bronchiolitis in a population-based cohort. *Pediatrics, 122*(6), 1196–1203.

Krahn, G., et al. (2007). Early clinical evaluation of the Edwards PediaSat™ oximetry catheter in pediatric patients. *Pediatric Critical Care Medicine, 8*(3), 18.2.152.

Laberge, J. M., & Flageole, H. (2007). Fetal tracheal occlusion for the treatment of congenital diaphragmatic hernia. *World Journal of Surgery, 31*(8), 1577–1586.

Lewis, S. A., Antoniak, M., Venn, A. J., Davies, L., Goodwin, A., Salfield, N., & Fogarty, A. W. (2005). Secondhand smoke, dietary fruit intake, road traffic exposures, and the prevalence of asthma: A cross-sectional study in young children. *American Journal of Epidemiology, 161*(5), 406–411.

Maggiorini, M. (2010). Prevention and treatment of high-altitude pulmonary edema. *Progress in Cardiovascular Diseases, 52*(6), 500–506.

Martell, M., Blasina, F., Silvera, F., Tellechea, S., Godoy, C., Vaamonde, L., & Olivera, W. (2007). Intratracheal sildenafil in the newborn with pulmonary hypertension. *Pediatrics, 119*(1), 215–216.

Martin, B. (2010). Family presence during resuscitation and invasive procedures: AACN practice alert. Retrieved from http://www.aacn.org

Medina, J., & Puntillo, K. (2006). *AACN protocols for practice: Palliative care and end-of-life issues in critical care.* Sudbury, MA: Jones and Bartlett.

Milgrom, H., & Dockhorn, R. J. (2008). Management of exercise-induced bronchospasm in children: Role of long-acting β2-adrenergic receptor agonists. *Pediatric Asthma, Allergy & Immunology, 21*(2), 59–72.

Mireku, N., Wang, Y., Ager, J., Reddy, R. C., & Baptist, A. P. (2009). Changes in weather and the effects on pediatric asthma exacerbations. *Annals of Allergy, Asthma & Immunology, 103*(3), 220–224.

Mohsen, T., Zeid, A. A., & Haj-Yahia, S. (2007). Lobectomy or pneumonectomy for multidrug-resistant pulmonary tuberculosis can be performed with acceptable morbidity and mortality: A seven-year review of a single institution's experience. *Journal of Thoracic and Cardiovascular Surgery, 134*(1), 194–198.

Mulkey, Z., Yarbrough, S., Guerra, D., Roongsritong, C., Nugent, K., & Phy, M. P. (2008). Postextubation pulmonary edema: A case series and review. *Respiratory Medicine, 102*(11), 1659–1662.

Murata, Y. (2009). Respiratory syncytial virus vaccine development. *Clinics in Laboratory Medicine, 29*(4), 725–739.

Murphy, M. F., Keller, M., et al. (2008). The young airway: Prehospital assessment and management of pediatric respiratory distress. *JEMS: A Journal of Emergency Medical Services, 33*(6), 58–71.

Ng, G., Derry, C., Marston, L., et al. (2008). Reduction in ventilator-induced lung injury improves outcome in congenital diaphragmatic hernia? *Pediatric Surgery International, 24*(2), 145–150.

Nishimura, T., Suzue, J., & Kaji, H. (2009). Breastfeeding reduces the severity of respiratory syncytial virus infection among young infants: A multi-center prospective study. *Pediatrics International: Official Journal of the Japan Pediatric Society, 51*(6), 812–816.

Northwestern University. (2009, January). Pulmonary hypertension: Research from Northwestern University, Department of Pediatrics provides new data about pulmonary hypertension. *Proteomics Weekly*, 837.

Oliveira, C. F., et al. (2007). An outcomes comparison of ACCM/PALS guidelines for pediatric septic shock with and without central venous oxygen saturation monitoring. *Pediatric Critical Care Medicine, 8*(3 suppl) A 2.

Parsons, J. P., & Mastronarde, J. G. (2009). Exercise-induced asthma. *Current Opinion in Pulmonary Medicine, 15*(1), 25–28.

Penaloza, D., Sime, F., & Ruiz, L. (2008). Pulmonary hemodynamics in children living at high altitudes. *High Altitude Medicine & Biology, 9*(3), 199–207.

Pichichero, M. E. (2010). Pertussis. In E. T. Bope, R. E. Rakel, & R. Kellerman (Eds.), *Conn's current therapy 2010* (pp. 144–146). Philadelphia, PA: Saunders Elsevier.

Prescribing reference. (2009, Summer). *NPPR: Nurse Practitioner's Prescribing Reference, 16*(2).

Pursnani, S. K., Amodio, J. B., Guo, H., et al. (2006). Localized persistent interstitial pulmonary emphysema presenting as a spontaneous tension pneumothorax in a full term infant. *Pediatric Surgery International, 22*(7), 613–616.

Roch, A., et al. (2007). Comparison of lung injury after normal or small volume optimized resuscitation in a model of hemorrhagic shock. *Intensive Care Medicine, 33*(9), 1645–1654.

Ruth-Sahd, L. A., & White, K. A. (2009). Bronchiolitis obliterans organizing pneumonia. *Dimensions of Critical Care Nursing, 28*(5), 204–208.

Sara, A., Hamdan, A., Hanaa, B., & Nawaz, K. A. (2008). Bronchiolitis obliterans organizing pneumonia: Pathogenesis, clinical features, imaging and therapy review. *Annals of Thoracic Medicine, 3*(2), 67–75.

Schmidt, B., Roberts, R. S., Davis, P., et al. (2007). Long-term effects of caffeine therapy for apnea of prematurity. *New England Journal of Medicine, 357*(19), 1893–1902.

Sedaghat-Yazdi, F., Torres, A. Jr., Fortuna, R., & Geiss, D. M. (2008). Pulse oximeter accuracy and precision affected by sensor location in cyanotic children. *Pediatric Critical Care Medicine, 9*(4), 393–397.

Senthil, R., Maskell, S., Hartley, B., & Aladangady, N. (2009). Blue episodes in a neonate. *Lancet, 373*(9676), 1734.

Short, E., Kirchner, H., Asaad, G., et al. (2008). Long-term sequelae of postnatal surfactant and corticosteroid therapies for BPD. *Journal of Perinatology, 28*(7), 498–504.

Slota, M. C. (Ed.). (2006). *Core curriculum for pediatric critical care nursing* (2nd ed.). St. Louis, MO: Saunders.

Spillers, J. (2010). PPHN: Is sildenafil the new nitric? A review of the literature. *Advances in Neonatal Care, 10*(2), 69–74.

Spooner, L. M., & Liu, E. (2009). Tuberculosis, CNS. In F. J. Domino, R. A. Baldor, A. M. Erlich, & J. Golding (Eds.), *The 5-minute clinical consult 2010* (18th ed., pp. 1358–1359). Philadelphia, PA: Lippincott Williams & Wilkins.

Spratto, G. R., & Woods, A. L. (2001). *PDR: Nurse's drug handbook.* Montvale, NJ: Delmar & Medical Economics.

Stenmark, K. R., & Rabinovitch, M. (2010). Emerging therapies for the treatment of pulmonary hypertension. *Pediatric Critical Care Medicine, 11*(2 suppl), S85–S90.

Sterling, Y. M., & El-Dahr, J. M. (2006). Wheezing and asthma in early childhood: An update. *Pediatric Nursing, 32*(1), 27–31.

Suntharalingam, J., Treacy, C. M., Doughty, N. J., Goldsmith, K., Soon, E., Toshner, M. R., & Pepke-Zaba, J. (2008). Long-term use of sildenafil in inoperable chronic thromboembolic pulmonary hypertension. *Chest, 134*(2), 229–236.

Syed, I., Tassone, P., Sebire, P., & Bleach, N. (2009). Acute management of croup in children. *British Journal of Hospital Medicine, 70*(1).

Trivits Verger, J., & Lebet, R. M. (Eds (2008). *AACN procedure manual for pediatric acute and critical care*. St. Louis, MO: Saunders.

Tsangaris, I., Galiatsou, E., Kostanti, E., & Nakos, G. (2007). The effect of exogenous surfactant in patients with lung contusions and acute lung injury. *Intensive Care Medicine, 33*(5), 851–55.

U.S. Organ Procurement and Transplantation Network (OPTN). (2005). Scientific Registry of Transplant Recipients (SRTR): OPTN/SRTR annual report. Retrieved February 20, 2005, from http://www.optn.org

Victoria, T., Mong, A., Altes, T., Jawad, A. F., Hernandez, A., Gonzalez, L., & Kramer, S. S. (2009). Evaluation of pulmonary embolism in a pediatric population with high clinical suspicion. *Pediatric Radiology, 39*(1), 35–41.

Wong, G. W., Leung, T. F., Ma, Y., Liu, E. K., Yung, E., & Lai, C. K. (2007). Symptoms of asthma and atopic disorders in preschool children: Prevalence and risk factors. *Clinical and Experimental Allergy, 37*(2), 174–179.

Young, T. E., & Magnum, B. (2009). *Neofax 2009.* Montvale, NJ: Thomson Reuters.

SECTION 5

Endocrine

1. What is the purpose of testing Hgb A_{1c} in patients with diabetes mellitus?

A. It is of little help in managing diabetes mellitus
B. It measures blood sugars over a 6 month period
C. It measures the effectiveness of diabetes mellitus therapy
D. It measures red blood cell activity in diabetes mellitus

2. The infant you are caring for has been diagnosed with central diabetes insipidus. The anticipated treatment for this condition is

A. Thyroid-stimulating hormone
B. Aldosterone
C. Sliding scale insulin
D. DDAVP

3. Your patient is a 16 year old who has been diagnosed with maternal hyperglycemia. Maternal hyperglycemia ultimately causes

A. Increased hepatic glucose uptake
B. Microsomia
C. Pierre Robin sequence
D. Decelerated lipogenesis

4. The anterior pituitary gland controls which of the following glands?

A. Parathyroid, adrenal medulla, and gonads
B. Thyroid, adrenal cortex, and gonads
C. Parathyroid, thyroid, gonads
D. Thyroid, adrenal medulla, and gonads

5. Which of the following statements is true regarding excess fetal insulin production?

A. Excess fetal insulin causes idiosyncratic hyperglycemia
B. Excess fetal insulin promotes the development of pulmonary surfactant
C. Excess fetal insulin may be the cause of delayed maturation of type II alveolar cells
D. Excess fetal insulin leads to pulmonary hypertension

6. Which of the following conditions would inhibit the release of thyroxine?

A. Hypocalcemia
B. Hyperthermia
C. Hypernatremia
D. Hypokalemia

7. **What is the function of antidiuretic hormone?**
   A. Aldosterone production
   B. Sodium balance
   C. Water balance
   D. Potassium balance

8. **Which of the following conditions inhibits antidiuretic hormone production?**
   A. Increased potassium levels
   B. Water intoxication
   C. Pelvic fracture
   D. Pituitary tumors

9. **Your patient has a tumor on her anterior pituitary gland. As a PICU nurse, you know stimulation of the anterior pituitary gland is from the hypothalamus by way of the**
   A. Sympathetic nervous system
   B. Feedback mechanism
   C. Vascular system
   D. Parasympathetic nervous system

10. **Calcitonin is released by the**
    A. Thyroid gland
    B. Adrenal medulla
    C. Hypothalamus
    D. Anterior pituitary gland

11. **Josh's serum calcium level is high. An increase in serum calcium, glucagon, or magnesium will stimulate the release of**
    A. Parathyroid hormone
    B. Calcitonin
    C. Endogenous epinephrine
    D. Aldosterone

12. **Which of the following statements is true regarding glucagon?**
    A. Glucagon promotes glycolysis
    B. Glucagon enables glucose to move into the cells
    C. Glucagon helps the body store glycogen
    D. Glucagon is released from the alpha cells in the pancreas

13. **Georgia has been diagnosed with SIADH. What is the most common presentation of a patient with SIADH (syndrome of inappropriate antidiuretic hormone)?**
    A. Excessive, dilute urine output
    B. Seizures
    C. Hypotension
    D. Tetany

14. **An increase in catecholamines and amino acids with a decrease in serum glucose will stimulate the release of**
    A. Calcitonin
    B. Insulin
    C. Aldosterone
    D. Glucagon

15. **A high serum magnesium or phosphate, a low serum calcium, and catecholamine release result in secretion of**
    A. Aldosterone
    B. Parathyroid hormone
    C. Glyceride
    D. Phosphates

16. **The most important nursing consideration in the infant patient with HHNS is**
    A. Prevention of dysrhythmias
    B. Administration of insulin
    C. Prevention of aspiration
    D. Monitoring electrolytes

17. **The most common cause of hypothyroidism is**
    A. Graves' disease
    B. Acromegaly
    C. Hashimoto's disease
    D. Decreased cortisol levels

18. **Which of the following conditions must be present for calcium to be optimally utilized by the body?**
    A. Increased oral calcium intake
    B. Increased phosphorus levels
    C. A euthyroid state
    D. Adequate vitamin D levels

19. **Your patient is having aldosterone levels monitored daily. Which of the following is a primary effect of aldosterone?**
    A. Aldosterone decreases renal potassium excretion
    B. Aldosterone increases renal potassium excretion
    C. Aldosterone decreases potassium excretion
    D. Aldosterone increases serum sodium levels

20. **Aldosterone is secreted by the**
    A. Zona reticularis of the adrenal cortex
    B. Zona glomerulus of the adrenal cortex
    C. Posterior pituitary gland
    D. Adrenal medulla

21. **Aldosterone secretion is regulated by**
    A. The anterior hypothalamus
    B. Potassium ions in the intracellular fluid
    C. Angiotensin II
    D. Hypercalcemia

22. **Your patient's aldosterone levels are low. As a PICU nurse, you know a factor that suppresses aldosterone production is**
    A. Hypocalcemia
    B. Hyperkalemia
    C. Stress
    D. Atrial natriuretic hormone

23. **Functions of the thyroid gland, adrenal gland, and male and female reproductive glands are regulated by the**
    A. Thyroid gland
    B. Pineal gland of the brain
    C. Pineal–pituitary axis
    D. Hypothalamic–pituitary axis

24. **Where is the pituitary gland located?**
    A. Superior to the hypothalamus gland near the optic chiasm
    B. Inferior to the hypothalamus and sits in the sella turcica of the skull
    C. Between the thalamus and hypothalamus in the midbrain
    D. Superior to the pons and brain stem

25. **Cortisol is a glucocorticoid. A major effect of cortisol in the body is to**
    A. Increase the loss of sodium from small intestines
    B. Lower blood pressure in times of stress
    C. Raise the level of free amino acids in the serum
    D. Stimulate urine loss

26. **Myron has been diagnosed with galactosemia. Galactosemia is a congenital disease transmitted as an**
    A. X-linked recessive disease
    B. Autosomal recessive disorder
    C. X-linked dominant trait
    D. Autosomal dominant disorder

27. **A disorder caused by a defect in copper excretion is known as**
    A. Cooper's disease
    B. Wilson's disease
    C. Brandon's chorea
    D. Meikle's chorea

28. **The lysosomal storage disease caused by glucocerebrosidase deficiency is known as**
    A. Meikle's disease
    B. Gaucher's disease
    C. Pompe's disease
    D. Tay-Sachs disease

29. **Randall is a 3 week old infant who appeared to be doing well at home until he began having seizures. On initial assessment, you note Randall is lethargic and has poor muscle tone. He appears to be having muscle spasms. Randall will not feed and has a "burned sugar" smell to his urine. You believe Randall is suffering from**
    A. Diabetic ketoacidosis
    B. Tyrosinemia
    C. Maple syrup urine disease
    D. Rhabdomyolysis

30. **How does hyperglycemic, hyperosmolar, nonketotic syndrome (HHNS) differ from diabetic ketoacidosis (DKA)?**
    A. HHNS has the same onset, higher blood sugars, and more dehydration than DKA
    B. HHNS has a slower onset, lower blood sugars, and less dehydration than DKA
    C. HHNS has a slower onset, much higher blood sugars, and more profound dehydration than DKA
    D. HHNS has the same onset as and lower blood sugars than DKA, but no dehydration

31. **Tyrone has been diagnosed with HHNS. Which of the following sets of lab test results would you anticipate for a patient with HHNS?**
    A. Glucose 550, positive ketones, serum osmolality 280 mOsm/L
    B. Glucose 1258, negative ketones, serum osmolality 375 mOsm/L
    C. Glucose 700, negative ketones, serum osmolality 270 mOsm/L
    D. Glucose 600, positive ketones, serum osmolality 240 mOsm/L

32. **Paul has congenital hypothyroidism. Congenital hypothyroidism is manifested by**
    A. A decreased TSH and a decreased T_4
    B. A euthyroid state
    C. An elevated TSH and a decreased T_4
    D. A decreased TSH and an elevated T_4

33. **Maternal thyroid disease can have a substantial influence on fetal and neonatal thyroid function because**
    A. Radiation will stimulate thyroid function
    B. Thioamides can stimulate thyroid growth
    C. Immunoglobulin G (IgG) autoantibodies can cross the placenta
    D. Thyroid function is enhanced

34. **Physical findings of congenital hypothyroidism include**
    A. Hyperthermia and poor feeding
    B. Erythema and diaphoresis
    C. Macroglossia and large fontanelles
    D. Diarrhea and irritability

35. **A nurse orienting to the PICU has an infant with a goiter and asks which position is best for this patient. An infant with a large goiter should be positioned**
    A. Supine with the legs slightly elevated
    B. In a side-lying position
    C. Prone with a small towel under the cheek
    D. Supine with the head slightly elevated and extended

36. Signs of vitamin D toxicity include

A. Seizures
B. Increased susceptibility to respiratory diseases
C. Azotemia
D. Hypocalcemia

37. Kayexalate is given as a treatment for hyperkalemia. What is the mechanism of action of this drug?

A. Kayexalate exchanges sodium ions for potassium ions
B. Kayexalate preserves the sodium pump
C. Kayexalate causes diarrhea, thereby removing potassium from the gastrointestinal tract
D. Kayexalate moves potassium into the intracellular space

38. Zack has a crush injury to his right thigh from falling off his bicycle. Why does this injury put Zack at risk for hyperkalemia?

A. There is more risk for hypokalemia
B. He is at no risk for hyperkalemia
C. Cellular destruction leads to increased circulating potassium levels
D. Wound infection decreases potassium levels

39. Functions of the thyroid gland, adrenal gland, and male and female reproductive glands are regulated by the

A. Hypothyroid gland
B. Pineal gland of the brain
C. Hypothalamic–pituitary axis
D. Thyroid gland

40. Infants with DiGeorge's syndrome may have which of the following electrolyte imbalances because of absent parathyroid glands?

A. Hyperkalemia
B. Hypercalcemia
C. Hypokalemia
D. Hypocalcemia

41. Which of the following conditions contributes to the development of acute hypoglycemia?

A. Insulinoma
B. Glucose consumption exceeds glucose production
C. Use of oral antihyperglycemic agents
D. Alcoholism

42. Greg has recurrent episodes of acute hypoglycemia. Which therapies may be used to treat acute hypoglycemia (blood sugar less than 50 mg/dL)?

A. Small, frequent meals, increased carbohydrate consumption
B. Intravenous D_{50} administration, oral glucose, and treat the cause
C. Increased carbohydrate diet, intravenous glucose
D. Treat the cause, increased carbohydrate consumption

43. What is the most common precipitating factor in the development of diabetic ketoacidosis (DKA)?

A. Hypoglycemia only
B. Hypoglycemia with obesity and family history
C. Hyperglycemia with concurrent illness or injury
D. Hyperglycemia only

44. What are some of the signs and symptoms associated with diabetic ketoacidosis (DKA)?

A. Polyuria, polydipsia, polyphagia, and dilute urine
B. Polyuria, polydipsia, polyphagia, fruity breath, dehydration, and marked fatigue
C. Hyperactivity, confusion, nausea, and vomiting
D. Kussmaul's respirations and dilute urine

45. Jane is 8 years old and has DKA. She has a blood glucose level of 460 mg/dL and a potassium level of 6.2. You have started an insulin drip. You know that the insulin drip

A. Will move potassium back into the intracellular space
B. Will not change the potassium level
C. Will draw more potassium from the intracellular space
D. Will draw more potassium from the extracellular space

46. Fran has been preliminarily diagnosed with Cushing syndrome. Which diagnostic tests do you anticipate the physician ordering for Fran?

A. Computerized tomography of the brain, chest, and abdomen, 24-hour urine cortisol levels, ACTH serum concentrations
B. Computerized tomography of the brain, chest, and abdomen, thyroid levels, basic metabolic panel
C. Serum and urine cortisol levels, thyroid panels, beta natriuretic peptide levels
D. Urine ACTH concentrations;, thyroid panel, C-reactive protein level

47. Which physical symptoms do you expect a patient to exhibit if diagnosed with Cushing syndrome?

A. Moon facies, edema, and weight loss
B. Moon facies, acne, and weight loss
C. Moon facies, purple striae on trunk, and buffalo hump
D. Moon facies, easy bruising, and weight loss

48. Which of the following hormones are produced by the anterior pituitary gland?

A. Vasopressin and oxytocin
B. FSH, LH, TSH, and ACTH
C. ADH, TSH, and FSH
D. GRF, TSH, and substance P

49. Where is the thyroid gland located?

A. Just below the hyoid bone
B. In the throat on either side of the trachea
C. Above the larynx
D. On top of the thymus gland

50. Where are the parathyroid glands located?

A. Anterior to the thyroid
B. Posterior to the thyroid gland
C. On top of the thyroid gland
D. Below the thyroid gland

51. Where is the pancreas located in the abdomen?

A. Right lower quadrant of the abdomen
B. Left upper quadrant of the abdomen
C. Right upper quadrant of the abdomen
D. Left lower quadrant of the abdomen

52. Why are hyperglycemia and hyperlipidemia seen concurrently in patients with diabetes mellitus?

A. Very-low-density lipoprotein (VLDL) production increases in response to increased insulin production
B. Insulin resistance promotes VLDL production
C. Lipid breakdown is hindered by hyperinsulinemia
D. Increases in the glucose level cause the liver to increase lipid production

53. Which of the following are risk factors for the development of diabetes mellitus?

A. Obesity (BMI of 42), blood pressure 160/95, HDL 28, and a brother with diabetes mellitus
B. Obesity (BMI of 27), blood pressure 120/70, HDL 42, and no family history of diabetes mellitus
C. Obesity (BMI of 26), Caucasian ancestry, blood pressure 190/100, and family history of diabetes mellitus
D. Obesity (BMI of 40), blood pressure 100/50, HDL 50, and no family history of diabetes mellitus

54. How is insulin secretion regulated?

A. Hormonal, exocrine gland secretion, glucose controls
B. Hormonal, insulin and neuronal controls
C. Chemical, glucagon and insulin controls
D. Chemical, hormonal and neuronal controls

55. What is the role of glucophage in the body?

A. Glucophage acts on the liver to decrease blood sugar
B. Glucophage acts on the liver to increase blood sugar
C. Glucophage acts on the pancreas to decrease blood sugar
D. Glucophage acts on the pancreas to increase blood sugar

56. What is nonalcohol steatohepatitis (NASH)?

A. Fatty liver from a poor diet
B. Fatty liver from a hepatitis B infection
C. Fatty liver infiltrates seen as a precursor to diabetes mellitus type 2
D. Fatty liver from obesity and excess consumption of dietary fats

57. What are the three major problems associated with macrovascular disease in a patient with diabetes mellitus?

A. Diabetic peripheral neuropathy, peripheral vascular disease, and cerebral vascular accident
B. Peripheral neuropathy, coronary artery disease, and cerebral vascular accident
C. Coronary artery disease, cerebral vascular accident, and peripheral vascular disease
D. Retinopathy, coronary artery disease, and cerebral vascular accident

58. What is the origin of microvascular disease in diabetes mellitus?

A. Vasoconstriction from hyperglycemia
B. Changes in the capillary basement membrane that cause hypoxia on the cellular level
C. Increased atherosclerotic plaques on the intima
D. Repeated hypoglycemic events

59. Where in the body are the catecholamines produced?

A. Liver
B. Kidneys
C. Adrenal cortex
D. Adrenal medulla

60. Which of the following hormone-related conditions is responsible for the symptoms of hypothyroidism?

A. Low levels of T_4 (thyroxine)
B. Low levels of T_3 (thriothyroxine)
C. Decreased thyrocalcitonin
D. Increased thyrocalcitonin

61. Which of the following signs may be elicited in a patient with hypocalcemia?

A. Short QT interval
B. Hyperparathyroidism
C. Chvostek's sign
D. Cullen's sign

62. Trousseau's sign is seen with which of the following conditions?

A. Increased serum calcium
B. Decreased serum calcium
C. Decreased serum phosphorus
D. Hypothyroidism

63. What is the treatment of choice once a diagnosis of pheochromocytoma is made?

A. Antihypertensive medications
B. Diuretics
C. Surgical removal of the tumor
D. Diet changes

64. **Which symptoms are to be expected when a patient is having a thyrotoxic crisis?**
    A. Hyperthermia and bradycardia
    B. Hypotension and bradycardia
    C. Flushing and hypoventilation
    D. Hypertension and hyperthermia

65. **Your patient is experiencing a thyrotoxic crisis. Which medication would you give to reduce the patient's symptoms?**
    A. Propranolol
    B. Levophed
    C. Adenosine
    D. Digoxin

66. **Which of the following conditions can cause a thyroid storm in a patient with hyperthyroidism?**
    A. An overdose of PTU (propylthyrouricil)
    B. Increased iodine intake
    C. Trauma or infection
    D. Decreased iodine intake

67. **Paula has been admitted to the pediatric intensive care unit with DKA. Her insulin drip is infusing at 4 units per hour. Her current blood sugar is 290 and her anion gap is 25. Which changes in her care should you anticipate?**
    A. Change the intravenous fluid to D_5W and continue the insulin drip
    B. Change the intravenous fluid to D_5NS and continue the insulin drip
    C. Discontinue the insulin drip and check stat blood sugars every four hours
    D. No changes in therapy

68. **Which of the following patients with diabetes is most likely to develop DKA?**
    A. Type 1, well controlled on 70/30 insulin
    B. Type 1, noncompliant, with cellulitis of the left leg
    C. Type 2, Hgb A_{1c} of 6.5, and minor surgery
    D. Type 2, noncompliant, with a mild upper respiratory tract infection

69. **Death in the hypothermic infant is caused by**
    A. The underlying disease process
    B. Aerobic metabolism
    C. Bradycardia
    D. Hypoglycemia and hypoxemia

70. **Temperature regulation in the infant is controlled by the hypothalamus through the release of which of the following hormones?**
    A. Dopamine
    B. Norepinephrine
    C. Cortisol
    D. Epinephrine

71. Gloria is a 13 year old admitted to the PICU following a cholecystectomy. Gloria is morbidly obese. She has a recent history of gastric bypass surgery for weight loss. You find her confused with slurred speech, and diaphoretic. Her BP is 94/40, pulse 116, and blood sugar 28. Your first action should be

A. Notify the physician and recheck the blood sugar
B. Open the intravenous fluid and give orange juice with sugar
C. Give one amp of D_{50} per hospital policy, notify the physician, and recheck her blood sugar in 30 minutes
D. Have the hospital lab recheck the patient's blood sugar

72. Sally is an 11 year old who has been admitted to the pediatric intensive care unit for new-onset diabetic ketoacidosis. You are teaching her about diabetes mellitus and Hgb A_{1c}. Which of the following Hgb A_{1c} values should be Sally's goal for good control of her diabetes mellitus?

A. 7–8%
B. 4–5%
C. 6–7%
D. 8–9%

73. Where is renin stored in the body?

A. Renal tubules
B. Loop of Henle
C. Juxtoglomerular cells of the nephron
D. Adrenal cortex

74. Which of the following conditions can trigger the renin–angiotensin mechanism?

A. Aldosterone and diuretics
B. Diuretics and decreased renal blood flow
C. Diuretics and adrenergic blockers
D. Increased renal blood flow and diuretics

75. What is the correct order in which the renin–angiotensin mechanism occurs when there is a decrease in blood flow to the kidneys?

A. Renin, aldosterone, angiotensin I, angiotensin I converting enzyme, angiotensin II
B. Increased ADH, renin, angiotensin I, angiotensin II
C. Renin, angiotensinogen, angiotensin I, angiotensin I converting enzyme, angiotensin II, aldosterone
D. Renin, ACTH, angiotensin I

76. Which changes are seen on the EKG of a patient with hyperkalemia?

A. Widening QRS, peaked T waves, and loss of P waves
B. Narrow QRS, peaked T waves, and U waves
C. Wide QRS, normal T waves, and U waves
D. Narrow QRS, normal T waves, and rapid rate

77. **Peter, who is 9 years old, was found unconscious in his backyard by his mother. His blood sugar is 1545, he has negative serum ketones, and his serum osmolality is 340. Which fluids do you anticipate giving Peter for medical treatment of this condition?**
    A. $D_5$1/2NS intravenous fluids 300 mL/hr and an insulin drip with sliding-scale coverage
    B. Normal saline at 100 mL/hr, subcutaneous insulin with sliding-scale coverage every 4 hours, and monitor potassium
    C. Intravenous fluids with normal saline in high volumes, insulin drip with sliding-scale coverage, and monitor electrolytes
    D. Normal saline intravenously, bicarbonate drip, and monitor electrolytes

78. **A fellow nurse asks you to explain the differences between the Somoygi effect and the dawn phenomenon. What are the major differences between the Somoygi effect and the dawn phenomenon?**
    A. They are essentially the same process
    B. The dawn phenomenon is nocturnal hypoglycemia, the Somoygi effect is greatly increased blood sugars in the early morning
    C. The Somoygi effect is nocturnal hypoglycemia with rebound hyperglycemia, the dawn phenomenon is increased morning glucose without nocturnal hypoglycemia
    D. The dawn phenomenon is morning hypoglycemia, the Somoygi effect is nocturnal hyperglycemia

79. **Your patient's thyroid-stimulating hormone (TSH) level is 0.001. Which condition does this value indicate?**
    A. Hypoactive anterior pituitary function
    B. Hyperactive anterior pituitary function
    C. Hypothyroidism
    D. Hyperthyroidism

80. **What is an important teaching point for a parent and a young patient with hypothyroidism?**
    A. Take the thyroid medication at the same time every day; there is no need to fast
    B. Take the thyroid medication at the same time every day, 30 minutes before breakfast
    C. Take the thyroid medicine each evening before bed
    D. Take the thyroid medicine daily with food

81. **Myra had a thyroidectomy yesterday for thyroid cancer. Today she is delirious, vomiting, hyperthermic, and tachycardic. It is imperative to notify the physician stat because**
    A. Myra has a postoperative infection
    B. Myra may have had a cerebrovascular accident
    C. Myra may have thyrotoxic crisis
    D. Myra is hypoxic and needs a tracheostomy

82. Treatment for thyrotoxic crisis includes

A. Nothing—there is no need for treatment, and the crisis will resolve spontaneously
B. Symptomatic care and waiting for symptoms to subside
C. Synthroid administration and supportive care
D. Administration of PTH and symptomatic care

83. Your patient's calcium level is 11.9 mg/dL. This value may be the result of which of the following conditions?

A. Hypoparathyroidism
B. Hyperparathyroidism
C. Excessive calcium intake
D. Recent fracture of a long bone

84. With which condition would you expect to see hypoparathyroidism develop?

A. Trauma
B. Hypercalcemia
C. Hypophosphatemia
D. After thyroid or neck surgery

85. Sam is admitted to the pediatric intensive care unit in hypertensive crisis. You notice large fluctuations in his blood pressure even without changing his nitroprusside drip. The physician orders a plasma catecholamine level. Sam's fractional epinephrine level is very high. What does this high level probably indicate?

A. Cocaine use
B. Pheochromocytoma
C. Adrenal cortex tumor
D. Hyperthyroidism

86. What is the treatment of choice once a diagnosis of pheochromocytoma is made?

A. Diet changes
B. Antihypertensive medications
C. Surgical removal of the tumor
D. Diuretics

87. Part of your patient education for the family of a patient with pheochromocytoma includes dietary restrictions. Which of the following foods should the patient avoid?

A. Cream cheese
B. Red meat
C. Chocolate
D. Aged cheddar cheese

88. Which glands regulate thyroid function?

A. Posterior pituitary and hypothalamus
B. Anterior pituitary and thalamus
C. Anterior pituitary and hypothalamus
D. Posterior pituitary and thalamus

89. Emily has end-stage renal disease (ESRD), stage IV, and undergoes hemodialysis every Monday, Wednesday, and Friday. Her calcium is 6.3 mg/dL and PTH is 70 pg/mL. What is happening to this patient?

A. Hypoparathyroidism
B. Secondary hyperparathyroidism
C. Secondary hyperthyroidism
D. Hypothyroidism

90. Aiden is admitted to the pediatric intensive care unit with myxedema coma. He is receiving intravenous thyroid replacement therapy when he suddenly develops hypotension, hypoglycemia, nausea, and vomiting. What has happened to Aiden?

A. He is having an allergic response to the thyroid medication
B. He needs an increased dose of thyroid medication
C. He needs a lower dose of thyroid medication
D. He is experiencing Addisonian crisis

91. The HCO_3 for your patient with diabetic ketoacidosis is 10 mEq/L. In addition to an insulin drip, you should anticipate performing which of the following actions?

A. Increasing the insulin drip to hasten the resolution of the metabolic acidosis
B. Giving a sodium bicarbonate bolus, and repeat every 4–6 hours
C. Establishing a sodium bicarbonate drip, and monitor the HCO_3 levels frequently
D. Decreasing the insulin drip, as the acidosis is resolving

92. Ryan is admitted to the pediatric intensive care unit for diabetic ketoacidosis. As his nurse, you know his insulin drip will be titrated by sliding scale and his anion gap. What does the anion gap measure?

A. An estimate of cations and anions
B. An estimate of unmeasured anions
C. An estimate of anions in the blood
D. Estimate of the correction of the acid–base balance

SECTION 5

Endocrine Answers

1. **Correct answer: C**
   Hgb A_{1c} measures the effectiveness of diabetes mellitus therapy. Hemoglobin and glucose have an affinity for each other, joining together to form a glycolated hemoglobin. The Hgb A_{1c} rises and falls in direct correlation with blood sugars. The American College of Endocrinologists recommends a Hgb A_{1c} of less than 6.5%, whereas the American Diabetes Association recommends a Hgb A_{1c} of less than 7%. Patients with Hgb A_{1c}'s less than 6% are considered nondiabetic.

2. **Correct answer: D**
   The traditional treatment for central diabetes insipidus involves the replacement of vasopressin or use of an analogue. The most effective analogue available is desmopressin (DDAVP).

3. **Correct answer: A**
   Maternal hyperglycemia ultimately causes increased hepatic glucose uptake secondary to fetal hyperinsulinemia and hyperglycemia. Increased glycogen synthesis, accelerated lipogenesis, and macrosomia will result.

4. **Correct answer: A**
   The anterior pituitary, or adenohypophysis, controls the function of the thyroid gland through its production of thyroid-stimulating hormone (TSH). The anterior pituitary also controls the adrenal cortex through release of antidiuretic hormone (ADH), and the gonads through production of luteinizing hormone (LH) or interstitial cell-stimulating hormone (ICSH).

5. **Correct answer: C**
   Excess fetal insulin may be the cause of delayed maturation of type II alveolar cells and pulmonary surfactant deficiency. The excess insulin may cause congenital cardiac anomalies such as cardiomyopathy and intraventricular septal hypertrophy.

6. **Correct answer: B**
   Hyperthermia would inhibit the release of thyroxine.

7. **Correct answer: C**
   Antidiuretic hormone (ADH), a hormone produced by the posterior pituitary gland, affects the functions of thirst and water balance. When the plasma becomes concentrated or the blood volume is reduced, the posterior pituitary gland releases ADH, causing water retention and concentration of urine. ADH production is regulated by a feedback mechanism within the pituitary gland.

8. **Correct answer: D**
   Pituitary tumors will inhibit ADH production. Antidiuretic hormone is controlled by a negative feedback system. Its production decreases when the osmoreceptors of the hypothalamus recognize hemodilution or hemoconcentration and adjust ADH production accordingly.

9. **Correct answer: C**
   Stimulation of the anterior pituitary gland comes from the hypothalamus by way of the vascular system.

10. **Correct answer: A**
    Calcitonin is released by the thyroid gland.

11. **Correct answer: B**
    An increase in serum calcium, glucagon, or magnesium will stimulate the release of calcitonin. Calcitonin release, in turn, will reduce serum calcium levels. Calcitonin targets bone and kidney cells to inhibit bone cell lysis, and it decreases calcium reabsorption by the kidney.

12. **Correct answer: D**
    Glucagon is released from the alpha cells in the pancreas. It inhibits glycolysis, increases lipolysis, and increases blood glucose by stimulating glycogenolysis and gluconeogenesis.

13. **Correct answer: B**
    Seizures are one of the most common presenting symptoms of syndrome of inappropriate antidiuretic hormone (SIADH). SIADH causes hemodilution and a relative decrease in serum sodium levels. Once the sodium falls below 120, the patient is at great risk for seizures. Excessive urine output and hypotension are both symptoms of diabetes insipidus.

14. **Correct answer: D**
    An increase in catecholamine and amino acid levels, accompanied by a decrease in serum glucose, will stimulate the release of glucagon. If the serum glucose becomes low following exercise, for example, glucagon is released to help produce an increase in blood glucose.

15. **Correct answer: B**
    A high serum magnesium or phosphate, low serum calcium, and catecholamine release result in secretion of parathyroid hormone. Bone breakdown is accelerated, releasing calcium into the blood. Calcium reabsorption is increased in the intestine, and kidney tubule reabsorption is decreased. Phosphate loss is increased in the urine, which decreases serum phosphate. Parahormone increases reabsorption of magnesium by the renal tubules. Renal calculi may develop.

16. **Correct answer: C**
    The most important nursing consideration in the infant patient with HHNS is to prevent aspiration. The severe hypokalemia that results from the lack of intracellular-to-extracellular shift is occurring because the patient is not usually acidotic. When the patient is hypokalemic, hypocalcemia and hypomagnesemia also occur. Muscle activity is compromised, and the patient is at high risk for aspiration because of a paralytic ileus.

17. **Correct answer: C**
Hashimoto's disease, also known as chronic lymphocytic thyroiditis, is the most common cause of hypothyroidism. Hashimoto's disease is an autoimmune disorder, the immune system makes antibodies against the thyroid and interferes with production of thyroid hormone.

18. **Correct answer: D**
Calcium cannot be utilized by the body without adequate vitamin D levels. Fifteen minutes' exposure to daylight on the skin without use of sunblock allows the body to create its own vitamin D. An increased phosphorus level would bind the calcium, making it unavailable.

19. **Correct answer: B**
The primary effect of aldosterone is increased reabsorption of water and sodium, which results in an increased extracellular fluid volume. Renal excretion of potassium is increased.

20. **Correct answer: B**
Aldosterone is secreted by the zona glomerulus of the adrenal cortex.

21. **Correct answer: C**
Aldosterone secretion is regulated by angiotensin II. When renal blood flow is decreased, angiotensin is released and stimulates aldosterone secretion. An increase in potassium ions in extracellular fluid will also stimulate the release of aldosterone. Adrenocorticotropic hormone will stimulate aldosterone production for short periods of time.

22. **Correct answer: D**
Atrial natriuretic hormone is a factor that suppresses aldosterone production. Hypercalcemia and hypokalemia also suppress aldosterone production.

23. **Correct answer: D**
The hypothalamic–pituitary axis releases a number of hormones that either inhibit or release several hormones that affect body functions.

24. **Correct answer: B**
The pituitary gland is inferior to the hypothalamus and sits in the sella turcica of the sphenoid bone. The other locations are incorrect. The correct order of these structures is the thalamus, hypothalamus, infundibulum, and pituitary gland.

25. **Correct answer: C**
Cortisol raises the concentration of free amino acids in serum by inhibiting collagen formation and protein synthesis. Cortisol stimulates gastric acid secretion, inhibits loss of sodium from the small intestines, acts as an antidiuretic hormone, and works with epinephrine and norepinephrine to increase blood pressure.

26. **Correct answer: B**
Galactosemia is a congenital disease transmitted as an autosomal recessive disorder. Because this disease is an autosomal recessive disorder, the parents of a child with galactosemia are unaffected, healthy carriers of the condition and have one normal gene and one abnormal gene.

27. **Correct answer: B**
Wilson's disease is caused by a defect in copper excretion. In this disorder, copper is deposited in the liver, brain, heart, and eyes. Hepatic dysfunction is common, along with elevated serum and urine copper. An infant with Wilson's disease may have seizures, dystonia, dysarthria, and tremors. Chelation therapy with oral penicillin and zinc salts may be prescribed. On occasion, a liver transplant may be necessary.

28. **Correct answer: B**
Gaucher's disease is a lysosomal storage disease caused by glucocerebrosidase deficiency. This disorder is autosomal recessive and may be managed by enzyme replacement therapy. Symptoms include thrombocytopenia and hepatosplenomegaly. On X-ray, a classic "Erlenmeyer flask shape" of the distal femur is seen.

29. **Correct answer: C**
Randall is probably suffering from maple syrup urine disease. His urine has the characteristic "burned sugar" or "sweet maple syrup" smell. Other symptoms of this disease include lethargy, poor feeding, muscle weakness, spasms, seizures, and poor weight gain. During acute episodes, the infant will exhibit hyperglycemia and profound acidosis.

30. **Correct answer: C**
HHNS develops slowly in type 2 diabetes, most often in elderly patients or those with undiagnosed diabetes mellitus. The blood sugars are generally more than 600 mg/dL and can exceed 1500 mg/dL. The other point of differentiation between HHNS and DKA is the lack of ketones noted with HHNS.

31. **Correct answer: B**
Blood sugars greater than 600 mg/dL with negative serum ketones and a serum osmolality greater than 310 mOsm/L are typical of hyperglycemic, hyperosmolar, nonketotic syndrome (HHNS). The pH is usually greater than 7.3, and the blood urea nitrogen may be elevated. With HHNS, osmolality is a better predictor of survivability than blood sugar levels.

32. **Correct answer: C**
Congenital hypothyroidism is manifested by an elevated TSH level and a decreased T_4 level. This disease is usually inherited in an autosomal recessive manner, but some cases are autosomal dominant. Congenital hypothyroidism occurs when the thyroid gland fails to develop or function properly. The thyroid gland may be absent, hypoplastic, or displaced. In a few cases, the gland is enlarged, but the production of thyroid hormones is deficient or absent.

33. **Correct answer: C**
Maternal thyroid disease can have a substantial influence on fetal and neonatal thyroid function because immunoglobulin G (IgG) autoantibodies can cross the placenta and inhibit thyroid function in the developing fetus. Thioamides used to treat maternal hyperthyroidism can obstruct fetal thyroid hormone synthesis. Most of these effects are transient. Radioactive iodine administered to a pregnant woman can destroy the fetus's thyroid gland.

34. **Correct answer: C**
Physical findings in congenital hypothyroidism include macroglossia, pallor, enlarged fontanelles, cool, dry skin, umbilical hernias, and coarse facial features. Not all infants

with congenital hypothyroidism display these characteristics, however. In addition, an infant with this condition may have an atrial or ventricular septal defect. Developmental delay is common.

35. **Correct answer: D**
An infant with a large goiter should be positioned supine with the head slightly elevated and extended. Maintaining a patent airway is a nursing priority. The goiter may impinge on the trachea, so correct positioning is essential.

36. **Correct answer: C**
Signs of vitamin D toxicity include azotemia, hypercalcemia, vomiting, and nephrocalcinosis. Vitamin D deficiency will result in hypocalcemia, increased susceptibility to respiratory diseases, lethargy, and seizures.

37. **Correct answer: C**
Kayexalate permanently exchanges 1 gram of medication for 1 mEq of potassium. Other therapies include IV insulin, $D_{50}W$, and sodium bicarbonate. These latter therapies allow quick, effective, short-term correction of the potassium level. Hemodialysis and Kayexalate are the only two treatments that permanently remove excess potassium.

38. **Correct answer: C**
Crush injuries can cause a massive release of potassium into the bloodstream. There is approximately 135–145 mEq of potassium in each cell.

39. **Correct answer: C**
Functions of the thyroid gland, adrenal gland, and male and female reproductive glands are regulated by the hypothalamic–pituitary axis. The hypothalamic–pituitary axis releases a number of hormones that either inhibit or release several hormones that affect body functions.

40. **Correct answer: D**
Infants with DiGeorge's syndrome may develop hypocalcemia because they lack parathyroid glands.

41. **Correct answer: B**
Lack of food or if the liver is unable to provide glucogenesis, it may cause a drop in blood glucose to less than 50 mg/dL. The other answers are risk factors for hypoglycemia.

42. **Correct answer: B**
D_{50}, oral glucose, and treating the cause are the most effective way to treat acute hypoglycemia. The other answers include increased carbohydrate consumption, which would be prohibited in patients with acute hypoglycemia. The optimal diet would consist of small, frequent meals and reduced consumption of carbohydrates.

43. **Correct answer: C**
DKA is seen with illness or injury such as infection, surgery, trauma, or UTI. DKA is defined as a fasting blood sugar greater than 250 mg/dL, ranging up to approximately 1000 mg/dL.

44. **Correct answer: B**
Signs and symptoms of DKA include polyuria, polydipsia, and polyphagia—collectively known as the "three P's." The fruity breath is caused by ketone production when fatty

acids are broken down. Dehydration is due to osmotic diuresis. Fatigue is due to potassium shifts from inside the cells to the intravascular space.

45. **Correct answer: A**
An insulin drip will move potassium back into the intracellular space. Potassium is pulled from the intracellular space due to metabolic acidosis. The insulin drip will help correct the metabolic acidosis by allowing the potassium to return to normal levels.

46. **Correct answer: A**
Cushing syndrome is usually seen in conjunction with Cushing disease. It is important to rule out tumors of the pituitary gland, chest tumors (i.e., small cell cancer of the lung), adrenal tumors, and pheochromocytomas. You should anticipate the physician ordering computerized tomography of the brain, chest and abdomen, a 24 hour urine cortisol level and ACTH serum concentrations. These tumors cause excessive ACTH production, leading to the physical changes seen with Cushing syndrome, such as moon facies, buffalo hump, truncal obesity, and purple striae on the abdomen.

47. **Correct answer: C**
Numerous physical changes occur with Cushing syndrome or Cushing disease, including thinning hair, acne, moon facies, increased body hair, buffalo hump on the upper back, purple striae on the trunk, truncal obesity with thin extremities, and easy bruising.

48. **Correct answer: B**
The anterior pituitary gland produces numerous hormones, including TSH, LH, FSH, ACTH, and melanocyte-stimulating hormone. Substance P is a hormone released by the hypothalamus. Vasopressin and oxytocin are released by the posterior pituitary gland.

49. **Correct answer: B**
The thyroid gland is located below the larynx, on either side of the trachea.

50. **Correct answer: B**
The parathyroid glands are located posterior to the thyroid gland and consist of four to six small glands. They produce parathyroid hormone (PTH), which regulates serum calcium, magnesium, and phosphorus levels. PTH also stimulates the kidney to produce bioavailable vitamin D.

51. **Correct answer: B**
The pancreas is located in the left upper quadrant of the abdomen and sits behind the stomach near the spleen and duodenum. This is a basic question—but one that has caught many an unwary nurse.

52. **Correct answer: B**
Insulin resistance predisposes the patient to elevated blood glucose and increased insulin production. Production of very-low-density lipoprotein (VLDL) increases with hyperinsulinemia.

53. **Correct answer: A**
Risk factors for the development of diabetes mellitus include blood pressure greater than 140/90 or higher than accepted for age, first-degree relative with diabetes mellitus, nonwhite ancestry, obesity (BMI greater than 30), and high-density lipoprotein (HDL) less than 35.

54. **Correct answer: D**
Insulin secretion is controlled by chemicals such as glucose and amino acids. Hormones such as GI hormones and prostaglandin will also control insulin secretion.

55. **Correct answer: A**
Glucophage (Metformin) serves as an antihyperglycemic agent by improving glucose tolerance in patients with type 2 diabetes. It decreases liver glucose production as well as intestinal absorption of glucose.

56. **Correct answer: C**
Nonalcohol steatohepatitis (NASH) is characterized by fatty liver infiltrates and is often seen in conjunction with insulin resistance, obesity, and increased triglycerides. NASH may progress to cirrhosis if the patient fails to make the appropriate lifestyle changes.

57. **Correct answer: C**
Coronary artery disease, cerebral vascular accident, and peripheral vascular disease are the three major problems associated with macrovascular disease and are often seen in type 2 diabetes mellitus. Mortality or morbidity in patients who experience these diabetic complications is typically due to macrovascular changes. Diabetes leads to early atherosclerosis and atherosclerotic heart disease. The other problems listed (retinopathy, peripheral neuropathy, and diabetic nephropathy) are microvascular diseases.

58. **Correct answer: B**
The origins of microvascular disease in diabetes mellitus are due to changes in the capillary basement membrane that cause hypoxia on the cellular level. Prolonged hyperglycemia thickens the capillary basement membrane, which in turn leads to decreased blood flow, hypoxia, and a lack of nutrients at the cellular level. The eye and kidney are the organs most susceptible to damage through this process.

59. **Correct answer: D**
The adrenal medulla produces 75–85% of the catecholamine epinephrine and 25% of the body's supply of norepinephrine (from phenylalanine).

60. **Correct answer: A**
Thyroxine is responsible for the symptoms of hypothyroidism. The decreased T_4 level leads to hypothyroid symptoms of cold, dry skin, hair loss, periorbital edema and possibly thyroid enlargement.

61. **Correct answer: C**
Chvostek's sign is seen with hypocalcemia. It is elicited by tapping the cheek over the zygomatic arch and causes facial twitching. The QT interval would be prolonged with hypocalcemia. Cullen's sign consists of ecchymosis around the umbilicus; it is often seen in conjunction with pancreatitis.

62. **Correct answer: B**
Trousseau's sign, which is also known as carpal-pedal spasm, is seen with decreased calcium levels. Hypocalcemia can occur with end-stage renal disease (which is associated with increased phosphorus levels) and decreased vitamin D levels. It is also seen in patients who receive three or more units of red blood cells that have been treated with calcium citrate.

63. **Correct answer: C**
The best treatment option for pheochromocytoma is surgical removal of the tumor. Alpha-adrenergic blockers or beta-adrenergic blockers may be used to treat hypertension until surgery can be performed.

64. **Correct answer: D**
Thyrotoxic crisis symptoms include hypertension, hyperthermia, flushing, tachycardia (especially atrial tachyarrhythmia), high-output heart failure, nausea and vomiting, psychosis, and delirium. Treatment includes supportive care and medications to block catecholamine effects.

65. **Correct answer: A**
Propranolol (Inderal) would be administered to a patient having a thyrotoxic crisis. This beta blocker decreases the effects of the sympathetic stimulation of thyrotoxic crisis. It controls heart rate, hypertension, and oxygen consumption.

66. **Correct answer: C**
Injury or infection as well as manipulation of the thyroid gland can trigger a thyroid storm and thyrotoxicosis.

67. **Correct answer: B**
Once the blood glucose is less than 300 mg/dL, D_5WNS should be added to slow the drop in glucose. Hourly monitoring of blood glucose levels should be continued. The anion gap should slowly be lowered to less than 20.

68. **Correct answer: B**
The patient who is most likely to develop DKA is the one who is noncompliant with the therapeutic regimen and has cellulitis. DKA is more common in patients with insulin-dependent diabetes, especially those who have another illness or infection such as cellulitis. Nevertheless, 20–30% of DKA patients have no identified precipitating factors. A patient with well-controlled diabetes is at low risk for DKA. Patients with type 2 diabetes are more likely to develop HHNS.

69. **Correct answer: D**
Infants experiencing severe hypothermia cannot provide a sufficient oxygen supply to meet the demand by the tissues; they also have hypoglycemia related to an increase in glycogen metabolism, which cannot be satisfied by their body's diminishing supply. In the absence of both oxygen and glucose, anaerobic metabolism is used to create energy. This metabolism is achieved at great cost to tissues, as lactic acid builds up in the body. As pH decreases and lactic acid increases, tissues throughout the body are destroyed. Bradycardia, apnea, renal failure, and altered neurologic function worsen as tissues are destroyed, and hypoxia and hypoglycemia continue.

70. **Correct answer: B**
Norepinephrine is released by the hypothalamus in response to chemical and temperature receptors in the skin, face, and along the spinal column. Norepinephrine triggers a cascade of actions within the body to retain or create heat in the core. The efficiency of this cascade is impaired by factors relating to the patient's weight, disease process, and respiratory function. Peripheral vasoconstriction shunts blood flow to internal organs in an effort to control heat loss through the massive surface area of the infant. Unfortunately, in attempting to raise temperature, the metabolic rate is also increased, resulting in a significant increase in consumption of oxygen and glycogen. The child's

body responds by burning brown fat or moving and flexing the extremities in an attempt to generate heat. Norepinephrine also causes pulmonary vasoconstriction that inhibits normal blood flow through the lungs, inhibiting blood oxygenation. The best treatment for hypothermia or cold stress is appropriate and timely prevention.

71. **Correct answer: C**
The most important issue is to increase the blood sugar and notify the physician. Orange juice and sugar should not be given to a new postoperative patient. Her gastric bypass and NPO status increase her risk for hypoglycemia. Other causes of acute hypoglycemia include alcohol abuse, insulinoma, medications, and adrenal insufficiency.

72. **Correct answer: C**
An Hgb A_{1c} of 6–7% indicates that Sally's glucose was 100–150 mg/dL over a 3-month period. An Hgb A_{1c} value of 4–5% is considered normal, whereas values of 7–8%, 8–9%, or more are indicative of poorly controlled diabetes mellitus.

73. **Correct answer: C**
Renin is stored in a crystalline form in the juxtoglomerular cells of the kidneys. When the kidneys perceive a decreased blood flow, the sympathetic response triggers the release of renin. The renin converts angiotensinogen to angiotensin I, a mild vasoconstrictor. If the problem is not resolved, the lungs release angiotensin I converting enzyme to create angiotensin II, a powerful vasoconstrictor. Angiotensin II triggers the release of aldosterone from the adrenal glands, which causes sodium and water retention, thereby increasing the blood pressure.

74. **Correct answer: B**
Anything that causes a perceived drop in renal blood flow triggers the renin–angiotensin mechanism. Renin release can also be triggered by sodium and volume depletion, such as that seen with diuretic use.

75. **Correct answer: C**
The kidneys perceive a drop in blood flow, leading to the release of renin from the juxtoglomerular cells of the nephron. The renin stimulates the release of angiotensinogen, which in turn stimulates the release of angiotensin I. If the blood pressure abnormality is not corrected, the lungs release angiotensin I converting enzyme, which in turn causes the secretion of angiotensin II. Angiotensin II stimulates the release of aldosterone from the adrenal glands, leading to greater retention of sodium and water and increased blood pressure.

76. **Correct answer: A**
A widening QRS, peaked T waves, and loss of P waves would be seen on an EKG if the patient was hyperkalemic. Hyperkalemia slows conduction, leading to these characteristic findings on the EKG. If the condition becomes severe, the patient can develop asystole.

77. **Correct answer: C**
Normal saline should be given in large volumes until the fluid depletion is corrected; D_5NS may then be administered once blood glucose is in the 250–300 mg/dL range. A sliding-scale insulin drip and hourly glucose monitoring would probably be ordered. Frequent electrolyte monitoring would also be performed. If the patient was given $D_5$1/2NS too early in the treatment, it could lead to cerebral edema.

78. **Correct answer: C**
The Somoygi effect consists of nocturnal hypoglycemia with rebound hyperglycemia. It is more common in patients with type 1 diabetes, especially children. The dawn phenomenon consists of morning hyperglycemia without nocturnal hypoglycemia. It is caused by growth hormone secretion in the early morning hours.

79. **Correct answer: D**
A thyroid-stimulating hormone (TSH) level of 0.001 indicates hyperthyroidism or thyrotoxicosis. Causes of this condition include goiter, Graves' disease, thyroid carcinoma, and TSH-secreting pituitary adenoma. Hyperthyroidism without toxicosis is most often related to excessive intake of thyroid hormones.

80. **Correct answer: B**
Thyroid medications should be taken on an empty stomach 30 minutes before breakfast. Other teaching points include the necessity for regular follow-up lab tests to assess TSH and T_4 levels, as well as symptoms of myxedema and hyperthyroidism. Taking thyroid medication in the evening can lead to insomnia.

81. **Correct answer: C**
It is imperative to notify the physician stat because thyrotoxic crisis is a rare but serious problem in post-thyroidectomy patients. It is also critical to report these symptoms if the patient has undertreated hyperthyroidism, has cardiopulmonary disease, or is undergoing hemodialysis.

82. **Correct answer: D**
Treatment of thyrotoxic crisis includes administration of PTH to decrease thyroid-stimulating hormone and thyroid hormone levels, plus symptomatic care.

83. **Correct answer: B**
A calcium level of 11.9 mg/dL indicates hyperparathyroidism. Hyperparathyroidism can be either primary or secondary in nature. Primary hyperparathyroidism is the excess secretion of parathyroid hormone (PTH) and may be related to a breakdown of the feedback system to the glands or overgrowth of the gland. Secondary hyperparathyroidism is generally related to a chronic disorder such as chronic renal failure or a malabsorption state.

84. **Correct answer: D**
Hypoparathyroidism is usually caused by damage (i.e., surgery) to the parathyroid gland. This damage leads to increased phosphatemia and lowered calcium levels.

85. **Correct answer: B**
A pheochromocytoma is a tumor of the adrenal medulla. These tumors are rarely malignant, but they stimulate the release of large amounts of catecholamines such as dopamine, epinephrine, and norepinephrine.

86. **Correct answer: C**
The best treatment option for pheochromocytoma is surgical removal of the tumor. Alpha-adrenergic blockers or beta-adrenergic blockers may be used to treat hypertension until surgery can be performed.

87. **Correct answer: D**
Hypertension in conjunction with a pheochromocytoma can be triggered by foods such as cheese, alcohol, yogurt, and caffeine. It is important to give the patient a list of foods to avoid. Crises often occur after life events where these foods might be consumed.

88. **Correct answer: C**
The anterior pituitary gland secretes thyroid-stimulating hormone (TSH). The hypothalamus regulates the anterior pituitary gland with thyrotropin-releasing hormone (TRH).

89. **Correct answer: B**
Emily has secondary hyperparathyroidism. In ESRD, vitamin D synthesis is decreased, which leads to hypocalcemia. The calcium is also bound to phosphorus, further reducing the calcium levels. This decrease stimulates the parathyroid glands to secrete parathyroid hormone in attempt to correct the calcium levels.

90. **Correct answer: D**
Aiden is having an Addisonian crisis. Subclinical adrenal insufficiency may coexist with myxedema. The treatment of choice is intravenous hydrocortisone therapy.

91. **Correct answer: C**
A sodium bicarbonate drip should be anticipated to replace the HCO_3. This intervention will help resolve the metabolic acidosis. Boluses would be given only if the patient's pH was very low. The insulin drip will not directly correct the HCO_3.

92. **Correct answer: B**
The anion gap measures anions not generally measured in routine labs. The anion gap is an estimate of the degree of lactic acidosis. The formula for figuring the anion gap is $Na - (HCO_3 + Cl)$. The normal level is 10–20 mEq/L. With diabetic ketoacidosis, the anion gap is greater than 30 mEq/L.

ENDOCRINE REFERENCES

Adam, A. C., Rubio-Texeira, M., & Polaina, J. (2004). Lactose: The milk sugar from a biotechnological perspective. *Critical Reviews in Food Science and Nutrition, 44*(7/8), 553–557.

Aehlert, B. (Ed.). (2005). *Comprehensive pediatric emergency care*. St. Louis, MO: Mosby.

Ahrens, T. (2006). *Critical care nursing certification*. Columbus, OH: McGraw-Hill.

Ala, A., Walker, A. P., Ashkan, K., Dooley, J. S., & Schilsky, M. L. (2007). Wilson's disease. *Lancet, 369*(9559), 397–408.

American Heart Association. (2010). Guidelines 2010 for cardiopulmonary resuscitation and emergency cardiovascular care. Retrieved from www.americanheart.org

Andresen, C., Moalli, M., Turner, C., Berryman, E., Pero, R., & Bagi, C. M. (2008). Bone parameters are improved with intermittent dosing of vitamin D_3 and calcitonin. *Calcified Tissue International, 83*(6), 393–403.

Balasubramanian, S., & Ganesh, R. (2008). Vitamin D deficiency in exclusively breast-fed infants. *Indian Journal of Medical Research, 127*(3), 250–255.

Bosch, A. M. (2006). Classical galactosaemia revisited. *Journal of Inherited Metabolic Disease, 29*(4), 516–525.

Bosch, A. M., IJlst, L., Oostheim, W., Mulders, J., Bakker, H. D., Wijburg, F. A., . . . Waterham, H. R. (2005). Identification of novel mutations in classical galactosemia. *Human Mutation, 25*(5), 502.

Brimioulle, S., Orellana-Jimenez, C., Aminian, A., & Vincent, J. L. (2008). Hyponatremia in neurological patients: Cerebral salt wasting versus inappropriate antidiuretic hormone secretion. *Intensive Care Medicine, 34*(1), 125–131.

Brodsky, D., & Martin, C. (2003). *Neonatology review*. Philadelphia, PA: Hanley & Belfus.

Burchett, M. L. R., Hanna, C. E., & Steiner, R. D. (2009). Endocrine and metabolic diseases. In C. E. Burns, A. M. Dunn, M. A. Brady, N. B. Starr, & C. G. Blosser (Eds.), *Pediatric primary care* (4th ed., pp. 584–611). St. Louis: Saunders Elsevier.

Burns, S. M. (Ed.). (2007). *American Association of Critical-Care Nurses (AACN): AACN protocols for practice: Healing environments* (2nd ed.). Sudbury, MA: Jones and Bartlett Learning.

Calonge, N., Teutsch, S., & Botkin, J. (2008). Expanding newborn screening: Process, policy, and priorities. *Hastings Center Report, 38*(3), 32–39.

Cardwell, C. R., Carson, D. J., Yarnell, J., Shields, M. D., & Patterson, C. C. (2008). Atopy, home environment and the risk of childhood-onset type 1 diabetes: A population-based case control study. *Pediatric Diabetes, 9*(3 pt 1), 191–196.

Chachkin, C. (2007). What potent blood: Non-invasive prenatal genetic diagnosis and the transformation of modern prenatal care. *American Journal of Law and Medicine, 33*(1), 9–53.

Chambers, M. A., & Jones, S. (Eds.). (2007). *Surgical nursing of children*. Philadelphia, PA: Elsevier.

Chernecky, C., & Berger, B. (2004). *Laboratory tests and diagnostic procedures* (4th ed.). Philadelphia, PA: Saunders.

Cheung, M., & Glorieux, F. (2008). Osteogenesis imperfecta: Update on presentation and management. *Reviews in Endocrine & Metabolic Disorders, 9*(2), 153–160.

Chiruvolu, A., Engle, W., Sendelbach, D., Manning, M. D., & Jackson, G. L. (2008). Serum calcium values in term and late-preterm neonates receiving gentamicin. *Pediatric Nephrology, 23*(4), 569–574.

Cloherty, J. P., Eichenwald, E. C., & Stark, A. R. (2004). *Manual of neonatal care* (5th ed.). Philadelphia, PA: Lippincott.

Crenner, C. (2008). The troubled dream of genetic medicine: Ethnicity and innovation in Tay-Sachs, cystic fibrosis, and sickle cell disease. *Journal of the History of Medicine and Allied Sciences, 63*(1), 124–126.

Cullen, K. W., & Buzek, B. B. (2009). Knowledge about type 2 diabetes risk and prevention of African-American and Hispanic adults and adolescents with family history of type 2 diabetes. *Diabetes Educator, 35*(5), 836–839.

Cunningham, F. G., Leveno, K. L., & Bloom, S. L. (2005). Obstetrical hemorrhage. In F. G. Cunningham, K. L. Leveno, S. L. Bloom, et al. (Eds.), *Williams obstetrics* (22nd ed.). New York: McGraw-Hill (pp. 619–670).

Drake Melander, S. (Ed.). (2004). *Case studies in critical care nursing: A guide for application and review* (3rd ed.). Philadelphia, PA: Saunders.

Dunn, J. P., & Jagasia, S. M. (2007). Case study: Management of type 2 diabetes after bariatric surgery. *Clinical Diabetes, 25*(3), 112–114.

Edwards, D. F. (1999). The Synergy Model: Linking patient needs to nurse competencies. *Critical Care Nurse. 19*(1), 88–98.

Eldin, W. S., Ragheb, A., Klassen, J., & Shoker, A. (2008). Evidence for increased risk of prediabetes in the uremic patient. *Nephron, 108*(1), c47–c55.

Emergency Nurses Association & Newberry, L. (2003). *Sheehy's emergency nursing: Principles and practice* (5th ed.). St. Louis, MO: Mosby/Elsevier.

Ensenauer, R. E., Michels, V. V., & Reinke, S. S. (2005). Genetic testing: Practical, ethical, and counseling considerations. *Mayo Clinic Proceedings, 80*(1), 63–73.

Enterovirus triggers type 1 diabetes mellitus. (2009). *Nurse Educator, 34*(4), 147.

Erdeve, M., Atasay, B., Arsan, S., Siklar, Z., Ocal, G., & Berberoglu, M. (2007). Hypocalcemic seizure due to congenital rickets in the first day of life. *Turkish Journal of Pediatrics, 49*(3), 301–303.

Figueiredo, B., & Costa, R. (2009). Mother's stress, mood and emotional involvement with the infant: 3 months before and 3 months after childbirth. *Archives of Women's Mental Health, 12*(3), 143–153.

Fingerhut, R., Simon, E., Maier, E., Hennermann, J. B., & Wendel, U. (2008). Maple syrup urine disease: Newborn screening fails to discriminate between classic and variant forms. *Clinical Chemistry, 54*(10), 1739–1741.

Fitzgerald Macksey, L. (2009). *Pediatric anesthetic and emergency drug guide.* Sudbury, MA: Jones and Bartlett Learning.

Gambol, P. (2007). Maternal phenylketonuria syndrome and case-management implications. *Journal of Pediatric Nursing, 22*(2), 129–138.

Gora-Harper, M. (1998). *The injectable drug reference.* Princeton, NJ: Bioscientific Resources.

Grabowski, G. (2008). Lysosomal storage disease 1: Phenotype, diagnosis, and treatment of Gaucher's disease. *Lancet, 372*(9645), 1263–1271.

Halliday, H. L., McClure, B. G., & Reid, M. (2002). *Handbook of neonatal intensive care* (4th ed.). Philadelphia, PA: Saunders.

Hay, W. W. Jr., Levin, M. J., Sondheimer, J. M., & Deterding, R. R. (Eds.). (2007). *Current diagnosis and treatment in pediatrics* (18th ed.). New York: McGraw-Hill.

Hernan, A., Lopez, M., Debes, J. D., & Dickstein, G. (2007). Wilson's disease: What lies beneath. *Digestive Diseases and Sciences, 52*(4), 941–942.

Hickey, J. V. (2008). *The clinical practice of neurological and neurosurgical nursing* (6th ed.). Philadelphia, PA: Lippincott Williams & Wilkins.

Hong, T., & Paneth, N. (2008). Maternal and infant thyroid disorders and cerebral palsy. *Seminars in Perinatology, 32*(6), 438–445.

Jones, K. L. (2006). *Smith's recognizable patterns of human malformation* (6th ed.). Philadelphia, PA: Elsevier.

Jones & Bartlett Learning (2011). *2011 nurse's drug handbook* (10th ed.). Sudbury, MA: Jones & Bartlett Learning.

Kalelioglu, I., Uzum, A. K., Yildirim, A., Ozkan, T., Gungor, F., & Has, R. (2007). Transient gestational diabetes insipidus diagnosed in successive pregnancies: Review of pathophysiology, diagnosis, treatment, and management of delivery. *Pituitary, 10*(1), 87–93.

Karlsen, K. (2006). *The S.T.A.B.L.E. program* (5th ed.). Park City, UT: American Academy of Pediatrics.

Karlsen, K., & Tani, L. Y. (2003). *S.T.A.B.L.E.: Cardiac module.* Park City, UT: American Academy of Pediatrics.

Kattwinkle, J. (Ed.). (2006). *Neonatal resuscitation textbook* (5th ed.). American Academy of Pediatrics & American Heart Association. Park City, UT: American Academy of Pediatrics.

Kenner, C., AmLung, S., & Flandermeyr, A. (1998). *Protocols in neonatal nursing.* Philadelphia, PA: Saunders.

Kenner, C., & Lott, J. (2004). *Neonatal nursing handbook.* St. Louis, MO: Elsevier.

Kenner, C., & Lott, J. (2007). *Comprehensive neonatal care* (4th ed.). St. Louis, MO: Elsevier.

Kenner, C., & McGrath, J. M. (Eds.). (2004). *Developmental care of newborns and infants: A guide for health professionals.* St. Louis, MO: Mosby.

Knoers, N. (2009). Inherited forms of renal hypomagnesemia: An update. *Pediatric Nephrology, 24*(4), 697–705.

Koch, R., Trefz, F., & Waisbren, S. (2010). Psychosocial issues and outcomes in maternal PKU. *Maternal Genetics and Metabolism, 99*(suppl 1), S68–S74.

Lambert, C., & Boneh, A. (2004). The impact of galactosaemia on quality of life: A pilot study. *Journal of Inherited Metabolic Disease, 27*(5), 601–608.

Leonard, J. V., & Morris, A. A. M. (2006). Diagnosis and early management of inborn errors of metabolism presenting around the time of birth. *Acta Paediatricia, 95*(1), 6–14.

Lewis, A., Courtney, C., & Atkinson, A. (2009). All patients with "idiopathic" hypopituitarism should be screened for hemochromatosis. *Pituitary, 12*(3), 273–275.

MacDonald, M. G., & Ramasethu, J. (2007). *Atlas of procedures in neonatology* (4th ed.). Philadelphia, PA: Lippincott Williams.

Mak, C., Lam, C., & Tam, S. (2008). Diagnostic accuracy of serum ceruloplasmin in Wilson disease: Determination of sensitivity and specificity by ROC curve analysis among ATP7B-genotyped subjects. *Clinical Chemistry, 54*(8), 1356–1362.

Malee, M. P. (2007). Pituitary and adrenal disorders in pregnancy. In S. G. Gabbe, J. R. Niebyl, & J. L. Simpson (Eds.), *Obstetrics: Normal and problem pregnancies* (5th ed.), (pp. 1038–1043). Philadelphia, PA: Elsevier Churchill Livingstone.

Markiewicz, M., & Abrahamson, E. (1999). *Diagnosis in color: Neonatology.* Philadelphia, PA: Mosby.

Martin, B. (2010). Family presence during resuscitation and invasive procedures: AACN practice alert. Retrieved from http://www.aacn.org

Merenstein, G. B., & Gardner, S. L. (2006). *Handbook of neonatal intensive care* (6th ed.). St. Louis, MO: Mosby.

Minniti, G., Gilbert, D., & Brada, M. (2009). Modern techniques for pituitary radiotherapy. *Reviews in Endocrine & Metabolic Disorders, 10*(2), 135–144.

Ng, P., Lee, C., Lam, C., Ma, K. C., Fok, T. F. Chan, I. H., & Wong, E. (2004, March). Transient adrenocortical insufficiency of prematurity and systemic hypotension in very low birthweight infants. *Archives of Disease in Childhood: Fetal and Neonatal Edition. 89*(2), F119–F126.

Packman, W., Henderson, S., Mehta, I., Ronen, R., Danner, D., Chesterman, B., & Packman, S. (2007). Psychosocial issues in families affected by maple syrup urine disease. *Journal of Genetic Counseling, 16*(6), 799–809.

Polin, R. A., & Spritzer, A. R. (2007). *Fetal and neonatal secrets* (2nd ed.). Philadelphia, PA: Mosby.

Poomthavorn, P., Lertbunrian, R., Preutthipan, A., Sriphrapradang, A., Khlairit, P., & Mahachoklertwattana, P. (2009). Serum free cortisol index, free cortisol, and total cortisol in critically ill children. *Intensive Care Medicine, 35*(7), 1281–1285.

Potter, S. J., Lu, A., Wilcken, B., Green, K., & Rasko, J. E. (2002). Hartnup disorder: Polymorphisms identified in the neutral amino acid transporter SLC1A5. *Journal of Inherited Metabolic Disease, 25*(6), 437–448.

Prescribing reference. (2009, Summer). *NPPR: Nurse Practitioner's Prescribing Reference, 16*(2).

Rennie, J. M., & Roberton, N. R. C. (2002). *A manual of neonatal intensive care* (4th ed.). New York: Arnold.

Sanchez, C. (2008). Mineral metabolism and bone abnormalities in children with chronic renal failure. *Reviews in Endocrine & Metabolic Disorders, 9*(2), 131–137.

Sarkar, S., Hagstrom, N. J., Ingardia, C. J., Lerer, T., & Herson, V. C. (2005). Prothrombotic risk factors in infants of diabetic mothers. *Journal of Perinatology, 25*(2), 134–138.

Sarkissian, C., Gámez, A., & Scriver, C. (2009). What we know that could influence future treatment of phenylketonuria. *Journal of Inherited Metabolic Disease, 32*(1), 3–9.

Shimshi, M., & Davies, T. F. (2010). Hypothyroidism. In R. E. Rakel & E. T. Bope (Eds.), *Conn's current therapy 2010* (pp. 672–676). Philadelphia: Saunders Elsevier.

Simon, E., Fingerhut, R., Baumkötter, J., Konstantopoulou, V., Ratschmann, R., & Wendel, U. (2006). Maple syrup urine disease: Favourable effect of early diagnosis by newborn screening on the neonatal course of the disease. *Journal of Inherited Metabolic Disease, 29*(4), 532–537.

Slota, M. C. (Ed.). (2006). *Core curriculum for pediatric critical care nursing* (2nd ed.). St. Louis, MO: Saunders.

Smeltzer, S., & Bare, B. G. (2003). *Brunner and Suddarth's textbook of medical–surgical nursing* (10th ed.). Philadelphia, PA: Lippincott Williams & Wilkins.

Spratto, G. R., & Woods, A. L. (2001). *PDR: Nurse's drug handbook.* Montvale, NJ: Delmar & Medical Economics.

Steyn, N. P., Lambert, E. V., & Tabana, H. (2009). Conference on "Multidisciplinary approaches to nutritional problems." Symposium on "Diabetes and health." Nutrition interventions for the prevention of type 2 diabetes. *Proceedings of the Nutrition Society, 68*(1), 55–70.

Summar, M. L., Dobbelaere, D., Brusilow, S., & Lee, B. (2008). Diagnosis, symptoms, frequency and mortality of 260 patients with urea cycle disorders from a 21-year, multicentre study of acute hyperammonaemic episodes. *Acta Paediatrica, 97,* 1420.

Suvarna, J., & Hajela, S. (2008). Cherry-red spot. *Journal of Postgraduate Medicine, 54*(1), 54–57.

Taeusch, H. W., Ballard, R. A., & Gleason, C. A. (2005). *Avery's diseases of the newborn* (8th ed.). Philadelphia, PA: Elsevier.

Tezer, H., Siklar, Z., Dallar, Y., & Dogankoç, S. (2009). Early and severe presentation of vitamin D deficiency and nutritional rickets among hospitalized infants and the effective factors. *Turkish Journal of Pediatrics, 51*(2), 110–115.

Trivits Verger, J., & Lebet, R. M. (Eds.). (2008). *AACN procedure manual for pediatric acute and critical care.* St. Louis, MO: Saunders.

U.S. Preventive Services Task Force. (2008). Screening for phenylketonuria (PKU): U.S. Preventive Services Task Force reaffirmation recommendation statement. *Annals of Family Medicine, 6*(2), 166.

Vandergheynst, F., & Decaux, G. (2008). Lack of elevation of urinary albumin excretion among patients with chronic syndromes of inappropriate antidiuresis. *Nephrology, Dialysis, Transplantation, 23*(7), 2399–2401.

Verklan, M. T., & Walden, M. (Eds.). (2004). *Certification and core review for neonatal intensive care nursing* (3rd ed.). St. Louis, MO: Elsevier.

Young, T. E., & Magnum, B. (2009). *Neofax 2009.* Montvale, NJ: Thomson Reuters.

Zaritzky, M., Ben, R., Zylberg, G., & Yampolsky, B. (2009). Magnetic compression anastomosis as a nonsurgical treatment for esophageal atresia. *Pediatric Radiology, 39*(9), 945–949.

SECTION 6

Hematology/Immunology

1. **The most prevalent type of anemia is known as**
   A. Chronic anemia
   B. Acute anemia
   C. Pernicious anemia
   D. Iron-deficiency anemia

2. **Acute post-hemorrhagic anemia develops after**
   A. Bone marrow is damaged
   B. The spleen is damaged
   C. Iron levels decrease by more than 15%
   D. A rapid loss of erythrocytes

3. **A decrease in the available number of erythrocytes caused by bone marrow production failure is known as**
   A. Chronic anemia
   B. Hemolytic anemia
   C. Aplastic anemia
   D. Pernicious anemia

4. **Your patient was admitted to the PICU for low H and H secondary to epistaxis, and bleeding into the diaphragm. She bleeds from the gums, even with only the lightest stimulus. Petechiae are noted on her chest and arms. Her platelet count is < 100,000. Her probable diagnosis is**
   A. ITP
   B. Pernicious anemia
   C. Aplastic anemia
   D. Hemolytic anemia

5. **High blood viscosity and low oxygen tension are the cause of which of the following types of anemia?**
   A. Pernicious anemia
   B. Aplastic anemia
   C. Sickle cell anemia
   D. Hemolytic anemia

6. **Your patient has been prescribed Epogen. As a PICU nurse, you know adverse effects of Epogen include**
   A. Decreased thrombosis
   B. Increased iron
   C. Hypertension
   D. Decreased BUN

7. **Which of the following types of cells would be considered nongranular leukocytes?**
   A. Eosinophils
   B. Neutrophils
   C. Monocytes
   D. Basophils

8. **Cellular humoral immunity is mediated by which of the following types of cells?**
   A. Eosinophils
   B. B lymphocytes
   C. T Lymphocytes
   D. Killer cells

9. **All of the clotting factors in blood are synthesized in the liver except**
   A. VIII and XII
   B. VII and IX
   C. IX and III
   D. IIa and IXa

10. **Hemoglobin is phagocytized primarily in the**
    A. Spleen
    B. Lungs
    C. Kidney
    D. Liver

11. **The synthesis of hemoglobin is regulated by**
    A. Myeloid stem cells
    B. Erythropoietin
    C. Thromboplastin
    D. Thrombopoietin

12. **There are four types of bilirubin. The type of bilirubin found in cord blood is called**
    A. Gestational bilirubin
    B. Unconjugated bilirubin
    C. Conjugated bilirubin
    D. Free bilirubin

13. **Your patient was born in a rural hospital. After a day in the hospital, mother and baby were discharged home last night. At home, the baby did not eat and cried continuously. The baby was just admitted to your PICU. The first thing you notice**

is that the baby is jaundiced and lethargic. As a PICU nurse, you know that if albumin binding sites are filled, increased amounts of free bilirubin are passed into the central nervous system and may result in

A. Cerebral hemorrhage
B. PPHN
C. Kernicterus
D. ITP

14. **One function of red blood cells is**
    A. Cell humoral mediation
    B. To function as macrophages
    C. Initiation of hemostasis
    D. Carbonic acid dissociation

15. **The physician has ordered an MCH test for your patient. This test evaluates**
    A. The average concentration of RBCs in a single sample
    B. The average amount (by weight) of hemoglobin in each RBC
    C. The average size and volume of a single RBC
    D. The average concentration of hemoglobin per single RBC

16. **Which of the following statements regarding ABO incompatibilities is true?**
    A. ABO incompatibility is more frequent in mothers with type O blood
    B. ABO incompatibility is more severe in mothers with type AB blood
    C. ABO incompatibility is more severe than Rh incompatibility
    D. ABO incompatibility does not protect against fetal Rh disease

17. **A positive result from a direct Coombs' test on an infant indicates**
    A. Antibodies are present in the maternal serum
    B. The blood type of the newborn
    C. Maternal IgG antibodies are present on the surface of the infant's red cells
    D. Antibodies against the infant's red cells are present in the mother's serum

18. **Your new patient was admitted for severe vitamin K deficiency, which is also known as hemorrhagic disease of the newborn. A factor that will negatively influence the production of vitamin K is**
    A. The presence of intracranial tumors
    B. A lack of sufficient intestinal flora
    C. Excess circulating extracellular calcium
    D. Overproduction of coagulation factors II and X

19. **Your patient has been diagnosed with DIC. Which of the following drugs is useful in the treatment of DIC to inhibit fibrinolysis?**
    A. Heparin
    B. Cryoprecipitate
    C. Prednisone
    D. Amicar

20. **Midori is 9 years old and has a history of hemolytic anemia. She was admitted today for chest pain, fever, and heart failure. These symptoms indicate Midori is probably suffering from**
    A. A hemolytic crisis
    B. Pulmonary edema
    C. DIC
    D. A myocardial infarction

21. **Immune-mediated HITT usually begins approximately _______ after the initiation of heparin therapy.**
    A. 24 hours
    B. 72 hours
    C. 3 days
    D. 5–7 days

22. **A definitive diagnosis of immune thrombocytopenic purpura may be made by**
    A. Platelet antibody screen
    B. Thrombin time
    C. PTT
    D. Prothrombin time

23. **Your patient has immune thrombocytopenic purpura that has worsened and become refractory to treatments, including plasmapheresis and injections of gamma globulin. Glucocorticoid therapy has also not been successful. The patient will be undergoing a splenectomy. One of the preoperative treatments to expect is**
    A. Interferon
    B. Anti-Rh immunoglobulin
    C. *Haemophilus influenzae* type B vaccination
    D. Colchicine

24. **Your patient requires an exchange transfusion. A major side effect of an exchange transfusion is**
    A. ABO incompatibility
    B. Necrotizing enterocolitis
    C. Urticaria
    D. Hematoma

25. **The Kleihauer-Betke test identifies**
    A. Sickle cell trait in utero
    B. Common blood group antigens
    C. Bone marrow lymphocyte precursors
    D. Fetal hemoglobin in maternal blood

26. **Your patient's mother carries the sickle cell trait. Which statement about sickle cell anemia is true?**
    A. Sickle cell anemia always results in death by age 40
    B. Sickle cell anemia causes a loss of protein intrinsic factor
    C. High blood viscosity and low oxygen tension may cause a sickle cell crisis
    D. Sickle cell disease is limited to the African American and Caucasian populations

27. A partial thromboplastin time (PTT) is used to assess

A. Intrinsic and common portions of the coagulation cascade
B. The number of fibrin degradation products present
C. The number of platelets
D. Increased use of clotting factors

28. Cheryl is 14 years old and plans to breastfeed her newborn. A mother's breastmilk contains the immunoglobulin known as

A. IgG
B. IgA
C. IgM
D. IgE

29. The major immunoglobulin found in serum and interstitial fluid is

A. IgG
B. IgA
C. IgE
D. IgM

30. Which of the following statements about human breastmilk is true?

A. Human breastmilk contains insoluble proteins
B. Human breastmilk is always the best choice for an infant
C. Human breastmilk is high in cytokines
D. Human breastmilk provides absolute protection against bronchopulmonary dysplasia

31. The extrinsic system of the coagulation cascade is initiated by

A. Exposure to cell membrane tissue factor
B. Vascular endothelial injury
C. Irritation of the intimal lining of blood vessels
D. Factor X activation

32. Which of the following tests is used to assess the extrinsic and common pathways of the coagulation cascade?

A. Split fibrin product
B. Prothrombin time
C. Partial thromboplastin time
D. Activated clotting time

33. Rhesus (Rh) hemolytic disease of the newborn is a severe, often fatal disease caused by

A. An Rh-negative mother alloimmunized during her first Rh-incompatible pregnancy
B. An Rh-positive mother with an Rh-negative fetus
C. An allergy to rhesus serum
D. The inability of IgG Rh antibodies to cross the placenta

34. If a teenage mother received an incompatible transfusion of Rh-positive platelets following a placental rupture, it would be appropriate to administer

A. Neostigmine
B. FFP
C. RhoGAM
D. CuroSurf

35. **A transfusion reaction that usually occurs within 5 to 30 minutes of the start of the transfusion is known as**
    A. An allergic reaction
    B. A febrile reaction
    C. An acute intravascular hemolytic reaction
    D. An acute extravascular hemolytic reaction

36. **Pernicious anemia results from a lack of**
    A. Vitamin B_6
    B. Vitamin A
    C. Vitamin B_{12}
    D. Vitamin E

37. **A pharmacologic antagonist to vitamin K is**
    A. Neostigmine
    B. Digoxin
    C. Amiodarone
    D. Phenobarbital

38. **Cyclosporine has significant adverse effects that include**
    A. Hepatotoxicity
    B. Hypertension
    C. Acute pancreatitis
    D. Hypokalemia

39. **Colin is 1 year old and was admitted to the PICU for respiratory difficulty. He has become increasingly restless and now has petechiae on his trunk, arms, and legs. His abdomen is slightly distended, and he is demonstrating increased respiratory effort. Colin is now obtunded. During your assessment, you note pink-tinged urine in the diaper, generalized ecchymosis, and oozing from the IV line insertion point. You suspect Colin may have**
    A. DIC
    B. Pulmonary emboli
    C. A fat embolism
    D. Meningitis

40. **Which of the following is an antirejection drug that is classified as an anti-metabolite?**
    A. Cyclosporine
    B. Terralimus
    C. Prednisolone
    D. Imuran

41. **Jane is 15 years old and was admitted for a liver transplant. A thorough history was obtained by the transplant coordinator prior to her admission to the PICU. Patients can become presensitized and are more likely to experience organ rejection if they have a history of**
    A. Multiple pregnancies
    B. Small or reduced lumens in the bile ducts

C. Destruction of small airways
D. Cytomegalovirus (CMV) infections

42. An absolute contraindication for a single-lung, double-lung, or heart–lung transplant is
A. Liver disease
B. Psychiatric illness
C. Previous cardiothoracic surgery
D. Kidney disease

43. Factor VIII deficiency is also known as
A. Hemophilia B
B. Sickle cell anemia
C. Von Willebrand's disease
D. Aplastic anemia

44. The blood component that contains factor VIII is
A. FFP
B. PRBCs
C. Salt-poor albumin
D. Cryoprecipitate

45. A fluid that causes decreased platelet aggregation and possible allergic reactions is
A. Hetastarch
B. Dextran
C. Lactated Ringer's
D. D_5/Isolyte M

46. Your patient is to receive two units of packed cells over the next 16 hours. When patients receive multiple transfusions, they are susceptible to increased
A. Bilirubin and amylase levels
B. BUN and creatinine levels
C. Serum potassium levels
D. Sodium and magnesium retention

47. Your patient has been diagnosed with immune thrombocytopenic purpura (ITP). Which of the following laboratory values would be expected for this patient?
A. Elevated PT and PTT
B. Capillary fragility test of 0.5
C. Platelet count of 11,000
D. Positive anti-RH immunosuppression

48. Your patient has been diagnosed with hemolytic anemia. She has been in the PICU for three days. You believe her condition was caused by
A. An inappropriate TPN solution
B. Reduced folate deficiency
C. Bone marrow aspiration
D. Intra-aortic balloon pump (IABP) counterpulsation

49. A medication that may cause hemolytic anemia is

A. Phenobarbital
B. Furosemide
C. Quinidine
D. Captopril

50. Your patient was admitted with a factor VIII deficiency. In addition to specific factor VIII, the blood component that carries factor VIII, factor XIII, and fibrinogen is

A. FFP
B. PRBC
C. Salt-poor albumin
D. Cryoprecipitate

51. In the pediatric critical care setting, patients with DIC are at a high risk of developing

A. Deficiencies in vitamin K and folate
B. Increased fibrinogen levels
C. A decreased D-dimer (less than 300)
D. Dependency on heparin to maintain hemostasis

52. Possible causes of thrombocytopenia in pediatric critical care patients could include

A. Alcoholism
B. Portal hypertension
C. Latex sensitivity
D. A low-protein diet

53. Nursing interventions by the pediatric critical care nurse should include which of the following to minimize risk to a patient with HIT?

A. Avoid the use of heparin flushes
B. Assess the need for manual blood pressure measurements
C. Monitor platelet counts
D. Observe for petechiae

54. Patients with type II HIT are at high risk for developing

A. Generalized bleeding
B. Pericarditis
C. Thrombosis
D. Limb amputation

55. Ian is a 13 year old who was thrown from the back of a truck onto a road; he suffered abdominal trauma with a splenic rupture and a fractured right humerus. While awaiting surgery in the PICU because the operating rooms were full, Ian received six units of PRBCs. As a PICU nurse, you know that Ian should also receive

A. FFP
B. Platelets
C. Whole blood
D. Heparin

56. **Keith is a 7 year old patient who was evenomated by a rattlesnake on the right lower leg this morning while crawling under a neighbor's porch. His entire right lower leg is ecchymotic. The best course of treatment would be**
   A. Clotting factors and antivenin
   B. Clotting factors and heparin
   C. IV at 100 mL/hr and antivenin
   D. IV at 100 mL/hr and heparin

57. **A snake bite will result in activation of which of the following responses to physiological insult to the body?**
   A. Fibrinolytic system
   B. Antithrombin system
   C. Intrinsic cascade
   D. Extrinsic cascade

58. **Following heart–lung transplants, prostaglandin (PGE_1) is used to**
   A. Promote wound healing
   B. Provide inotropic support
   C. Promote pulmonary vasodilation
   D. Augment the heart rate

59. **Rowena had a renal transplant approximately one year ago. She was admitted to your unit for severe flu-like symptoms. Which sign or symptom would lead you to suspect that Rowena is having an acute rejection episode?**
   A. Hypotension
   B. Pelvic pain
   C. Increased urine output
   D. Decreased urine osmolality

60. **Organ rejection that occurs 3–5 days post transplant, is antibody mediated, and is accompanied by fever and oliguria is known as**
   A. Chronic rejection
   B. Acute rejection
   C. Accelerated acute rejection
   D. Hyperacute rejection

61. **Rejection of a transplanted organ usually occurs as a result of**
   A. Cellular immunity
   B. Humoral immunity
   C. Delayed hypersensitivity reaction
   D. Complement cascade

62. **What is the most common cause of a fatal transfusion reaction?**
   A. Immunocompromised recipient
   B. Volume overload
   C. Mismatched blood
   D. Severe hyperkalemia

63. **Which antirejection agent is used for induction therapy for lung transplants and lowers the number of circulating T cells?**
    A. Daclizumab
    B. Muromonab
    C. Polyclonal antibody
    D. Paroxetine

64. **The activated coagulation time (ACT) is more sensitive to ______ and _______ than whole blood clotting time.**
    A. Oxygenation, hemofiltration
    B. Factor VIII, heparin
    C. Warfarin, leukemia
    D. Liver disease, calcium

65. **Your patient had a previous transplant two years ago. She is now experiencing severe back pain. Back pain or abdominal pain with itching can be indicators of acute rejection in which organ?**
    A. Pancreas
    B. Lung
    C. Liver
    D. Kidney

66. **Tamika was stung by a bee and had an anaphylactic reaction. She has received epinephrine both via Epi-Pen and intravenously. Tamika is now intubated because she had severe airway obstruction due to swelling. Epinephrine is given for anaphylactic reactions because**
    A. It prevents localized edema
    B. It promotes temporary changes in ST segments
    C. It prevents third space fluid loss
    D. It promotes bronchodilation and inhibits additional mediator release

67. **Why is DIC usually fatal if left untreated?**
    A. Exsanguination
    B. Intracranial hemorrhage
    C. Myocardial infarction
    D. Cerebral thrombosis

68. **Ginger has been diagnosed with an oat-cell carcinoma. Oat-cell carcinomas are primarily found in**
    A. The central airways
    B. The genital area
    C. The bronchial wall
    D. The pancreas

69. **Which of the following lab tests would support a diagnosis of acute liver failure?**
    A. Decreased creatinine and BUN
    B. Increased serum glucose
    C. Negative hepatitis serology
    D. Factors V and VII levels less than or equal to 20% of normal levels

70. Mike has been treated in your unit for an exacerbation of his thalassemia. Patient and family teaching for a patient with thalassemia would include

A. Keeping the limbs flat to avoid a stasis ulcer
B. Avoiding oral stimulants (e.g., caffeine)
C. Eating fewer, larger, high-protein meals
D. Using warm water to cleanse the skin

71. How does low-molecular-weight heparin (LMWH) differ from unfractionated heparin?

A. LMWH is more difficult to administer
B. LMWH has more side effects
C. LMWH is more stable
D. Unfractionated heparin is easier to administer

72. Clopidogrel may interfere with the metabolism of which of the following drugs?

A. Phenobarbital
B. Phenytoin
C. Cimetidine
D. Estrogen

73. Kim was admitted to your unit for anemia due to chronic renal failure. She is receiving Epogen. Adverse effects of Epogen include

A. Hypertension
B. Increased iron
C. Decreased thrombosis
D. Decreased BUN

74. Scott is a 16 year old who has not been eating correctly for about two weeks because he is stressed out about asking a girl to their junior prom. He eats a diet of toaster pastries, pastas, and high-calorie, high-sugar foods. Scott collapsed at home today after becoming dyspneic. His EKG shows sinus tachycardia without ectopy. He is pale, somewhat irritable, and complains of a headache. His initial diagnosis is folic acid deficiency. Tomorrow Scott is scheduled for more tests to determine if there is an underlying disease process. You suspect that he simply has a dietary deficiency and prepare to instruct him about foods that contain high amounts of folic acid. These foods would include

A. Green beans
B. Peanut butter
C. Oranges
D. Fish

75. Blood component replacement therapy for DIC may include all of the following except

A. FFP
B. Cryoprecipitate
C. Amicar
D. Platelets

76. Quinn is an 8 year old admitted to the PICU with chest pain and respiratory distress. He weighs approximately 60 pounds. During your assessment, you note that he is short of breath and has a dry cough. On Quinn's chest, you find irregularly shaped lumps near the left infraclavicular border. Which of the following questions should you ask Quinn and his mother?

A. "Have you suddenly gained weight in the last two months?"
B. "Have you noticed skin patches that are itchy and with a green cast?"
C. "Have you noticed any stomach pain or swelling?"
D. "Has your appetite increased over the last few months?"

77. Mabel is a 16 year old diagnosed with Hodgkin's lymphoma. Which of the following techniques is important to teach her about skin care?

A. Use an alcohol-based cleaner to treat acne
B. Use a moisturizer containing lidocaine
C. Use ice packs directly on the skin to decrease swelling
D. Scrub daily with a pumice-based soap

78. Hodgkin's lymphoma is primarily associated with which pediatric age range?

A. 0–5 years old
B. 3–8 years old
C. 8–15 years old
D. > 15 years old

79. Non-Hodgkin's lymphomas (NHL) account for what percentage of the total lymphoma cases in the pediatric population?

A. 20%
B. 40%
C. 60%
D. 80%

80. Garrett is a 3 year old with chronic myelogenous leukemia (CML). Which of the following lab results would you expect to see with this disease?

A. A platelet count of 600,000
B. WBC of 4.2
C. Chromosome studies with abnormal chromosomes 10 and 20
D. An absence of blast cells

81. Which of the following is the most common form of leukemia in children?

A. Acute lymphoblastic leukemia
B. Acute myelogenous leukemia
C. Acute nonlymphoid leukemia
D. Chronic myelogenous leukemia

82. Whitney is a 10 year old diagnosed with acute lymphoblastic leukemia. During your assessment, you note that she is confused, hypotonic, and starts having generalized seizures. You would anticipate receiving orders for which of the following tests?

A. A spinal tap
B. CT scan
C. MRI
D. PET scan

83. Terrell is receiving mechlorethamine intravenously to treat his chronic myelogenous leukemia. He complains of a slight burning sensation 10 minutes after the infusion begins. What should you do?

A. This is normal, so no action is required

B. Raise the arm and place warm compresses on the infusion site

C. Continue the infusion while you start a second IV line

D. Stop the infusion immediately and establish a second IV site

84. Asayo is a 7 year old being admitted for chemotherapy. When discussing Asayo's nutritional needs with her parents, which of the following statements is correct?

A. The parents and staff should be strict regarding intake and pressure Asayo to eat

B. Include Asayo in the process of making food choices and bring her favorite foods from home

C. Promise a special toy if Asayo will eat two large meals a day

D. When she is hungry, allow Asayo to eat as much as she wants

85. Jacob is a 12 year old with non-Hodgkin's lymphoma. Which action is important to include daily in Jacob's care?

A. Schedule family time whenever possible

B. Avoid telling Jacob of upcoming diagnostic procedures until just before the testing

C. Post a daily schedule of tests, nursing care times, and medications

D. Limit visitors to those who are more than 14 years old and allow them to come only once a week

86. Which of the following statements is true about hepatitis D?

A. Hepatitis D is detectable only when the patient has concurrent HBV infection

B. IgM rises late in the course of infection

C. IgG rises slowly and the increase is limited to the acute phase of infection

D. Hepatitis D is an RNA virus that is able to self-replicate when it is present concurrently with HBV

SECTION 6

Hematology Answers

1. **Correct answer: D**
   Iron-deficiency anemia is the most frequently occurring anemia seen around the world. It can be caused by either consumption of an iron-poor diet or an excessive loss of iron. Trauma is a primary cause of acute loss, with the anemia then resulting from bleeding. Blood donations, menses, GI bleeding, malabsorption syndromes, pica, and excessive diarrhea are all potential causes of this type of anemia. If you could view the erythrocytes under a microscope, they look kind of "puny": They are pale from lack of hemoglobin and tend to be smaller than normal red blood cells.

2. **Correct answer: D**
   Acute posthemorrhagic anemia may be the result of hemorrhage, cancerous lesion, an ulcerative lesion that erodes an arterial wall, trauma to a major vessel, or rupture of an aneurysm. After hemorrhage, plasma is lost and vasoconstriction takes place. The concentration of erythrocytes is increased because the volume is low. In other words, the same number of cells are not diluted in the usual amount of fluid, so the count is artificially high. It can take approximately six weeks for hemoglobin levels to return to normal.

3. **Correct answer: C**
   A decrease in the available number of erythrocytes caused by bone marrow production failure is known as aplastic anemia. Approximately 50% of all cases of aplastic anemia are caused by toxins; the other 50% have an unknown cause. Among the known causes are radiation (e.g., X-rays, radioactive isotopes, radium), benzene, streptomycin, carbon tetrachloride, DDT, chloramphenicol, and sulfonamides. In addition, many types of pesticides other than DDT are thought to contribute to aplastic anemia.

4. **Correct answer: A**
   Idiopathic thrombocytopenia purpura (ITP) is the result of a low platelet count. Sometimes platelets are destroyed early and systematically. The cause of ITP is thought to be an autoimmune response. Hemorrhages may occur in the brain, which may then lead to stroke and an increased intracranial pressure.

5. **Correct answer: C**
   Sickle cell anemia occurs primarily in the African American population. Affected individuals are homozygous for HgS and have more HgS than HgA. As a consequence, some of the cells develop a "sickle" shape—curved with rough edges. It is postulated that a crisis occurs when the low oxygen tension causes a proliferation of these abnormal cells. When these cells travel through the microcirculation, their sharp edges damage capillaries. A simple condition like cold weather can precipitate massive sickling.

Other identified risk factors include dehydration, vomiting, diarrhea, high altitude, excessive exercise, and stress. When the sickled cells break apart, they occlude the microcirculation and lower oxygen tension, which initiates more sickling. Sickle cell crisis is a very painful time for the patient, and oxygen, pain management, and fluids are very important components of treatment.

6. **Correct answer:** C
   Epogen and Procrit are both forms of recombinant erythropoietin; they are used to correct the anemia that can occur with chronic renal failure. Adverse effects include clotting at the site of vascular access, depletion of iron, and potential increases in potassium, creatinine, and BUN.

7. **Correct answer:** C
   A monocyte would be considered a nongranular leukocyte. Both monocytes and lymphocytes are classified as agranulocytes. Monocytes are the largest leukocytes, but account for only a small portion of the total cell count for WBCs. When the monocytes mature, they become tissue macrophages and work as phagocytes. When a phagocyte lives in the liver, it is called a Kupffer cell. When it is in the lungs, it is called an alveolar macrophage. When it is found in connective tissues, it is a histiocyte.

   Macrophages contain lysosomal enzymes and chemicals that can destroy bacteria. If a macrophage is activated by an antigen, it will secrete monokines, which control communication between all the cells involved in the immune response.

8. **Correct answer:** B
   Cellular humoral immunity is mediated by B lymphocytes. B lymphocytes originate and mature in the bone marrow. They form antibodies (immunoglobulins) that regulate a response to a specific antigen that has bound itself to the B cell's receptor sites. The B cell then forms a specific antibody for that particular antigen. Five different types of immunoglobulins exist: IgG, IgA, IgM, IgE, and IgD. After the antibodies are synthesized, the specific antibody can attach itself to its antigen and trigger the reaction that allows for phagocytosis. These cells retain a "memory" for the specific antigen; thus, if another exposure occurs, the response will be quicker and stronger than the original response.

9. **Correct answer:** A
   All factors except VIII and XII are synthesized in the liver, which explains why liver injuries can bleed so much and are so dangerous. (As an aside, while we were researching and confirming the answer to this question, we found out that the factors in the clotting cascades were numbered by order of discovery, not order of use.) Just FYI!

10. **Correct answer:** D
    Hemoglobin is phagocytized primarily in the liver. Hemoglobin consists of two parts. The first part, known as "heme," causes the reddish color and contains iron and porphyrin. The second part, a protein called "globin," combines with oxygen to form oxyhemoglobin. Hemoglobin also binds with CO_2 and carries it to alveoli to be expired. When the hemoglobin is phagocytized, it breaks down into the heme and globin components. The iron in the hemoglobin is processed and reused to manufacture new hemoglobin. The porphyrin is converted to bilirubin and is excreted in urine and feces.

11. **Correct answer: B**
Erythropoietin is a hormone responsible for the synthesis of hemoglobin. Erythropoietin levels increase in response to anemia and low oxygen states, and levels decrease in response to hypertransfusion. Levels are also increased in infants with Down syndrome and intrauterine growth restriction. Erythropoietin levels may also be elevated in infants born to mothers with pregnancy-induced hypertension or diabetes.

12. **Correct answer: B**
The type of bilirubin found in cord blood is called unconjugated bilirubin. All cord blood found in a fetus is unconjugated; it is eventually metabolized, conjugated, and excreted by the maternal gallbladder and liver. If an infant is unaffected by hemolytic disease, the mean cord blood bilirubin concentration is 1.8 mg/dL. This value is independent from and unaffected by the infant's gestational age or weight.

13. **Correct answer: C**
If albumin binding sites are filled, increased amounts of free bilirubin pass into the central nervous system and may result in kernicterus. Free bilirubin crosses the blood–brain barrier and lodges in the brain cells. The patient is usually affected in the first five days of life. Symptoms include lethargy, irritability, hypotonia, a high-pitched cry, and poor eating. The infant may also demonstrate spasticity and opisthotonic posturing. If bilirubin levels rise slowly, phototherapy might be able to reduce the bilirubin level and prevent kernicterus. If the bilirubin level rises quickly, exchange transfusion may be required.

14. **Correct answer: D**
A red blood cell has multiple functions, including carbonic acid dissociation to form bicarbonate ions. The RBC provides oxygen transport via hemoglobin and carbon dioxide transport via carboxyhemoglobin. It buffers protons by binding with hemoglobin to form acid hemoglobin.

15. **Correct answer: B**
A mean corpuscular hemoglobin (MCH) test measures the average amount (by weight) of hemoglobin in each RBC. A mean corpuscular hemoglobin concentration (MCHC) test measures the average concentration of hemoglobin per single RBC. A mean corpuscular volume (MCV) test measures the average size and volume of a single RBC.

16. **Correct answer: A**
ABO incompatibility is most often seen in mothers with type O blood, which has an absence of antigens. If the mother is exposed to A and B antigens from the fetus, an ABO incompatibility will result. The mother can also be exposed to A and B antigens carried in food, bacteria, and pollen. This can make the first pregnancy perilous. ABO incompatibility is less severe than Rh incompatibility and occurs more frequently. ABO incompatibility protects the fetus from Rh disease through rapid destruction of A and B cells. This rapid destruction prevents Rh antigen exposure and resultant maternal antibody production.

17. **Correct answer: C**
A positive result from a direct Coombs' test indicates the presence of maternal IgG antibodies on the surface of the infant's red blood cells. Cord blood that is contaminated by Wharton's jelly may produce unreliable results. Cold agglutinins may cause

false-positive results. Heparin sodium and heparin calcium may cause false-negative results. Many diseases and drugs (e.g., quinidine, methyldopa, procainamide) can lead to production of these antibodies.

A positive indirect Coombs' test indicates that antibodies against the infant's red cells are present in the mother's serum.

18. **Correct answer: B**
A more appropriate term for hemorrhagic disease of the newborn is vitamin K deficiency bleeding (VKDB) disease. Vitamin K production depends on sufficient intestinal flora. Vitamin K is necessary for the production of calcium and various coagulation factors.

Newborns are relatively deficient in vitamin K. Contributing factors to this deficiency include low vitamin K stores at birth, poor placental transfer of vitamin K, low levels of vitamin K in breastmilk, and sterility of the gut. The basic commercial infant formulas contain supplemental vitamin K, so VKDB is almost exclusively a condition found in breastfed infants. Infants with inadequate intake are at higher risk.

The most common sites of bleeding are the umbilicus, mucous membranes, GI tract (melena), circumcision, and venipuncture sites. The infant may also present with a distended abdomen, jaundice, and signs of increased intracranial pressure. Hematomas, such as large cephalohematomas, along with bruising, are also common findings. Intracranial hemorrhage (ICH) is responsible for nearly all deaths from VKDB.

19. **Correct answer: D**
Aminocaproic acid (Amicar) interferes with plasmin and inhibits fibrinolysis. Synthetic antithrombin III inhibits thrombin and can be very useful in treating DIC.

20. **Correct answer: A**
Patients who have hemolytic anemia may remain healthy until they are exposed to a major stressor such as infection, trauma, or surgery. A psychological stressor such as divorce of the child's parents or a change in school may also initiate a crisis. The patient may be overwhelmed, allowing hemolysis to accelerate and may cause tissue hypoxia and ischemia and progress to necrosis and infarction. Treatment is supportive and targeted to the presenting symptoms.

21. **Correct answer: D**
Immune-mediated HITT usually begins five to seven days after the initiation of heparin therapy. If a severe reaction develops, the patient will have chest pain due to cardiac ischemia, neurologic impairment, and LOC changes and paresthesias due to cerebral ischemia. The patient may develop pulmonary emboli, dyspnea, extremity pain, and pallor due to thrombosis; arterial thrombosis is also possible.

22. **Correct answer: A**
A definitive diagnosis of immune thrombocytopenic purpura may be made by a platelet antibody screen. The PT, PTT, and thrombin time are normal with ITP, because these tests measure only nonplatelet factors in the coagulation cascade. The platelet antibody screen measures the presence of IgG and IgM antiplatelet antibodies.

23. **Correct answer: C**
Preoperative treatment would include a *Haemophilus influenzae* type B vaccination. Interferon is not applicable. Anti-Rh immunoglobulin and colchicine are treatments for ITP that will have probably been tried prior to the decision to perform a splenec-

tomy. The patient should also be vaccinated for pneumococcal and meningococcal organisms to lower the risk of postoperative infection.

24. **Correct answer: B**
Serious side effects of exchange transfusions include necrotizing enterocolitis, air embolism, volume and pressure changes, thromboembolism, bradycardia, and bacterial contamination. Hypothermia, volume overload, transfusion-mediated lung injury, and death are additional serious side effects of exchange transfusions.

25. **Correct answer: D**
The Kleihauer-Betke test identifies fetal hemoglobin in maternal blood. The results of this test allow for calculations to determine the amount of fetal–maternal hemorrhage and the amount of immune globulin (RhoGAM) necessary to prevent sensitization. If a patient has a positive test, follow-up testing at a postpartum check-up should be done to rule out the possibility of a false-positive result. For example, a false-positive result in the mother could be caused by sickle cell trait, which causes persistent elevation of fetal hemoglobin.

26. **Correct answer: C**
Sickle cell crisis is thought to occur when low oxygen tension causes a proliferation of the sickled cells.

27. **Correct answer: A**
A partial thromboplastin time (PTT) is used to assess intrinsic and common portions of the coagulation cascade. Its results may be affected by an absence of clotting factors, anticoagulants, low levels of clotting factors, inhibitors, and increased use of clotting factors.

28. **Correct answer: B**
A mother's breastmilk contains the immunoglobulin known as immunoglobulin A (IgA). This immunoglobulin is also secreted in human colostrum. IgA, which does not cross the placental barrier, is the most common immunoglobulin in the gastrointestinal and respiratory tracts.

    During pregnancy and lactation, because of hormonal stimuli, IgA B lymphocytes colonize mammary glands and produce a specific secretory IgA that may bind to pathogens, thereby preventing infection. The antimicrobial effects of IgA antibodies are thought to be related to immune exclusion, interference, or an inhibited ability to adhere to the epithelial cell wall, all of which help provide protection to the neonate. Agglutination, neutralization, and immune elimination by phagocytosis and cytotoxicity may also enhance the antimicrobial effects. HIV-infected mothers do not demonstrate the same type of protection, so IgA antibodies may enhance transmission of HIV infection.

29. **Correct answer: A**
The major immunoglobulin in serum and interstitial fluid is immunoglobulin G (IgG), which provides immunity against viral and bacterial pathogens. IgG is transferred to the fetus either actively or passively, and its level increases somewhat gradually until 40 weeks of gestation. In postmature infants, the levels of IgG are decreased, just as they are in premature infants. However, in the preterm infant, the level is proportionate to the gestational age.

30. **Correct answer: C**
Human breastmilk is high in cytokines. Cytokines are soluble proteins that stimulate the chemotaxis of neutrophils and assist in epithelial cell propagation. Of all the factors associated with immunity—immunological, hormonal, and enzymatic—cytokines are believed to play a significant role in the immune modulation and immune protection afforded by breastmilk. Most of the cytokines that are known to be deficient in the neonate, particularly in preterm infants, have been found in significant amounts in breastmilk.

31. **Correct answer: A**
Activation of the extrinsic system of the coagulation cascade is initiated by exposure of cell membrane tissue factor from tissue injury. Activation of the intrinsic system is initiated by vascular endothelial injury.

32. **Correct answer: B**
The prothrombin time (PT) is used to assess the extrinsic and common pathways of the coagulation cascade. The partial thromboplastin time (PTT) is used to assess the intrinsic and common pathways of the coagulation cascade.

33. **Correct answer: A**
Rhesus (Rh) hemolytic disease of the newborn (HDN) is a severe, often fatal disease caused by incompatibility between an Rh-negative mother and her Rh-positive fetus. The mother becomes alloimmunized to the D antigen present on fetal red blood cells (RBCs) during the first Rh-incompatible pregnancy. The first pregnancy is rarely affected because the number of Rh antibodies produced by the mother is low and the antibodies usually consist of IgM. When the mother is exposed to D-positive fetal RBCs during a subsequent Rh-incompatible pregnancy, the mother develops a secondary immune response. At this point, a large number of IgG Rh antibodies are produced that cross the placenta and make fetal red cells susceptible to attack by antibodies. The mother may also become alloimmunized as a result of fetal–maternal hemorrhage, bleeding that occurs during normal delivery, ectopic pregnancies, spontaneous or induced abortions, and abdominal trauma.

34. **Correct answer: C**
If the mother received an incompatible transfusion of Rh-positive platelets following a placental rupture, it would be appropriate to administer RhoGAM. This medication may be used for prevention of Rh immunization in any Rh-negative person after transfusion of Rh-positive blood or blood products such as platelets or red blood cells.

35. **Correct answer: C**
An intravascular hemolytic reaction is a transfusion reaction that usually occurs within 5–30 minutes of the start of the transfusion. The patient may experience chills, fever, tachycardia, hypotension, hematuria, back pain, and may exhibit additional signs of shock. The extravascular hemolytic reaction may manifest as fever, low H and H even after transfusion, and elevated bilirubin.

36. **Correct answer: C**
Pernicious anemia results from a lack of vitamin B_{12}. This disease results from lack of a protein intrinsic factor in the stomach that normally helps the body absorb vitamin B_{12}. This stress on the heart from the resultant hypoxia can cause heart murmurs, tachycardias, arrhythmias, hypertrophy, and heart failure. A lack of vitamin B_{12} raises

the homocysteine level; these high levels of homocysteine, in turn, add to the buildup of fatty deposits. A lack of vitamin B_{12} can damage nerve cells and cause problems such as paresthesias in the hands and feet and problems with ambulation and balance. Memory loss, visual disturbances, and confusion may develop. This type of anemia was termed "pernicious" because it was often fatal before the cause was discovered to be a lack of vitamin B_{12}.

37. **Correct answer: D**
Pharmacologic antagonists to vitamin K include phenobarbital and hydantoin (anticonvulsants) and heparin and warfarin (anticoagulants). These drugs induce hepatic enzymes and increase vitamin K degradation. Vitamin K transport across the placenta is inhibited, and vitamin K–dependent clotting factors are depressed.

38. **Correct answer: B**
Cyclosporine is associated with significant adverse effects, including nephrotoxicity, hypertension, hyperkalemia, leg cramps, headache, seizures, and development of neoplasms.

39. **Correct answer: A**
Colin probably has DIC. Disseminated intravascular coagulation is an overstimulation of the clotting cascade. Both the intrinsic and extrinsic pathways are activated at the same time, which accelerates the clotting process. When the clots lyse, the fibrin split products are anticoagulants. Eventually, all of the clotting factors are used up, and no further clots can form. Neonates are at increased risk for DIC secondary to inappropriate levels of anticoagulants and fibrinolytics, along with decreased levels of antithrombin and protein. One treatment for DIC is antithrombin III, which sometimes attenuates organ failure and reverse coagulopathy.

40. **Correct answer: D**
Imuran is an antirejection drug that is classified as an antimetabolite. Antimetabolites interfere with RNA and DNA synthesis and inhibit T- and B-lymphocyte proliferation.

41. **Correct answer: A**
Patients can be presensitized and are more likely to develop organ rejection if they have a history of multiple pregnancies. It is becoming more common in some areas for teenagers to have had multiple pregnancies by age 15. Other possible causes of organ rejection include transfusions, previous organ transplants, and blood type incompatibilities. Small lumens in the bile ducts, destruction of small airways, and CMV infections are the results of organ rejection, not causes.

42. **Correct answer: B**
An absolute contraindication for a single-lung, double-lung, or heart–lung transplant is psychiatric illness. Patients with a history of psychiatric illness may be unable to comprehend or follow through with a complicated postoperative medication regimen.

43. **Correct answer: C**
Factor VIII deficiency is also known as von Willebrand's disease. Hemophilia A and B are factor IX deficiencies.

44. **Correct answer: D**
The blood component that contains factor VIII is cryoprecipitate (which means "quick frozen"). Cryoprecipitate does have some disadvantages—notably, its high cost. Use of

cryoprecipitate is also associated with a risk of transmission of hepatitis A, hepatitis C, hepatitis G, and HIV. Several newer recombinant factor VIII products are available that avoid these problems.

45. **Correct answer: B**
Dextran is a fluid that causes decreased platelet aggregation and possible allergic reactions. Sometimes Dextran causes acute tubular necrosis because it is made of polymers consisting of high-molecular-weight polysaccharides.

46. **Correct answer: C**
When patients receive multiple transfusions, they are susceptible to increased serum potassium levels. When blood is transfused, sometimes the cells lyse and the intracellular potassium is released. This outcome can also occur when the cells strike the floating ball in the infusion chamber. It is sound practice to monitor the patient's electrolytes after each two units of blood given. In addition, the patient should be monitored for dysrhythmias.

47. **Correct answer: C**
ITP usually occurs after a viral infection. The first symptom may be purpura and petechiae on the distal extremities. The PT and PTT results are normal because they test for nonplatelet parts of the coagulation pathway. The result of the capillary fragility test will be greater than 1. Anti-RH immunoglobulin is a treatment for the disease. Continually monitor the patient for signs and symptoms of intracranial hemorrhage.

48. **Correct answer: D**
Usually at about the third day following admission, PICU patients tend to develop anemia. The IABP could cause cells to lyse, as could prosthetic heart valves, heart–lung bypass, and bacterial endotoxins. A reduced folate level would lead to megaloblastic anemia. Bone marrow aspiration is a diagnostic procedure. TPN solutions do not produce anemia.

49. **Correct answer: C**
Quinidine is a medication that may cause hemolytic anemia; procainamide and acetaminophen are other medications that may have this effect. Phenobarbital may cause aplastic anemia, whereas furosemide may cause a generalized anemia. Captopril causes pancytopenia.

50. **Correct answer: D**
Cryoprecipitate carries factor VIII, factor XIII, and fibrinogen. There is a risk of disease transmission and transfusion reactions with its use.

51. **Correct answer: A**
In the pediatric critical care setting, patients with DIC are at a high risk of developing deficiencies in vitamin K and folate. DIC often leads to nutritional deficits.

52. **Correct answer: B**
Possible causes of thrombocytopenia in pediatric critical care areas include portal hypertension, as well as sepsis, viral infection, burns, and radiation therapy. Medications such as thiazides, furosemide, penicillins, sulfonamides, ranitidine, and heparin may also cause thrombocytopenia. Chemotherapy is another cause.

53. **Correct answer: A**
HIT is heparin-induced thrombocytopenia, so it is best to eliminate the use of heparin in this case.

54. **Correct answer: B**
Patients with type II HIT are at great risk for developing pericarditis. Type II HIT is sometimes called "white clot syndrome." With this condition, thrombi are primarily venous in origin, and their formation can lead to DVT, pulmonary emboli, thrombotic stroke, limb ischemia, and myocardial infarction.

55. **Correct answer: B**
Ian should also receive platelet infusions. PRBCs contain no platelets, and platelets must be given to promote hemostasis.

56. **Correct answer: A**
Rattlesnakes evenomate their bite victims with an enzyme called hyaluronidase, which breaks down the hyaluronic acid barriers on cells. The cells lyse, and the resulting exudative products enter the bloodstream. Treatment of snake bite patients is very similar to that for patients with DIC, because fibrin split products (anticoagulants) are released in both instances. The patient may require multiple vials of antivenin and clotting factors to counteract this cascade of events.

57. **Correct answer: D**
Damage to the tissues and vessels as a result of a snake bite initiates the extrinsic cascade. Thromboplastin and factor VII are released and will be activated in the presence of calcium.

58. **Correct answer: C**
Following heart–lung transplants, prostaglandin (PGE_1) is given to promote pulmonary vasodilation. Prostaglandin relaxes the smooth muscles within the pulmonary airways and promotes vasodilation within the arteries. Inotropic support is usually accomplished with epinephrine. The heart rate is usually augmented with isoproterenol. Wound healing is promoted with a single small dose of methylprednisolone.

59. **Correct answer: B**
The transplanted kidney is placed in the pelvic area, so pelvic pain is an ominous sign. Patients who have undergone kidney transplants should be educated to notify their physicians immediately if they begin suffering from pelvic pain, as it is a symptom of rejection.

60. **Correct answer: C**
Accelerated acute rejection is defined as organ rejection that occurs three to five days post transplant, is antibody mediated, and is characterized by fever and oliguria.

61. **Correct answer: A**
Rejection of a transplanted organ usually occurs as a result of cellular immunity. The function of T cells is cellular immunity. These cells recognize the transplanted organ cells as foreign and mount an attack against the "invaders," resulting in rejection. Immunosuppressive drugs suppress this normal response.

62. **Correct answer: C**
The most common cause of a fatal transfusion reaction is mismatched blood. Mismatched blood causes a hemolytic reaction that results in systemic cellular lysis. The overwhelming destruction of cells cannot be corrected rapidly enough by the bone marrow, and the patient ultimately dies.

63. **Correct answer: C**
Polyclonal antibodies are antirejection agents that are used for induction therapy for patients receiving lung transplants; they lower the number of circulating T cells in organ recipients. Polyclonal antibodies are also used for episodes of acute rejections. Daclizumab and muromonab are monoclonal antibodies. They can also be used for induction therapy—they alter the T cells so they cannot recognize antigens. Paroxetine (Paxil) is an antidepressant.

64. **Correct answer: B**
The ACT is more sensitive to factor VIII and heparin than whole blood clotting time. The ACT test measures the ability of the blood to clot; it is easy to perform and is highly reliable. In this test, fresh, whole blood is added to a test tube that contains an activator (e.g., glass particles, kayolin, diatomaceous earth). The result indicates the time it takes for a clot to form.

65. **Correct answer: C**
Back pain or abdominal pain with itching can be indicators of acute rejection of the liver. Additional indicators would include elevated liver enzymes, elevated bilirubin, jaundice, and elevated ammonia levels (a late sign). The itching is a result of bilirubin deposits in the skin.

66. **Correct answer: D**
Epinephrine is given for anaphylactic reactions because it promotes bronchodilation and inhibits additional mediator release. Epinephrine counteracts the bronchoconstrictive and vasodilator actions of histamine by stimulating alpha, $beta_1$, and $beta_2$ receptors. Epinephrine is also useful in treating hay fever and urticaria.

67. **Correct answer: A**
DIC is most often fatal because of exsanguination.

68. **Correct answer: C**
Oat-cell carcinomas (a type of small-cell carcinoma) are primarily found in the bronchial wall. On CXR, a central mass will be seen. This type of carcinoma readily spreads to the brain, bone, liver, and adrenal glands. The prognosis for patients with this disease is very poor.

69. **Correct answer: D**
As the liver becomes compromised, symptoms reflect inefficient liver functioning, with levels of clotting factors V and VII becoming less than or equal to 20% of the normal levels. In acute liver failure, creatinine and BUN values will be increased, while serum glucose levels will be decreased. Any patient with new-onset, acute hepatic failure should be tested for all hepatitis forms. Hepatitis is one of the most common causes of acute liver failure and may be first diagnosed when liver failure presents.

70. **Correct answer: B**
In thalassemia, the erythrocytes—known as "target cells"—are very thin and fragile. Thus use of oral stimulants could lead to vasoconstriction. The serum bilirubin is elevated in this disease, so you should caution the patient against scratching. Cool water and lotion may be used for skin care. The integrity of the skin is weakened, so careful positioning is paramount. The patient may require ongoing transfusions. Multiple transfusions may actually lead to the presence of too much iron, which might then have to be removed through chelation.

71. **Correct answer: C**
Low-molecular-weight heparin is more stable than unfractionated heparin. LMWH (i.e., Lovenox) is so stable and predictable that PTT tests are not required. It is also easy to administer at home.

72. **Correct answer: B**
Clopidogrel (Plavix) will interfere with phenytoin, tamoxifen and tolbutamide, fluvastin, toresemide, and warfarin. It also may alter the effectiveness of nonsteroidal anti-inflammatory drugs. Plavix does not seem to affect estrogen, cimetidine, or phenobarbital.

73. **Correct answer: A**
Epogen and Procrit are both forms of recombinant erythropoietin. They are used to correct the anemia that can occur with chronic renal failure. Potential adverse effects of these medications include hypertension, clotting at the site of vascular access, depletion of iron, and increases in potassium, creatinine, and BUN.

74. **Correct answer: B**
Peanut butter contains large amounts of folic acid. Other foods that are high in folic acid include red beans, broccoli, asparagus, liver, and beef.

75. **Correct answer: C**
Blood component replacement therapy for DIC may include Amicar, a medication used to inhibit fibrinolysis. Unfortunately, its administration may change a simple bleeding issue into DIC. For this reason, Amicar must be used in combination with heparin. DIC is usually treated with FFP, cryoprecipitate, and platelets. Cryoprecipitate contains 5 to 10 times more fibrinogen than FFP. A good rule of thumb is to give 10 units of cryoprecipitate for each 3 units of FFP. If the patient is actively bleeding, platelets are commonly used.

76. **Correct answer: C**
An irregularly shaped lump near the infraclavicular border, accompanied by respiratory distress with dry cough, is suspicious for lymphoma. The PICU nurse should ask if there has been any abdominal pain or distention that might be indicative of hepatosplenomegaly. Rapid tumor growth is associated with Burkitt's (non-Hodgkin's) lymphoma. Additional questions will assist in determining which type of lymphoma may be present. A sudden weight loss, fever, and nausea and vomiting with decreased appetite have been associated with lymphomas. The nurse's findings and history assessment should be reported to the physician immediately. Given that this patient is reporting respiratory distress, the physician may perform a biopsy to determine the type of lymphoma and order additional tests to determine spread of the disease.

77. **Correct answer: B**
Mabel is 16 years old and may have body image issues related to her Hodgkin's lymphoma and treatment. Patients with Hodgkin's lymphoma often have severe itching and bruising. The itching is caused by an increase of eosinophils in the bloodstream. If liver impairment and hepatomegaly are present, patients may have difficulty clotting and present with bruising and petechiae. Skin care should focus on maintaining skin integrity and soothing itching. A moisturizer containing lidocaine may sooth itching and prevent skin compromise. Alcohol-based cleaners and soaps with pumice will dry the skin and be too abrasive. Ice may be used to sooth itching, but the patient should use a barrier when it is applied to prevent damage to the dermal layer.

78. **Correct answer: D**
Hodgkin's lymphoma is most often seen in children older than 15. It is very rarely seen in children younger than 5 years old. Boys are more commonly affected by Hodgkin's lymphoma. Increased risk has been noted in children with an existing immunologic disorder such as HIV or AIDS.

79. **Correct answer: C**
Non-Hodgkin's lymphoma (NHL) accounts for 60% of lymphoma cases. NHL includes several different diseases—namely, Burkitt's and non-Burkitt's lymphoma, large-cell lymphomas, and lymphoblastic lymphoma.

80. **Correct answer: A**
A patient with chronic myelogenous leukemia (CML) will present with a high platelet count, an abnormal WBC count (elevated), and a high blast count. CML has been associated with genetic abnormalities affecting chromosomes 9 and 22, also called Philadelphia chromosome. This genetic abnormality further increases the growth and longevity of the abnormal immature white blood cells.

81. **Correct answer: A**
Acute lymphoblastic leukemia (ALL) is the most common form of leukemia found in children. It is also the most common type of cancer. Acute myelogenous leukemia (AML) is a type of acute nonlymphoid leukemia (ANLL). Chronic myelogenous leukemia (CML) is another type of leukemia. Leukemia results in overgrowth of immature white blood cells (blasts) in the bone marrow, bloodstream, and lymph system. The spleen may also become engorged with blast cells, which inhibits its filtering capabilities. If the blast growth continues, neurologic symptoms may appear.

82. **Correct answer: A**
Whitney's presentation of confusion, hypotonia, and seizures is indicative of spinal cord involvement. A spinal tap would provide proof of the presence of blast cells in the spinal fluid. Rapid, aggressive chemotherapy treatment is indicated.

83. **Correct answer: D**
Mechlorethamine (Mustargen) is a highly necrotic chemotherapeutic agent. The IV site should be monitored closely for pain, swelling, burning, stinging, or site redness. Orders should be in place to treat infiltration whenever Mustargen is ordered. Treatment may include sodium thiosulfate injection, cool compresses for 6–12 hours after infusion has been stopped, sodium chloride injection, or lidocaine 1% injections.

84. Correct answer: D

Children undergoing chemotherapy may not receive sufficient caloric intake due to side effects of chemotherapy such as oral mucosal ulcerations, nausea and vomiting, rectal ulcerations, and fatigue. Asayo should be included in the process of making food choices, and her favorite foods should be brought from home to stimulate her hunger and intake. Parents and staff should anticipate a decrease in nutritional intake and provide any desired food on request. When the patient is hungry, encourage small frequent meals to limit nausea and vomiting. Never use food as a route for reward or punishment, as this produces unnecessary pressure and may indicate family stress and a need for intervention.

85. Correct answer: A

It is vital to normal growth and development and family health to schedule family time when no procedures, medications, or medical/nursing interference occurs. This practice provides the family with time to be a family and function more normally. Jacob is old enough to understand diagnostic testing and be involved in the scheduling of tests. Waiting until just before a procedure to tell him about it may not allow Jacob to psychologically prepare for the procedure and will likely increase his stress. Posting all medical and nursing treatments may impede the patient's ability to feel normal. Discuss the plan of care at the beginning of the shift and as needed. Patients will need frequent interactions with their peers and family so that they can feel more like normal children. Limiting interaction and socialization will depress normal development and stunt psychological growth and coping mechanisms. It is important to maintain a sense of normalcy despite a medical diagnosis.

86. Correct answer: A

Hepatitis D (HDV) can replicate only when hepatitis B (HBV) is present. When HDV is present, either as a co-infection or as a superinfection, liver disease and progression are more rapid and severe. IgM levels rise early in infection and may remain chronically high. IgG levels rise more slowly during infection, but will continue to be elevated for the remainder of the patient's life.

HEMATOLOGY/IMMUNOLOGY REFERENCES

Aehlert, B. (Ed.). (2005). *Comprehensive pediatric emergency care.* St. Louis, MO: Mosby.

Ahrens, T. (2006). *Critical care nursing certification.* Columbus, OH: McGraw-Hill.

American Association of Critical-Care Nurses. (2006). *Core curriculum for critical care nursing* (6th ed.). Philadelphia, PA: Saunders.

American Association of Critical-Care Nurses. (2007). *AACN certification and core review for high acuity and critical care* (6th ed.). Philadelphia, PA: Saunders.

American Heart Association. (2010). Guidelines 2010 for cardiopulmonary resuscitation and emergency cardiovascular care. Retrieved from www.americanheart.org

Arbelaez, A. M., Vyas, A. K., & Shepard, S. P. (2009). Endocrine diseases. In S. M. Dusenbery & A. J. White (Eds.), *The Washington manual of pediatrics* (pp. 210–212). Philadelphia: Wolters Kluwer Health/Lippincott Williams & Wilkins.

Aster, R. H., & Bougie, D. W. (2007). Drug-induced immune thrombocytopenia: Current concepts. *New England Journal of Medicine, 357*(6), 580–587.

Bacigalupo, A., & Passweg, J. (2009). Diagnosis and treatment of acquired aplastic anemia. *Hematology/Oncology Clinics of North America, 23*(2), 159–170.

Bhullar, I. S., Braman, R., & Block, E. F. J. (2007). Recombinant factor VII as an adjunct to control of hemorrhage from chest trauma in a Jehovah's Witness. *American Surgeon, 73*(8), 818–819.

Biagini, E., Spirito, P., Leone, O., Picchio, F. M., Coccolo, F., Ragni, L., . . . Raperzzi, C. (2008). Heart transplantation in hypertrophic cardiomyopathy. *American Journal of Cardiology, 101*(3), 387.

Bolton-Maggs, P. H. (2009). Factor XI deficiency: Resolving the enigma? *Hematology, 33(2),* 97–105.

Burns, S. M. (Ed.). (2007). *American Association of Critical-Care Nurses (AACN): AACN protocols for practice: Healing environments* (2nd ed.). Sudbury, MA: Jones and Bartlett.

Chambers, M. A., & Jones, S. (Eds.). (2007). *Surgical nursing of children.* Philadelphia, PA: Elsevier.

Chernecky, C., & Berger, B. (2004). *Laboratory tests and diagnostic procedures* (4th ed.). Philadelphia, PA: Saunders.

Chierakul, W., Tientadakul, P., Suputtamongkol, Y., Wuthiekanun, V., Phimda, K., Limpalboon, R., . . .Day, N. P. (2008). Activation of the coagulation cascade in patients with leptospirosis. *Clinical Infectious Diseases, 46*(2), 254.

Chowdhury, T., Barnacle, A., Haque, S., Sebire, N., Gibson, S., Anderson, J., & Roebuck, D. (2009). Ultrasound-guided core needle biopsy for the diagnosis of rhabdomyosarcoma in childhood. *Pediatric Blood & Cancer, 53*(3), 356–360.

Clark, N., Witt, D., & Delate, T. (2008). The clinical consequence of subtherapeutic anticoagulation: The low INR study (LINeRS). *Journal of Thrombosis and Thrombolysis, 25*(1), 127–128.

Curley, M. A. Q. (1998). Patient–nurse synergy: Optimizing patients' outcomes. *American Journal of Critical Care, 7,* 64–72.

Danes, A. F., Cuenca, L. G., Rodriguez Bueno, S., Mendarte-Barrenechea, L., & Ronsano, J. B. (2008). Efficacy and tolerability of human fibrinogen concentrate administration to patients with acquired fibrinogen deficiency and active or in high-risk severe bleeding. *Vox Sanguinis, 94*(3), 221–226.

Dhaliwal, G., Cornett, P. A., & Tierney, L. M. (2004). Hemolytic anemia. *American Family Physician, 69*(11), 2599–2606.

Domen, R. E., & Hoeltge, G. A. (2003). Allergic transfusion reactions: An evaluation of 273 consecutive reactions. *Archives of Pathology & Laboratory Medicine, 127*(3), 316–320.

Dossey, B. M., Keegan, L., & Guzzetta, C. (2003). *Holistic nursing: A handbook for practice* (3rd ed.). Sudbury, MA: Jones and Bartlett.

Doyle, P., Sajid, M., O'Brien, T., Dubois, K., Engel, J. C., Macksey, Z. B., & Reed, S. (2008). Drugs targeting parasite lysosomes. *Current Pharmaceutical Design, 14*(9), 889–900.

Drake Melander, S. (Ed.). (2004). *Case studies in critical care nursing: A guide for application and review* (3rd ed.). Philadelphia, PA: Saunders.

Dvorak, C. C., & Cowan, M. J. (2008). Hematopoietic stem cell transplantation for primary immunodeficiency disease. *Bone Marrow Transplantation, 41*(2), 119–126.

Edwards, D. F. (1999). The Synergy Model: Linking patient needs to nurse competencies. *Critical Care Nurse, 19*(1), 88–98.

Emergency Nurses Association & Newberry, L. (2003). *Sheehy's emergency nursing: Principles and practice* (5th ed.). St. Louis, MO: Mosby/Elsevier.

Eyre, R., Feltbower, R. G., Mubwandarikwa, E., Eden, T. O., & McNally, R. J. (2009). Epidemiology of bone tumors in children and young adults. *Pediatric Blood & Cancer, 53*(6), 941–952.

Finch, R. (2009). Antimicrobials: Past, present and uncertain future. *Clinical Medicine, 9*(3), 257–258.

Finkelmeier, B. A. (2000). *Cardiothoracic surgical nursing* (2nd ed.). Philadelphia, PA: Lippincott Williams & Wilkins.

Fitzgerald-Macksey, L. (2009). *Pediatric anesthetic and emergency drug guide*. Sudbury, MA: Jones and Bartlett.

Goldstein, G., Toren, A., & Nagler, A. (2007). Transplantation and other uses of human umbilical cord blood and stem cells. *Current Pharmaceutical Design, 13*(13), 1363–1373.

Goodhue, C. J., & Brady, M. A. (2009). Atopic and rheumatic disorders. In C. E. Burns, M. A. Brady, A. M. Dunn, N. B. Starr, & C. G. Blosser (Eds.), *Pediatric primary care* (4th ed., pp. 575–577). St. Louis: Saunders Elsevier.

Gora-Harper, M. (1998). *The injectable drug reference*. Princeton, NJ: Bioscientific Resources.

Gurm, H. S., & Eagle, K. A. (2008). Use of anticoagulants in ST-segment elevation myocardial infarction patients: A focus on low-molecular-weight heparin. *Cardiovascular Drugs and Therapy, 22*(1), 59–69.

Hardin, S. R., & Kaplow, R. (Eds.) (2004). *Synergy for clinical excellence: The AACN Synergy Model for Patient Care*. Sudbury, MA: Jones and Bartlett.

Hay, W. W. Jr., Levin, M. J., Sondheimer, J. M., & Deterding, R. R. (Eds.). (2007). *Current diagnosis and treatment in pediatrics* (18th ed.). New York: McGraw-Hill.

Hedner, U., & Brun, N. C. (2007). Recombinant factor VIIa (rFVIIa): Its potential role as a hemostatic agent. *Neuroradiology, 49*(10), 789–793.

Heparin-induced thrombocytopenia: A quick review of recent studies. (2007). *Journal of Respiratory Diseases, 28*(9), 396.

Hickey, J. V. (2008). *The clinical practice of neurological and neurosurgical nursing* (6th ed.). Philadelphia, PA: Lippincott Williams & Wilkins.

Hirohata, A., Nakamura, M., Waseda, K., Honda, Y., Lee, D. P., Vagelos, R. H., . . . Fearon, W. F. (2007). Changes in coronary anatomy and physiology after heart transplantation. *American Journal of Cardiology, 99*(11), 1603.

Johnsen, P., Townsend, J., Bøhn, T., Simonsen, G. S., Sundsfjord, A., & Nielsen, K. M. (2009). Factors affecting the reversal of antimicrobial-drug resistance. *Lancet Infectious Diseases, 9*(6), 357–364.

Jones & Bartlett Learning (2011). *2011 nurse's drug handbook* (10th ed.). Sudbury, MA: Jones & Bartlett Learning.

Kamoun, M., & Grossman, R. A. (2008). Kidney-transplant rejection and anti-MICA antibodies. *New England Journal of Medicine, 358*(2), 196; author reply, 196.

Kramer, B. (2008). Antenatal inflammation and lung injury: Prenatal origin of neonatal disease. *Journal of Perinatology, 28*(S1), S21–S27.

Krishnamoorthy, P., Alyaarubi, S., Abish, S., Gale, M., Albuquerque, P., & Jabado, N. (2006). Primary hyperparathyroidism mimicking vaso-occlusive crises in sickle cell disease. *Pediatrics, 118*(2), 786–787.

Labbé, E., Herbert, D., & Haynes, J. (2005). Physicians' attitude and practices in sickle cell disease pain management. *Journal of Palliative Care, 21*(4), 246–251.

Lee, G. M., Lorick, S. A., Pfoh, E., Kleinman, K., & Fishbein, D. (2008). Adolescent immunizations: Missed opportunities for prevention. *Pediatrics, 122*(4), 711–717.

Levi, M., & Cate, H. T. (1999). Disseminated intravascular coagulation. *New England Journal of Medicine, 341*(8), 586–592.

Lipson, J. G., Dibble, S. L., & Minarik, P. A. (Eds.). (1996). *Culture and nursing care: A pocket guide.* San Francisco, CA: UCSF Nursing Press.

Lisman, T., & Leebeek, F. W. G. (2007). Hemostatic alterations in liver disease: A review on pathophysiology, clinical consequences, and treatment. *Digestive Surgery, 24*(4), 250–258.

Maloney, K., Foreman, N. K., Giller, R. H., Greffe, B. S., Graham, D. K., Quinones, R. R., & Keating, A. K. (2009). Neoplastic disease. In W. W. Hay, Jr., M. J. Levin, J. M. Sondheimer, & R. R. Deterding (Eds.), *Current diagnosis and treatment in pediatrics* (19th ed., pp. 871–873). New York: McGraw-Hill Medical.

Martin, B. (2010). Family presence during resuscitation and invasive procedures: AACN practice alert. Retrieved from http://www.aacn.org

McNally, P. (2001). *GI/liver secrets* (2nd ed.). Philadelphia, PA: Hanley & Belfus/Elsevier.

Medina, J., & Puntillo, K. (2006). *AACN protocols for practice: Palliative care and end-of-life issues in critical care*. Sudbury, MA: Jones and Bartlett.

Meyer, J. S., Nadel, H. R., Marina, N., Womer, R. B., Brown, K. L., Eary, J. F., . . . Kailo, M. D. (2008). Imaging guidelines for children with Ewing sarcoma and osteosarcoma: A report from the Children's Oncology Group Bone Tumor Committee. *Pediatric Blood & Cancer, 51*(2), 163–170.

Mitka, M. (2007). Dual antithrombotic therapy's increased risks not always offset by benefit. *Journal of the American Medical Association, 298*(13), 1504.

Mongardon, N., Bruneel, F., Henry-Lagarrigue, M., Legriel, S., Revault, D. L., Guezennic, P., . . . Bedos, J. P. (2007). Shock during heparin-induced thrombocytopenia: Look for adrenal insufficiency! *Intensive Care Medicine, 33*(3), 547–548.

Murphy, S. B. (2008). Tailoring treatment to prognosis for childhood localized non-Hodgkin's lymphoma. *Journal of Clinical Oncology, 26*(7), 1020–1021.

Norris, W. E. (2004). Acute hepatic sequestration in sickle cell disease. *Journal of the National Medical Association, 96*(9), 1235–1239.

Nursing care of the child with an immunologic disorder. (2008). In T. Kyle, *Essentials of pediatric nursing* (pp. 912–915). Philadelphia, PA: Wolters Kluwer/Lippincott Williams & Wilkins.

Olson, J. D., Brandt, J. T., Chandler, W. L., Van Cott, E. M., Cunningham, M. T., Hayes, T. E., . . . Wang, E. C. (2007). Laboratory reporting of the International Normalized Ratio: Progress and problems. *Archives of Pathology & Laboratory Medicine, 131*(11), 1641–1617.

Pagana, K. D., & Pagana, J. (2005). *Mosby's Manual of diagnostic and laboratory tests* (3rd ed.). St. Louis, MO: Mosby/Elsevier.

Perry, S. E., Hockenberry, M. J., Lowdermilk, D. L., & Wilson, D. (Eds.). (2010). Musculoskeletal or articular dysfunction. In *Maternal child nursing care* (4th ed., pp. 1705–1708). Philadelphia, PA: Mosby/Elsevier.

Prasad, V. K., & Kurtzberg, J. (2008). Emerging trends in transplantation of inherited metabolic diseases. *Bone Marrow Transplantation, 41*(2), 99–108.

Prescribing reference. (2009, Summer). *NPPR: Nurse Practitioner's Prescribing Reference, 16*(2).

Pulte, D., Gondos, A., & Brenner, H. (2008). Trends in 5- and 10-year survival after diagnosis with childhood hematologic malignancies in the United States, 1990–2004. *Journal of the National Cancer Institute, 100*(18), 1301–1309.

Punyko, J. A., Gurney, J. G., Scott Baker, K., Hayashi, R. J., Hudson, M. M., Liu, Y., . . . Mertens, A. C. (2007). Physical impairment and social adaptation in adult survivors of childhood and adolescent rhabdomyosarcoma: A report from the Childhood Cancer Survivors Study. *Psycho-Oncology, 16*(1), 26–37.

Rodeberg, D. A., Stoner, J. A., Hayes-Jordan, A., Kao, S. C., Wolden, S. L., Qualman, S. J., . . . Hawkins, D. S. (2009). Prognostic significance of tumor response at the end of therapy in group III rhabdomyosarcoma: A report from the Children's Oncology Group. *American Society of Clinical Oncology, 27*(32), 3705–3711.

Shorr, A. K., Helman, D. L., Davies, D. B., & Nathan, S. D. (2004). Sarcoidosis, race, and short-term outcomes following lung transplantation. *Chest, 125*(3), 990–996.

Skidmore-Roth, L. (2004). *Mosby's 2004 nursing drug reference.* St. Louis, MO: Mosby/Elsevier.

Slota, M. C. (Ed.). (2006). *Core curriculum for pediatric critical care nursing* (2nd ed.). St. Louis, MO: Saunders.

Spratto, G. R., & Woods, A. L. (2001). *PDR: Nurse's drug handbook.* Montvale, NJ: Delmar & Medical Economics.

Stewart, L. J., Johnston, R. B. Jr., & Liu, A. H. (2009). Immunodeficiency. In W. W. Hay, Jr., M. J. Levin, J. M. Sondheimer, & R. R. Deterding (Eds.), *Lange current diagnosis and treatment in pediatrics* (19th ed., pp. 891–910). New York: McGraw–Hill Medical.

Swanson, K., Dwyre, D. M., Krochmal, J., & Raife, T. J. (2006). Transfusion-related acute lung injury (TRALI): Current clinical and pathophysiologic considerations. *Lung, 184*(3), 177–185.

Swartz, M. K. (2009). Hematologic disorders. In C. E. Burns, M. A. Brady, A. M. Dunn, N. B. Starr, & C. G. Blosser (Eds.), *Pediatric primary care* (4th ed., pp. 631–633). St. Louis, MO: Saunders Elsevier.

Trivits Verger, J., & Lebet, R. M. (Eds.). (2008). *AACN procedure manual for pediatric acute and critical care.* St. Louis, MO: Saunders.

Unkle, D. W. (2007). Heparin-induced thrombocytopenia. *Orthopaedic Nursing, 26*(6), 383–387.

Urden, L. D., Stacy, K. M., & Lough, M. E. (2007). *Thelan's critical care nursing: Diagnosis and management* (5th ed.). St. Louis, MO: Mosby.

von Köckritz-Blickwede, M., & Nizet, V. (2009). Innate immunity turned inside-out: Antimicrobial defense by phagocyte extracellular traps. *Journal of Molecular Medicine, 87*(8), 775–783.

Young, N. S., Scheinberg, P., & Calado, R. T. (2008). Aplastic anemia. *Current Opinion in Hematology, 15*(3), 162–168.

Zhang, D., Zhang, F., Zhang, Y., Gao, X., Li, C., Ma, W., & Cao, K. (2007). Erythropoietin enhances the angiogenic potency of autologous bone marrow stromal cells in a rat model of myocardial infarction. *Cardiology, 108*(4), 228–236.

SECTION 7

Neurology

1. **Which of the following statements is true regarding scoliosis?**
   A. Scoliosis is congenital in origin
   B. The first sign of scoliosis is a prominent scapula
   C. Most cases have a juvenile onset
   D. A severe form of scoliosis has a curve from 20 to 40 degrees

2. **You are caring for Angie, a 6 month old with hydrocephalus. The baby had a ventriculo-peritoneal (VP) shunt placed earlier today. Over the past few hours you have noticed that she has become increasingly lethargic. As the pediatric ICU nurse, you know that**
   A. The shunt may be occluded
   B. It is not unusual for babies with hydrocephalus to fatigue easily
   C. The shunt is functioning well
   D. It is the baby's usual naptime

3. **The most common cause of acquired hydrocephalus is**
   A. HIV infection
   B. Idiopathic
   C. A maternal rubella infection
   D. Bacterial meningitis

4. **Common symptoms of hydrocephalus in a 4 month old infant would include**
   A. Macewen's sign, fused fontanelles
   B. Macrocrania, rapid skull growth, failure to thrive
   C. Flat scalp veins, split sutures
   D. Microcrania, hyperreflexia, bulging fontanelles

5. **Your 3 year old male patient with hydrocephalus received a ventriculo-peritoneal shunt 2 days ago. On your initial assessment, you find him febrile, tachycardic, and lethargic. You should anticipate which of the following orders from the physician?**
   A. CBC with differential, CRP, sedimentation rate, ceftazidime, cooling measures
   B. CSF cultures, acetaminophen, azithromycin
   C. CT scan, CSF cultures, ciprofloxacin
   D. Levofloxacin, CT scan, CRP

6. **Syringomyelia is most often seen in conjunction with which other neurologic problem?**
   A. Syringomyelia occurs as a unique entity
   B. Myoclonic seizures
   C. Chiari II malformation
   D. Schizencephaly

7. **Which assessments should be done for a 4 month old infant with hydrocephalus after a ventriculo-peritoneal shunt placement?**
   A. Frequent NS, HOB at 30 degrees, head midline
   B. VS Q15 minutes, HOB flat, positioned on the left side
   C. NS hourly, HOB 30 degrees, positioned on the right side
   D. Head midline, prone positioning

8. **Which nursing diagnoses should be addressed for a child after a ventriculo-peritoneal shunt is placed?**
   A. Increased ICP, potential for inadequate oxygenation, potential for infection, pain
   B. Decreased ICP, potential for inadequate oxygenation, potential for infection, pain
   C. Potential for infection, pain management, potential for dehydration
   D. Potential for infection, pain management, alteration in nutrition

9. **What is the most common cause of hearing loss among children in the United States?**
   A. Syphilis
   B. Loud music
   C. CMV infection
   D. Herpes simplex infection

10. **Which of the following signs is used to help diagnose hydrocephalus in an infant?**
    A. Battle's sign
    B. Macewen's sign
    C. Lhermitte's sign
    D. Trendelenberg's sign

11. **What are the two most common causes of a comatose state in a child younger than 5 years of age?**
    A. Falls and drowning
    B. Inappropriate use of car seats and trauma
    C. Nonaccidental trauma and near-drowning
    D. Accidental overdose and head injury

12. **Ingestion of which of the following drugs may lead to coma?**
    A. Diet pills, opiates, phencyclidine piperidine
    B. Scopolamine, opiates, ethanol
    C. Cocaine, lithium, atropine
    D. Ethanol, lysergic acid diethylamide, atropine

13. **What does the Pediatric Glasgow Coma Scale measure?**
    A. Eye opening, deep tendon reflexes, verbal response
    B. Eye opening, motor response, verbal response
    C. Eye opening, motor response, cranial nerve response
    D. Eye opening, cranial nerve response, verbal response

14. **Susan, who is 14, was an unrestrained passenger in a motor vehicle accident. She is admitted to the pediatric ICU after suffering a basilar skull fracture. Which of the following signs is indicative of a fracture of the middle fossa?**
    A. Rhinorrhea
    B. Raccoon's eyes
    C. Battle's sign
    D. Subconjunctival hemorrhage

15. **Tom, a 15 year old baseball player, is admitted to the PICU after being struck by a baseball bat during a game. He has blunt force trauma to the left side of his head. Nursing management of this patient includes frequent assessments. The PICU nurse knows which of the following conditions is the most sensitive indicator of Tom's neurological status?**
    A. Vital signs
    B. Pediatric Glasgow Coma Scale
    C. Level of consciousness
    D. Intracranial pressure monitoring

16. **While assessing a patient with a basilar skull fracture, the PICU nurse notices a stain on the patient's pillow. The stain consists of a small amount of blood encircled by a pale yellow ring. It is called**
    A. A halo sign
    B. Battle's sign
    C. Grey-Turner's sign
    D. Ludwig's sign

17. **The most accurate method of measuring intracranial pressure is placement of a(n)**
    A. Subarachnoid bolt
    B. Intraventriculostomy
    C. Epidural catheter
    D. Subdural catheter

18. **Normal intracranial pressure in a 3 year old child is**
    A. 0–5 mmHg
    B. 3–7 mmHg
    C. 16–20 mmHg
    D. 20–40 mmHg

19. **What is the function of the myelin sheath in the central nervous system?**
    A. It protects the dendrites from injury
    B. It allows for faster transmission of nerve impulses
    C. Its purpose has not yet been determined
    D. It creates the gray matter in the brain and spinal cord

20. **Mary is a 12 year old patient in your pediatric ICU. She suffered an acute hemorrhagic stroke from a ruptured arteriovenous malformation (AVM) and is not expected to survive long. You know that Mary's intracranial pressure is rising, as she now is developing Cushing syndrome. Which signs and symptoms do you expect to see in a patient with Cushing syndrome?**
    A. Increased systolic blood pressure, widening pulse pressure, bradycardia
    B. Elevated blood pressure, narrow pulse pressure, tachycardia
    C. Bradycardia, low blood pressure, narrow pulse pressure
    D. Tachycardia, increased systolic blood pressure, widening pulse pressure

21. **When should a lumbar puncture be done on a patient with increased intracranial pressure?**
    A. Once the patient has completed a CT or MRI scan
    B. A lumbar puncture should always be done to check intracranial pressure
    C. The decision to do a lumbar puncture should be made on a case-by-case basis
    D. Never

22. **Decreased intracranial pressure may be due to**
    A. CO_2 retention
    B. PaO_2 less than 50 mmHg
    C. Increased cerebrospinal fluid absorption
    D. Increased metabolic activity

23. **Frank, a 16 year old, has a closed head injury secondary to a fall during a Rave party. As a pediatric ICU nurse, you know the most important indicator of neurologic deterioration in this patient is**
    A. His blood pressure
    B. Cranial nerve testing
    C. His level of consciousness
    D. The Pediatric Glasgow Coma Scale

24. **Trevor has a closed head injury. He also has an indwelling Foley catheter. In one hour, his urine output increased from 30 mL/hr to 1000 mL of very pale, clear urine. Trevor is probably suffering from**
    A. A volume shift from the third space
    B. Syndrome of inappropriate antidiuretic hormone
    C. Diabetes insipidus
    D. Diuresis from steroids

25. **The pediatric ICU nurse knows the treatment of diabetes insipidus includes**
    A. Fluid restriction
    B. Intravenous replacement to cover the increased urine output
    C. Diuretics
    D. Demeclocycline

26. **Why is it important to stop seizure activity in a patient with status epilepticus?**
    A. Oxygen depletion may occur due to an impeded airway
    B. There is an increased risk of cerebrovascular accident
    C. Continued seizure activity causes lactic acidosis and cerebral edema
    D. Injury risk increases with continued seizures

27. What is the correct formula for calculating cerebral perfusion pressure (CPP)?

A. CPP = SBP – MAP – ICP
B. CPP = MAP – ICP
C. CPP = ICP – MAP
D. CPP = MAP – CVP – ICP

28. What is the ideal range for cerebral perfusion pressure for a 4 year old child?

A. 50–60 mmHg
B. 20–40 mmHg
C. 10–20 mmHg
D. 70–90 mmHg

29. Joy is a 6 year old girl who had a small basilar skull fracture after a motor vehicle accident. Which of the cranial nerves (CN) are affected by a basilar skull fracture?

A. I, VII, VIII
B. I, II, III
C. I, V, VIII
D. II, III, VIII

30. Your 12 year old patient has a head injury and has just developed nystagmus. The pediatric ICU nurse knows nystagmus is

A. Eyes deviated to the side of the injury
B. Convergent gaze
C. Rhythmic tremor or shaking of the eyes
D. Divergent gaze

31. What are the most common causes of the syndrome of inappropriate antidiuretic hormone?

A. Bronchogenic (oat-cell) carcinoma, pneumonia, head injury
B. Pneumonia, COPD, tuberculosis
C. Brain tumors, pneumonia, polycystic kidney disease
D. Polycystic kidney disease, cerebrovascular accident, oat-cell carcinomas

32. Intact spinal reflexes indicate

A. Functional upper motor neurons
B. Nonfunctional lower motor neurons
C. Nonfunctional upper motor neurons
D. Functional lower motor neurons

33. You are caring for Gene, a 14 year old boy who is a new paraplegic. The neurologist wants to test Gene's spinothalamic tract responses. How is the spinothalamic tract tested?

A. Deep tendon reflexes
B. Babinski reflex
C. Pinprick or monofilament testing
D. Patellar tendon reflex

34. **What is autonomic hyperreflexia?**
    A. A malfunction of the autonomic nervous system seen with a head injury
    B. A malfunction of the autonomic nervous system seen with a spinal cord injury
    C. A malfunction of the autonomic nervous system seen with pituitary tumor removal
    D. A malfunction of the autonomic nervous system seen with epidural bleeds

35. **The pediatric ICU nurse should anticipate which of the following treatments for the syndrome of inappropriate antidiuretic hormone (SIADH)?**
    A. Fluid replacement, potassium chloride, declomycin
    B. Fluid restriction, diuretics, sodium replacement, declomycin
    C. Declomycin, vasopressin, diuretics
    D. Fluid restriction, potassium chloride, diuretics

36. **Part of the criteria for brain death is an absent Doll's Eyes reflex. A normal response to the Doll's Eyes maneuver would be**
    A. Disconjugate gaze with head turn
    B. Conjugate gaze in the opposite direction as the head is turned
    C. Conjugate gaze in the same direction as the head is turned
    D. Nystagmus with head turning

37. **Melanie, a 15 year old, was injured in a motor vehicle accident. A few minutes ago, she began to exhibit decerebrate posturing. As the pediatric ICU nurse, you know the manifestation of this type of posturing would involve**
    A. One arm flexed, one flaccid, legs flaccid
    B. Both arms fully extended and internally rotated, legs flaccid
    C. Both arms fully extended and internally rotated, legs fully extended with toes pointed
    D. Flaccid arms and legs extended

38. **Felix has been transferred from the ED to the pediatric ICU after a gunshot wound to his T11–T12 spine. Upon initial assessment, you find motor paralysis on the same side as the gunshot wound but loss of pain and temperature sensation on the opposite side. This finding is known as**
    A. Grey-Turner syndrome
    B. Cushing syndrome
    C. Syndrome X
    D. Brown-Sequard syndrome

39. **Your PICU patient with a right-side head injury suddenly develops right pupil dilation. What does this change probably indicate?**
    A. Basilar skull fracture
    B. Uncal herniation
    C. Brain stem herniation
    D. Cerebral vascular accident

40. **What is the most common bacteria that causes meningococcal meningitis?**
    A. *Streptococcus pneumoniae*
    B. *Neisseria meningitidis*
    C. *Staphylococcus aureus*
    D. *Haemophilius influenzae*

41. What are the common risk factors for the development of meningococcal meningitis?

A. Adolescent, immunodeficiency, living in close quarters
B. Youth, splenectomy, living in a dormitory
C. Infant, HIV infection, living at home
D. Youth, only child status, recent upper respiratory tract infection

42. What is the hallmark symptom of meningococcal meningitis?

A. Headache
B. Petechiae
C. Malaise
D. Vomiting

43. Ted, a 12 year old, was ill 4 days ago with a slight cold. Now he is experiencing ascending weakness in both legs. This symptom is suggestive of which of the following illnesses?

A. Guillain-Barré syndrome
B. Chronic fatigue syndrome
C. Tetanus
D. *Clostridium botulinum* infection

44. In a child older than 6 years of age, a positive Babinski or plantar reflex indicates

A. A reflex elicited with a reflex hammer to the Achilles tendon
B. Normal neurologic functioning
C. An upper motor neuron lesion of the pyramidal tract
D. A lower motor neuron lesion of the pyramidal tract

45. What is the proper technique for eliciting a Babinski response?

A. Stroke the sole of the foot from side to side
B. Stroke the sole of the foot along the lateral sole from the heel up toward the toes and across the ball of the foot
C. Strike the heel and the ball of the foot
D. Strike the Achilles tendon with a reflex hammer

46. Your patient has just returned from placement of a ventriculo-peritoneal shunt. The burr hole is located on the right parieto-occipital side because

A. The right side provides easier access to the surgeon during placement
B. The left side is near the speech comprehension center
C. The left side is near the personality center
D. The right side provides easier access to the posterior horn

47. Dane, a 10 year old boy with meningitis, is having a lumbar puncture. As his pediatric ICU nurse, you know the cerebral spinal fluid (CSF) should be

A. Hazy with a glucose level of 85
B. Clear with RBCs present
C. Clear and colorless with less than 45 mg/dL of protein
D. Clear and colorless with a white blood cell count greater than 150 cells/mm^2

48. **When performing a neurologic examination, the PICU nurse knows that the six cardinal eye directions for eye movement are testing**
   A. CN II, III, and IV
   B. CN III, IV, and VI
   C. CN II, V, and VII
   D. CN V, VI, and VII

49. **Your 12 year old patient has had a hemorrhagic left-sided stroke. What is the most common cause of stroke in children in the United States?**
   A. Uncontrolled diabetes mellitus
   B. Ventricular septal defects
   C. Uncontrolled hypertension
   D. Arteriovenous malformation (AVM)

50. **Your priority in caring for a pediatric patient with a cerebrovascular accident is**
   A. Preventing decubitus ulcers
   B. Preventing aspiration of food or fluid
   C. Preventing contractures
   D. Preventing depression

51. **Jeremy has had a stroke and is unable to communicate. Which area in the cerebrum controls verbal expression?**
   A. Wernicke's area
   B. Broca's area
   C. Limbic area
   D. Pontine area

52. **What is the homunculus?**
   A. A strip of the frontal lobe that affects motor skills
   B. A strip of the parietal lobe that affects sensory reception
   C. A strip in the cerebellum that affects balance and fine motor coordination
   D. A strip of cerebral cortex that controls the sensory and motor functioning

53. **Georgia, a 15 year old, has Guillain-Barré syndrome. What is the most important parameter to monitor for this patient?**
   A. Blood pressure
   B. Negative inspiratory force (NIF)
   C. Pain level
   D. Cerebrospinal fluid study results

54. **Which results would you expect in the evaluation of the cerebrospinal fluid in a patient with Guillain-Barré syndrome?**
   A. Increased white blood cells
   B. Increased protein levels
   C. Increased glucose levels
   D. Anaerobic bacteria

55. Which of the following nursing diagnoses would be the most appropriate for a patient with Guillain-Barré syndrome?

A. Impaired motor weakness, impaired respiratory function, acute pain
B. Impaired respiratory function, impaired nutrition, acute pain
C. Impaired motor weakness, impaired bowel function, acute pain
D. Impaired respiratory function, impaired bowel function, acute pain

56. Your patient with Guillain-Barré syndrome is experiencing a great deal of pain. Why is this pain occurring?

A. Parasympathetic function
B. Sympathetic inactivity
C. Autonomic dysfunction
D. Sympathetic function

57. Nursing management of a pediatric patient with Guillain-Barré syndrome must be prioritized to constantly monitor

A. Lab results and neurologic signs
B. Respiratory status and neurologic signs
C. Respiratory status and lab results
D. Lab results and urinary output

58. A relative contraindication for administration of methylprednisolone following a spinal injury would be

A. A spinal cord injury less than 4 hours old
B. Pregnancy
C. A patient younger than the age of 8 years
D. An intubated patient

59. Fredrick, an 18 year old, was injured while skateboarding. He suffered a T8 spinal cord injury one month ago. He had been diagnosed with spinal shock while in the pediatric intensive care unit. As Frederick's nurse, you know the symptoms of spinal shock include

A. Areflexia, autonomic dysfunction, loss of sensation, eliminatory dysfunction
B. Areflexia, peripheral vasodilatation, decreased SVR, loss of sensation
C. Areflexia, heightened sensation, cardiovascular shock
D. Areflexia, bowel and bladder dysfunction, bradycardia

60. McKenzie has a C6 spinal cord injury for which she has spent 35 days in the PICU due to sequelae from neurogenic shock. How does neurogenic shock differ from spinal shock?

A. Neurogenic shock is a less severe form of shock with spinal cord injury that causes a brief decrease in blood pressure
B. Neurogenic shock is a more severe form of shock that causes cardiovascular collapse in patients with a spinal cord injury above T6
C. Neurogenic shock is a more severe form of shock that increases paralysis and death
D. Neurogenic shock is a more severe form of shock that occurs within hours after a spinal cord injury and causes increased sympathetic outflow

61. **A patient's family member asks you about the arteriovenous malformation that caused her brother's stroke. You explain that arteriovenous malformations (AVMs) are**
   A. Commonly found misshapen blood vessels
   B. More common in women than in men
   C. A complex tangle of misshapen blood vessels that are susceptible to hemorrhage
   D. Never seen in children

62. **Spinal reflexes indicate**
   A. Functional upper motor neurons
   B. Nonfunctional lower motor neurons
   C. Nonfunctional upper motor neurons
   D. Functional lower motor neurons

63. **Your response to a stressful situation such as resuscitation of a patient causes a sympathetic nervous system response. A sympathetic response to stimulus results in**
   A. Heightened awareness, increased blood pressure, bronchial constriction, increased glucogenosis
   B. Dilated pupils, bronchial relaxation, increased gastric motility, normal urine output
   C. Vasodilation, increased blood pressure, decreased gastric secretions, pupils at 3 mm
   D. Increased respiratory depth, increased heart rate, decreased gastric motility, sphincter dilation

64. **Amy, a 16 year old patient, is transferred to the pediatric ICU after recovering from surgery for a subarachnoid hemorrhage due to a ruptured anterior communicating artery aneurysm. Cerebral aneurysms are most often found in the**
   A. Internal carotid arteries
   B. Bifurcations of the anterior–posterior Circle of Willis
   C. Temporal artery
   D. Vertebral arteries

65. **A child would be expected to complain of or exhibit which of the following symptoms if he had a ruptured cerebral aneurysm?**
   A. Nuchal rigidity
   B. Fever
   C. Nausea and vomiting
   D. Explosive headache, often described as "the worst headache of my life"

66. **Nursing management of a patient with a cerebral aneurysm includes**
   A. Ambulation, monitoring of vital and neurologic signs
   B. Pediatric GCS assessments and monitoring for cerebral vascular spasm
   C. Maintaining normal intracranial pressure
   D. Maintaining systolic blood pressure at less than 120 mmHg

67. Greg is a 5 year old patient who recently had influenza and developed ataxia. He was admitted to the pediatric ICU for observation. What are some of the clinical signs expected in children with ataxia?

A. Refusal to walk, afebrile, nystagmus
B. Tremors, fever, myalgias
C. Slurred speech, febrile seizures
D. Refusal to walk, tremors, afebrile

68. You are caring for Evan, a 10 year old admitted to the pediatric ICU after surgery for a ruptured appendix. Evan also has Tourette syndrome, which causes him to exhibit multiple motor and vocal tics. He often blurts out obscenities when you walk in the room. Which of the following statements is true concerning Tourette syndrome?

A. The symptoms will get worse as Evan grows older
B. The symptoms will fade as Evan grows older
C. Evan's symptoms will remain the same as he grows older
D. You have frightened Evan and will get this same response each time he sees you

69. Dasan is an 11 year old with focal neurologic deficits, papilledema, and increased intracranial pressure. He is being admitted to the pediatric ICU. Dasan has no petechiae or nuchal rigidity. His only significant medical history is recent otitis media, which was not treated with antibiotics. Which of the following tests would you anticipate to be ordered for Dasan?

A. Lumbar puncture
B. PET scan
C. CT or MRI
D. CBC, CMP, blood cultures

70. Which type of brain tumor is most common in children?

A. Medulloblastoma
B. Astrocytoma
C. Lymphoma
D. Metastatic bone tumor

71. Jerry is a 6 year old who had a subarachnoid hemorrhage after being struck by a car while riding his bicycle. Which of the following conditions is most likely to occur with this injury?

A. Communicating hydrocephalus
B. Diabetes mellitus
C. Seizure disorder
D. Nystagmus

72. Which cranial nerve is most often affected by basilar skull fracture?

A. Cranial nerve II (optic)
B. Cranial nerve III (oculomotor)
C. Cranial nerve IV (trochlear)
D. Cranial nerve I (olfactory)

73. **What is an early sign of uncal herniation?**
    A. Contralateral pupil dilation
    B. Ipsilateral pupil dilation
    C. Contralateral pupil constriction
    D. Ipsilateral pupil constriction

74. **Janey, an 8 year old, has just been diagnosed with myasthenia gravis after developing bilateral ptosis. Which test is performed to confirm or rule out myasthenia gravis?**
    A. Teflon test
    B. Tensilon test
    C. Serum myoglobin test
    D. CT scan of the brain

75. **What is the "purple glove syndrome"?**
    A. A complication of intravenous phenytoin administration
    B. A complication of intravenous lopressor administration
    C. A complication of intravenous adenosine administration
    D. A complication of intravenous phenobarbital administration

76. **Which type of seizure is treated with topiramate?**
    A. Grand mal seizure
    B. Absence seizure
    C. Partial seizure
    D. Febrile seizure

77. **How do partial seizures differ from grand mal seizures?**
    A. In grand mal seizures, the patient does not lose consciousness
    B. In a partial seizure, the patient loses consciousness
    C. In partial seizures, the patient does not lose consciousness
    D. In partial seizures, the patient goes into a postictal state for 4–6 hours

78. **In children, in which age range are febrile seizures most likely to occur?**
    A. Newborn infants to 6 months
    B. 6 months to 6 years of age
    C. 10 months to 10 years of age
    D. Infants up to 1 year of age

79. **Which triptans are used in children younger than 10 years of age for treatment of migraine headaches?**
    A. Imitrex is the drug of choice for childhood migraines
    B. Frovia is the drug of choice of childhood migraines
    C. Maxalt is the drug of choice for childhood migraines
    D. Triptans are not recommended for children younger than 10 years of age for migraines

80. Lian, a 9 year old patient, has ADHD and is taking dextroamphetamine/amphetamine (Adderall). She was admitted to the pediatric ICU for viral cardiomyopathy. Which dose of Adderall should she receive while hospitalized?

A. 30 mg of Adderall
B. 20 mg of Adderall
C. Adderall is contraindicated in this case
D. The dose is adjusted per patient response

81. You are to administer mannitol to your patient with cerebral edema. Which precautions should you take when giving this drug?

A. No precautions are necessary
B. Mannitol must be administered quickly over 1–2 minutes
C. Mannitol must be administered slowly through an in-line 5-micron filter
D. Mannitol is contraindicated in children

82. How quickly should phenobarbital sodium be administered intravenously to a 15 year old patient?

A. Phenobarbital should be given at less than 30 milligrams per minute
B. Phenobarbital should be given via rapid intravenous push
C. Phenobarbital should be given in a drip chamber over 1 hour
D. Phenobarbital should not be given to children

83. Tess is a 14 year old patient with newly diagnosed grand mal seizures. You are teaching Tess's parents about seizures. Which of the following actions has the highest priority for the parents if Tess has a seizure?

A. Placing a bite block in Tess's mouth when the seizure starts
B. Calling 911 every time Tess seizes
C. Making sure Tess takes her birth control pill at the same as her antiepileptic drug
D. Protecting the airway during a seizure

84. You are teaching Geoff's parents about his closed head injury suffered in a motor vehicle accident. You explain that the term "coup–contra-coup brain injury" means

A. It is a mild concussion that resolves quickly
B. It is a complicated brain injury that may have lasting effects
C. It is a moderate concussion that will resolve in 4–6 months
D. It is a complicated brain injury that will resolve completely

85. Which of the following conditions is not a symptom of a cerebellar tumor?

A. Truncal ataxia
B. Nystagmus
C. Impaired coordination
D. Ataxia

86. Deep cerebral hemispheric tumors cause

A. Hemiplegia
B. Motor dysfunction
C. Speech dysfunction
D. Irritability

87. **The type of supratentorial tumor that causes metabolic dysfunctions, eating dysfunctions, and autonomic seizures is known as a(n)**
    A. Frontal lobe tumor
    B. Occipital lobe tumor
    C. Sella-turcica area tumor
    D. Parietal lobe tumor

88. **The type of hydrocephalus that results from a loss of brain parenchyma is known as**
    A. Noncommunicating hydrocephalus
    B. Normal-pressure hydrocephalus
    C. Hydrocephalus ex vacuo
    D. Communicating hydrocephalus

89. **Separation of cranial sutures may occur in infants and children and is known as**
    A. A concussion
    B. Basilar skull fracture
    C. "Ping-Pong" depression
    D. Diastasis

90. **Roger has sustained a head injury and is demonstrating blood collection behind the tympanic membrane. This symptom usually indicates a**
    A. Skull base fracture
    B. Temporal bone fracture
    C. Middle fossa basilar fracture
    D. Parietal skull fracture

91. **Your patient has sustained a middle fossa basilar skull fracture and exhibits damage to the olfactory verve. Which of the following symptoms would help confirm this diagnosis?**
    A. Rhinorrhea
    B. Anosmia
    C. Otorrhea
    D. Nystagmus

92. **Thomas is 8 years old and has an epidural hematoma. His symptoms include hemiplegia, hemiparesis, and an inequality of his pupils greater than a 1-mm difference. This inequality in the pupils is known as**
    A. Miosis
    B. Ford's sign
    C. Anisocoria
    D. Hill's sign

93. **An injury to the sacral cord and lumbar nerve roots resulting in areflexia of the lower limbs, bowel, and bladder is known as**
    A. Brown-Sequard syndrome
    B. Spinal atresia
    C. Areflexic hypertonia
    D. Conus medullaris

94. Depressed skull fractures in infants may result in indentation or pliable skull bone(s) without loss of bone integrity. This condition is known as

A. "Ping-Pong" depression
B. Diastasis
C. Medullary bulge
D. Walker fracture

95. The type of aneurysm that results from a bacterial embolic arteritis is called a(n) ______ aneurysm

A. Fusiform
B. Saccular
C. Atherosclerotic
D. Mycotic

96. The type of ICP monitoring device that is inserted below the skull and above the dura mater is a(n)

A. Subdural catheter
B. Epidural catheter
C. Subarachnoid bolt
D. Intraventricular catheter

97. The P_2 wave on a normal ICP waveform represents

A. A dicrotic wave
B. Percussion
C. Decreased intracranial compliance
D. Diastolic pressure

98. Which of the following statements about the B waves on an abnormal ICP waveform is true?

A. B waves represent hypovolemia
B. B waves indicate decreased level of consciousness
C. B waves are fluctuations in system pulses
D. B waves are related to respirations

99. A sustained, rapid, and moderately deep hyperpnea is known as

A. Cheyne-Stokes respirations
B. Ataxic respirations
C. An apneustic respiratory pattern
D. Central neurogenic hyperventilation

100. A completely irregular breathing pattern with deep and shallow breaths is known as

A. Cheyne-Stokes respirations
B. Ataxic respirations
C. An apneustic respiratory pattern
D. Pyrogenic respiration

101. Normal ICP in children ranges from

A. 1.5 to 6 mmHg
B. 3 to 7.5 mmHg
C. 8 to 10 mmHg
D. 11 to 15 mmHg

102. In an older child, approximately what percentage of cardiac output is delivered to the brain?

A. 5%
B. 10%
C. 15%
D. 20%

103. A moderate reduction in alertness, increased sleeping, and decreased interest in the environment is called

A. Obtundation
B. Coma
C. Clouding of consciousness
D. Stupor

104. A child who is unresponsive except to repeated stimuli is

A. Lethargic
B. Obtunded
C. Stuporous
D. Posturing

105. Jugular venous oxygen saturation (SjO_2) is used to

A. Identify patients at risk for cerebral ischemia
B. Monitor brain temperature
C. Measure the balance between cerebral oxygen delivery and cerebral oxygen consumption
D. Identify complications of catheter insertion

106. The normal range for SjO_2 is between

A. 60% and 75%
B. 70% and 85%
C. 80% and 90%
D. 85% and 97%

107. Which of the following statements about SjO_2 monitoring is true?

A. SjO_2 monitoring should be used for patients older than age 8 and/or who weigh 30 kg
B. SjO_2 monitoring is not used in conjunction with ICP or CPP monitoring
C. SjO_2 values may be abnormally low in patients with nonviable brain tissue
D. The SjO_2 catheter does not need to be calibrated

108. The intravenous fluid of choice to help lower cerebral hypertension is

A. D_5W
B. Lactated Ringer's solution
C. 3% saline
D. $D_{10}W$

109. Phenytoin (Dilantin) was prescribed for your patient. As a PICU nurse, you know long-term effects of anticonvulsive therapy with phenytoin include

A. Drowsiness
B. Abdominal distress
C. Hyperkinesis
D. Gingival hyperplasia

110. An abnormal connection between arteries and veins with no common capillary bed is known as

A. A Chiari malformation
B. A canal of Landers
C. An arteriovenous malformation
D. A cavae malforma

111. A grade III periventricular intraventricular hemorrhage is

A. A subependymal hemorrhage
B. An intraventricular hemorrhage with ventricular dilation
C. An intraventricular and parenchymal hemorrhage
D. An intraventricular hemorrhage without ventricular dilation

112. Your patient has a periventricular intraventricular hemorrhage. She is exhibiting hypotonia, a decreased hematocrit, and a decreased level of consciousness. This patient has which of the following clinical syndromes?

A. A silent syndrome
B. A catastrophic syndrome
C. A vasospastic syndrome
D. A salutatory syndrome

113. A patient with stage II Reye syndrome will present as

A. Stuporous, agitated, delirious
B. Lethargic, confused
C. Decerebrate posturing, dilated pupils
D. Unresponsive, coma, decorticate posturing

114. Patients who sustain spinal injuries above the T1 level are at risk for

A. Brown-Sequard syndrome
B. Autonomic hyperreflexia
C. Impaired temperature regulation
D. Spinal shock

115. Which of the following signs or symptoms will differentiate a generalized seizure from syncope?

A. Incontinence
B. Sense of an impending loss of consciousness
C. A headache
D. An actual loss of consciousness

116. Where is cerebrospinal fluid formed in the brain?

A. In the lateral ventricles
B. In the third ventricle
C. In the fourth ventricle
D. In the foramen of Monroe

117. Henry is an 18 year old with Guillain-Barré syndrome. When you are teaching him about his condition, you explain that there are four variations of this disease. What are the four types of Guillain-Barré syndrome?

A. Ascending, progressive, relapsing–remitting, pure motor
B. Ascending, descending, Miller-Fischer variant, pure motor
C. Ascending, descending, relapsing, pure sensory
D. Ascending, relapsing–remitting, pure motor, pure sensory

118. How are tumors that arise in the brain different from other cancers?

A. There is no difference
B. They are not as aggressive as other tumors
C. They do not metastasize
D. Brain tumors are the most aggressive type of tumor

119. Your 11 year old patient suffered a severe head injury in a motor vehicle accident. She exhibits a downward deviation of both eyes. This most likely means the ________ is being compressed

A. Parietal area
B. Midbrain
C. Basal ganglia
D. Middle fossa

120. An infratentorial herniation that produces decerebrate posturing and small, reactive pupils is known as a

A. Midbrain compression
B. Cingulate herniation
C. Pontine compression
D. Central herniation

121. When a nerve is not conducting an impulse, this phase is known as the

A. Simple reflex
B. Polysynaptic reflex
C. Resting membrane potential
D. Monosynaptic phase

122. The response of a neuron to depolarization is called the

A. Action potential
B. The affector impulse
C. Polysynaptic reflex
D. Monosynaptic phase

123. Arterial circulation to the skin and muscle of the face and scalp (the extracerebral structures) is provided by the

A. Vertebral arteries
B. External carotid arteries
C. Internal carotid arteries
D. Posterior cerebral arteries

124. The basal ganglia and the lateral portion of the cerebral hemispheres are supplied with blood from the

A. Circle of Willis
B. Posterior cerebral arteries
C. Vertebral arteries
D. Middle cerebral artery

125. The primary respiratory and cardiac centers, along with the vasomotor centers, are controlled by the

A. Pons
B. Medulla oblongata
C. Midbrain
D. Reticular formation

126. The connective tissue layers that cover the brain are called meninges. The specific membrane that attaches directly to the roots of the spinal cord and brain is called the

A. Dura mater
B. Arachnoid
C. Choroid layer
D. Pia mater

127. Normal cerebral spinal fluid (CSF) flow in a toddler should be approximately ______ per hour

A. 3–5 mL
B. 10–15 mL
C. 5–10 mL
D. 15–20 mL

128. Hypoxia may cause cerebral edema. The type of edema that usually occurs in gray matter due to water quickly shifting into cells is known as

A. Cytotoxic edema
B. Intestinal edema
C. Vasogenic edema
D. Hypercellular edema

129. When a child suffers an arteriovenous malformation (AVM), the most common presenting symptom is

A. Severe headache
B. Spontaneous hemorrhage
C. Seizures
D. A cranial systolic bruit

130. Elliot is a 5 year old who has suffered a ruptured intracranial aneurysm. Because of the possibility of vasospasm, surgery has been postponed for a week. Elliot should be stable enough for surgery if he attains which of the following physiological parameters?

A. BP 70/40 mmHg, MAP 50 mmHg, PaO_2 80%
B. MAP < 80 mmHg, CVP 25 mmHg, BP $< 60/40$ mmHg
C. CPP > 70 mmHg, MAP > 70 mmHg, ICP < 20 mmHg
D. MAP > 50 mmHg, CVP 20 mmHg, CPP 40 mmHg

131. Your patient has been diagnosed with bacterial meningitis following a lumbar puncture and subsequent CSF analysis. CSF results for bacterial meningitis will show

A. Normal glucose levels
B. Normal or slightly increased protein levels
C. A slightly elevated WBC count
D. Decreased glucose

132. Which of the following statements is true about Becker muscular dystrophy (BMD)?

A. BMD is more severe than Duchenne muscular dystrophy (DMD)
B. BMD is not X-linked; DMD is X-linked
C. In BMD, children lose the ability to walk by the time they reach 20 or more years of age
D. Pseudohypertrophy of the calves is more prevalent in BMD than in DMD

133. Your patient has been diagnosed with Tourette syndrome. She often utters obscenities directed at the staff. This symptom of Tourette syndrome is called

A. Halopheria
B. Coprolalia
C. Sydenham chorea
D. Lacrea

134. A primary cause of an intracranial headache is

A. Tension
B. A subdural hematoma
C. A brain tumor
D. Meningitis

135. Absence seizures are characterized by

A. No postictal state
B. Discharge of neurons in one hemisphere
C. Loss of posture
D. Increased thoracic muscle tone

136. Bilateral cortical injury results in

A. Asymmetric responses
B. Flaccidity
C. Decerebrate posturing
D. Decorticate posturing

137. A decrease in facial strength indicates a lesion in

A. Cranial nerve III
B. Cranial nerve V
C. Cranial nerve VII
D. Cranial nerve IX

138. Bell's palsy is a viral inflammatory disease that causes demyelination of cranial nerve

A. V
B. VII
C. X
D. XII

139. The neurologist has been called to evaluate your patient for a possible brain tumor. The physician places a fork in the patient's hand and asks the patient to identify the object while the patient's eyes are closed. The physician is assessing

A. Kinesthetic sensation
B. Graphesthesia
C. Two-point discrimination
D. Stereognosis

140. Which of the following conditions would not be an extrapyramidal side effect of an antipsychotic medication?

A. Dystonia
B. Hallucinations
C. Hypertension
D. Akathisia

141. The ability to discriminate between sweet, sour, salt, and bitter tastes is known as

A. Agnosia
B. Anosmia
C. Hyposmia
D. Ageusia

142. Ella was admitted to the PICU for pain and paresthesias in her feet and hands. Her physician wanted her evaluated for Guillain-Barré syndrome. It is more likely that Ella is suffering from

A. Vitamin B_{12} deficiency
B. A thiamine deficiency
C. Vitamin E overdose
D. Vitamin A overdose

143. Jeffrey is 17 years old and has been diagnosed with trigeminal neuralgia (tic douloureux). He is scheduled for surgery in the morning. Although this condition usually appears later in life, Jeffrey has been suffering with the pain for the past two years. The surgical procedure Jeffrey will undergo is known as a

A. Surgical decompression
B. Fulton procedure
C. Trigeminal decompression
D. Rhizotomy

144. The Salter-Harris classification system is used to

A. Classify growth plate fractures
B. Classify types of seizures in children
C. Classify the severity of compartment syndrome in children
D. Classify the levels of nonstructural scoliosis

SECTION 7

Neurology Answers

1. **Correct answer: C**
   Most cases of scoliosis have a juvenile onset. Congenital scoliosis is an embryologic malformation. The first sign of scoliosis is usually uneven hips and shoulders. A severe form of scoliosis is characterized by a curve of greater than 40 degrees and will require a spinal fusion.

2. **Correct answer: A**
   The shunt may be occluded. This is a medical emergency. The neurosurgeon needs to be notified immediately. When any infant with a ventriculo-peritoneal shunt becomes lethargic, it means the shunt is not working for some reason and there is an increase in the ICP.

3. **Correct answer: D**
   The most common cause of acquired hydrocephalus is bacterial meningitis. Bacterial meningitis, which may be caused by several different organisms, can damage the CSF system, leading to an acquired hydrocephalus. While HIV infection can be spread to the neonate, it is not as common as bacterial meningitis. Idiopathic causes of hydrocephalus are congenital in nature. Maternal rubella infections cause deafness, cataracts, and cardiac disease.

4. **Correct answer: B**
   Common symptoms of hydrocephalus in a 4 month old infant would include macrocrania, rapid skull growth, and failure to thrive. Many symptoms are associated with hydrocephalus, including bulging fontanelles, split cranial sutures, apnea, bradycardia, distended scalp veins, failure to thrive, vomiting, drowsiness, Macewen's sign, head bobbing, and transcranial illumination.

5. **Correct answer: A**
   The symptoms of lethargy, tachycardia, and an increased temperature suggest the patient has an infection. Establishing the presence of an infection via CBC with differential, CRP and sedimentation rate is important. Antibiotics such as ceftazidime are used due to their broad-spectrum coverage. Cooling measures and acetaminophen are important to reduce the fever and, therefore, reduce the risk of febrile seizures. The other three options suggest administration of fluoroquinolones. These antibiotics have a narrow antibacterial spectrum and are not appropriate for this child.

6. **Correct answer: C**
   Syringomyelia is most often seen with Chiari II malformation. It creates cysts called syrinx that grow to produce long cavities within the spinal cord. These cavities damage the afferent spinal cord causing interruption of nerve conduction from the brain to the

extremities, which in turn results in weakness and pain. Chiari II malformation is best identified via MRI.

7. **Correct answer: A**
   Frequent neurologic checks are strongly recommended. Raising the HOB to 30 degrees promotes drainage of CSF, and placing the head at the midline position maintains optimal CSF drainage. It is imperative to notify the neurosurgeon at once if the patient experiences a change in the neurologic signs, especially if the baby becomes lethargic.

8. **Correct answer: A**
   The four nursing diagnoses of increased ICP, potential for inadequate oxygenation, potential for infection, and pain are the most appropriate for a baby with a new ventriculo-peritoneal shunt. There is at least one inappropriate option in all of the other answers.

9. **Correct answer: C**
   CMV (Cytomegaly virus) is the leading cause of hearing loss in children in the United States. CMV is a beta herpesvirus that can cause a myriad of neurologic problems for the neonate and children. CMV is the most common congenital infection in humans and it has the most serious sequelae.

10. **Correct answer: B**
    Macewen's sign is diagnostic for hydrocephalus. This sign can be elicited by tapping the junction of the frontal, parietal, and temporal lobes. A strong resonant sound is produced with hydrocephalus and is also seen in brain abscesses. Battle's sign consists of ecchymosis behind the ear over the mastoid area and is seen with a basilar skull fracture. Lhermitte's sign is a sudden neck pain produced with flexing of the neck. Trendelenberg's sign is associated with a hip abnormality, causing the pelvis to sag opposite the affected hip when the patient stands on one leg.

11. **Correct answer: C**
    Among children younger than 5 years of age, nonaccidental trauma and near-drowning are the two most common reasons for a comatose state. Nearly 6 million cases of child abuse are reported each year in the United States, according to Child Help. In children older than 5 years of age, the most common causes of coma are drug overdose and accidental head injury.

12. **Correct answer: B**
    The drugs most commonly identified in children who overdose and may become comatose are those readily found in the home. These substances may include atropine, scopolamine, benzodiazepines, barbiturates, ethanol, lithium, opiates, and tricyclic antidepressants. Drugs such as phencyclidine piperidine (PCP), cocaine, diet pills, and lysergic acid diethylamide (LSD) cause agitated behaviors and hallucinations.

13. **Correct answer: B**
    The Pediatric Glasgow Coma Scale (GCS) is commonly used to assess a patient's neurologic status. It also gives clues about survivability. The scale assesses the patient's ability to open their eyes spontaneously, to react to voice commands, to react to painful stimuli, or not to react at all. The motor response tests the patient's ability to follow commands, localize to pain, flexion withdraw from pain, demonstrate decorticate or decerebrate posturing, or show no response to pain. The verbal response assesses orien-

tation or appropriateness or responses, disorientation, inappropriate speech, incomprehensible words, or no response. The lower the GCS score, the worse the outlook for the patient. A consistent score of 6–7 indicates coma.

14. **Correct answer: C**
    Battle's sign is indicative of a fracture of the middle fossa. It is seen as ecchymosis over the mastoid bone and appears 12–24 hours after the injury. Rhinorrhea, raccoon's eyes, and subconjunctival hemorrhage are signs of an anterior fossa fracture.

15. **Correct answer: C**
    Level of consciousness is the most sensitive indicator of neurologic status in a patient. The brain tissue is extremely sensitive to even minute changes in oxygen and glucose levels. When cerebral edema occurs, as in a closed head injury, these levels very quickly affect the level of consciousness of a patient.

16. **Correct answer: A**
    The halo sign is indicative of a basilar skull fracture. This leakage of fluid may be a dangerous sign for the patient, as meningitis can easily develop due to a pathway that allows bacteria to invade from the oropharynx.

17. **Correct answer: B**
    The most accurate method of measuring intracranial pressure is placement of an intraventriculostomy. Because the catheter is inserted directly into one of the lateral ventricles, it is the most direct and accurate method of measuring intracranial pressure. The drain is inserted on the right side of the head. The ventriculostomy allows for not only drainage of excess CSF, but also sampling of CSF to monitor the patient for infection.

18. **Correct answer: B**
    Normal intracranial pressure for a young child is 3–7 mmHg. Sustained intracranial pressures greater than 10 mmHg may lead to severe neurologic damage or herniation.

19. **Correct answer: B**
    The myelin sheath is produced by oligodendrocytes in the brain and Schwann cells in the peripheral nervous system. Myelin is responsible for the rapidity with which nerve impulses move from neuron to neuron and from the brain to the spinal cord. Impulses can travel as fast as 25,000 miles per second along an axon coated with myelin. This phenomenon explains why diseases that destroy myelin, such as multiple sclerosis, affect mobility.

20. **Correct answer: A**
    Increased systolic blood pressure, widening pulse pressure, and bradycardia are symptoms of Cushing syndrome (also known as Cushing's triad). These symptoms are late indicators of a serious deterioration of neurologic status. This patient is at very high risk for herniation and imminent death.

21. **Correct answer: D**
    Lumbar puncture in a patient with increased intracranial pressure can lead to herniation of the tentorium or brain stem and, subsequently, death.

22. **Correct answer: C**
Cerebrospinal fluid absorbed at an increased rate decreases intracranial pressure. CO_2 retention, a PaO_2 less than 50 mmHg, and increased metabolic activity contribute to increased intracranial pressure.

23. **Correct answer: C**
The most important indicator of neurologic deterioration in this patient is his level of consciousness. Level of consciousness changes are seen before other symptoms develop because the cerebral cortex is extremely sensitive to oxygen pressure changes. Signs of this change may be subtle at first, such as mild confusion.

24. **Correct answer: C**
Trevor probably has diabetes insipidus. Diabetes insipidus (DI) is a serious decrease in antidiuretic hormone (ADH). The most common causes of neurogenic DI are closed head injury and posterior pituitary tumor removal. ADH is produced by the posterior pituitary gland. Closed head injury and cerebral edema place increased pressure on the pituitary gland, which in turn decreases ADH production. Other common causes of DI are lung cancer (small- or oat-cell carcinoma), leukemia, and lymphoma. Try to think of the patient with diabetes insipidus (DI) as the opposite of a patient with the syndrome of inappropriate antidiuretic hormone (SIADH): DI is "dry." SIADH is "wet."

25. **Correct answer: B**
Treatment of diabetes insipidus usually includes intravenous replacement with D_5W/ ½ NS and 20 mEq of potassium, titrated to replace hourly urine output. Other therapies include DDAVP (desmopressin) nasal spray or a pitressin infusion. Strict I&O and daily weights, monitoring electrolytes, and monitoring serum and urine osmolalities are additional possible nursing actions.

26. **Correct answer: C**
Seizure activity should be stopped in a patient with status epilepticus because continued seizures deplete glucose and oxygen in the brain. The hypoxia causes cerebral edema, and the increased lactic acidosis can lead to damage of the neurons.

27. **Correct answer: B**
The correct formula for cerebral perfusion pressure is CPP = MAP – ICP. Cerebral perfusion pressure is a calculated measurement of the pressure gradient that allows blood to flow to the brain. The goal is a CPP of 50–80 mmHg. The CPP may also be calculated using the CVP instead of the ICP, because it is a measure of vascular resistance.

28. **Correct answer: A**
The ideal range of CPP for a 4 year old child is 50–60 mmHg. This value actually applies to all children in the 2 to 4 year old age range. In children, the CPP goal is 40–70 mmHg, and the goal ranges are higher in older children and teens. The CPP may also be calculated using the CVP instead of the ICP, because it is a measure of vascular resistance.

29. **Correct answer: A**
The cranial nerves affected by a basilar skull fracture are CN I, VII, and VIII. Cranial nerve I, the olfactory nerve, is the most frequently affected cranial nerve in a basilar skull fracture and leads to a loss of sense of smell. CN VII (facial nerve) and CN VIII (acoustic nerve) are less likely to be affected unless the patient experiences a severe

head injury. CN VII (facial nerve) injury causes ipsilateral or same-side paralysis. CN VIII (acoustic nerve) injury can interrupt balance and hearing.

30. **Correct answer: C**
Nystagmus is a rhythmic tremor or shaking of the eyes. Nystagmus indicates pressure or damage to cranial nerve VIII (acoustic) in the vestibular portion. Shaking is usually stronger on one side and may occur in any of the cardinal eye directions.

31. **Correct answer: A**
Syndrome of inappropriate antidiuretic hormone (SIADH) has many causes. The most common causes include bronchogenic (oat-cell) cancer, pneumonia, and head injury. Other less common causes include stroke, tuberculosis, Guillain-Barré syndrome, meningitis, encephalitis, multiple sclerosis, subarachnoid hemorrhage, pancreatic cancer, and lymphoma. The patient with SIADH produces very little urine and can quickly become fluid overloaded. Therefore, the SIADH patient is "wet," while the patient with diabetes insipidus is "dry" due to their high urine output.

32. **Correct answer: D**
The knee jerk, also known as the patellar reflex, demonstrates a functional lower motor neuron. Such reflexes are also known as deep tendon reflexes. The nerve impulse makes an arc from the tendon to the sensory portion of the spinal cord to the motor root and back to the patella, causing extension of the lower leg.

33. **Correct answer: C**
The spinothalamic tract is tested by a pinprick or monofilament sensation. The spinothalamic tract carries impulses from the spine to the thalamus. Thus it is a sensory motor tract. The lateral spinothalamic senses pain and temperature, whereas the anterior tract senses light touch and pressure. The spinal tracts can be identified by their names—for example, in *spinothalamic,* "spino" means the tract starts in the spinal cord and "thalamic" means it terminates in the thalamus. Likewise, a *cerebrospinal* tract goes from the cerebral cortex to the spinal cord.

34. **Correct answer: B**
Autonomic hyperreflexia is a malfunction of the autonomic nervous system seen with spinal cord injury. This potentially life-threatening response to minor stimuli is seen after spinal cord injury at T6 or higher. It occurs after the initial spinal shock has resolved. Symptoms can include severe hypertension, dysrhythmias, severe headache, and photophobia.

35. **Correct answer: B**
Treatment for SIADH includes fluid restriction, diuretics, sodium replacement, and declomycin. Because SIADH causes hemodilution, its treatment centers on normalizing serum and urine osmolality.

36. **Correct answer: B**
The normal Doll's Eyes, or oculocephalic reflex, results in the eyes appearing to move to the opposite direction from the head turn. For example, if the head is turned quickly to the patient's left, the eyes normally appear to move to the far right side. If the reflex is absent, the eyes appear fixed and do not move. This is a poor neurologic sign, which indicates the presence of pontine and midbrain damage. This test may be utilized in determining brain death.

37. **Correct answer: C**
If Melanie was exhibiting decerebrate posturing, you would observe both arms fully extended and internally rotated and both legs fully extended with toes pointed. Decerebrate posturing demonstrates pressure on the midbrain and pons. It is a very poor neurologic sign, especially if it continues for more than 4 hours. The neurologist needs to be notified at once of this change in the patient's status.

38. **Correct answer: D**
Brown-Sequard syndrome causes ipsilateral (same-side) motor paralysis and contralateral (opposite-side) loss of pain and temperature sensation. This syndrome occurs because of the way the pyramidal tracts cross in the spinal column. Grey-Turner syndrome consists of flank ecchymosis and is seen with pancreatitis. Cushing syndrome is seen with chronic high cortisol levels. Syndrome X is a term used in the past to describe prediabetes.

39. **Correct answer: B**
Ipsilateral (same-side) pupil dilation is the symptom seen with uncal herniation across the tentorium. The tentorium is a fold of dura mater that supports the temporal and occipital lobes. Herniation puts pressure directly on CN III, causing pupil dilation. This is a very poor sign with regard to the patient's survival.

40. **Correct answer: B**
Neisseria meningitidis is the causative agent for meningococcal meningitis. *Streptococcus pneumoniae* causes pneumococcal meningitis. *Haemophilius influenzae* causes *Haemophilius* meningitis. *Staphylococcus aureus* is not likely to cause meningitis but can cause infection in the brain if the patient has had ventriculostomy drains or bolts placed there.

41. **Correct answer: B**
Common risk factors for the development of meningococcal meningitis are young age, decreased immune status (such as after a splenectomy or with HIV infection), and close living quarters. Lack of immunization puts children of any age at risk for meningococcal meningitis. Outbreaks are often seen in school dormitories, especially among those children who have not received the proper immunizations, such as meningococcal conjugate vaccine (MCV4).

42. **Correct answer: B**
Petechiae are the hallmark symptom of meningococcal meningitis. The other symptoms can be seen with any form of meningitis.

43. **Correct answer: A**
Guillain-Barré syndrome is a demyelenating autoimmune process that affects the spinal and cranial nerves. It is seen after viral infections. The most common form is the ascending variety, which is associated with bilateral ascending weakness. The myelin helps transmit motor responses at a speed of 25,000 miles per second from the brain. In Guillain-Barré syndrome, the myelin is interrupted or destroyed, causing loss of motor function. The severity of GBS may vary from mild symptoms that resolve in a few days to complete loss of motor function including the cranial nerves and respiratory muscles. It can take many months to years for GBS to resolve, and in a few cases the patients may experience residual neurologic deficits. The patient with GBS does not lose sensory functioning and may have a great deal of pain.

44. **Correct answer: C**
A positive Babinski or plantar reflex is a sign of an upper motor neuron lesion in children who are older than 6 years of age. Prior to the child reaching 6 years of age, the nervous system has not fully matured and the Babinski reflex elicited may be positive without being a pathologic sign. In contrast, a positive Babinski or plantar reflex in an older child may be seen with spinal cord compression, head injury, and stroke. It is a pathologic sign.

45. **Correct answer: B**
The proper technique to elicit a Babinski response is to follow the lateral sole of the foot from the heel up to and across the ball of the foot. It should be done in one motion with a relatively sharp instrument such as the end of a reflex hammer.

46. **Correct answer: B**
Ventriculo-peritoneal (VP) shunts are placed via a burr hole on the right parieto-occipital side because the left side is too near the speech comprehension center (Wernicke's area). The personality center is located in the frontal (judgment) and temporal (intellectual and emotional functions) lobes. The VP shunt is inserted into the right anterior horn, not the posterior horn.

47. **Correct answer: C**
The cerebral spinal fluid should be clear and colorless, with a protein count of 16–45 mg/dL. The WBC count should be 0–5 cells/mm2, and the glucose level is approximately 80% of serum glucose.

48. **Correct answer: B**
The six cardinal eye movements test CN III (oculomotor), CN IV (trochlear), and CN VI (abducens). CN III is assessed by having the patient follow the examiner's finger or a light up and out, up and in, down and out, and inward toward the nose. CN IV is assessed by having the patient follow the examiner's finger down and in toward the tip of the nose. CN VI is assessed by following the examiner's finger out toward the ear.

49. **Correct answer: D**
The most common cause of hemorrhagic stroke in children is an arteriovenous malformation (AVM). Other family members should be evaluated for AVM as well, because this condition may be caused by an inherited trait.

50. **Correct answer: B**
Prevention of aspiration should be the priority of the pediatric ICU nurse. The other answers are also part of caring for a patient with a cerebrovascular accident, but the ABCs (airway, breathing, circulation) are always the first priority.

51. **Correct answer: B**
Broca's area, which is located at the lower edge of the frontal lobe, is responsible for verbal expression. A deficit in this area produces expressive aphasia, in which the patient can comprehend what is said but lacks the ability to form the words due to loss of motor skills.

52. **Correct answer: D**
The homunculus is the outer strip of the cerebral cortex, which governs the motor functioning of the frontal lobe and the sensory functioning of the parietal lobe. It demonstrates how much of the cortex controls each body part. For example, in the

parietal lobe, very large sections of the cortex are devoted to the face, hands, and feet due to the complexity of the sensations necessary for protection. In the frontal lobe, a larger portion of the motor cortex is devoted to the face, hands, and tongue.

53. **Correct answer: B**
The most important parameter to monitor in a patient with Guillain-Barré syndrome is the negative inspiratory force. The negative inspiratory force measures the ability of the patient to take a deep breath to minus 28 mmHg. Once the effort is less than 28 mmHg, the patient should be evaluated for possible intubation to prevent respiratory arrest.

54. **Correct answer: B**
Protein in the CSF is always increased with Guillain-Barré syndrome due to the destruction of the myelin sheath. Because Guillain-Barré syndrome is an autoimmune disorder, WBCs, abnormal glucose levels, and bacteria would not be expected in the CSF.

55. **Correct answer: A**
The most appropriate nursing diagnoses would be impaired motor weakness, impaired respiratory function, and acute pain. Patients with Guillain-Barré syndrome experience motor weakness due to the loss of the myelin sheath. Loss of motor function leads to impaired respiratory function. Many patients with Guillain-Barré syndrome have acute pain due to the increased sensitivity of the sympathetic nervous system.

56. **Correct answer: C**
Autonomic dysfunction in Guillain-Barré syndrome is caused by lack of balance in the autonomic nervous system. The sympathetic nervous system is unopposed, which leads to heightened sensitivity and overresponse to even minor stimuli.

57. **Correct answer: B**
Respiratory status and neurologic signs are the most important nursing management issues, especially in the early onset of the demyelination process. It is imperative to protect the airway in these patients, because the symptoms may advance quickly, requiring mechanical ventilation. Monitoring the neurologic and respiratory status will also indicate the recovery status of the patient with Guillain-Barré.

58. **Correct answer: B**
A relative contraindication for administration of methylprednisolone following a spinal injury would be pregnancy. Additional relative contraindications would be an injury more than 8 hours old, mediation allergy, and uncontrolled diabetes mellitus.

59. **Correct answer: A**
The symptoms of spinal shock include areflexia, autonomic dysfunction, loss of sensation, and eliminatory dysfunction. Spinal shock occurs hours to weeks after a cord injury causing autonomic loss, and the severity of a spinal cord injury cannot be fully assessed until the shock has resolved. The level of function for a patient with a spinal cord injury to T8 would include no abdominal reflexes and spastic paraplegia of the lower limbs, but the patient could still be functionally independent.

60. **Correct answer: B**
Neurogenic shock is a much more severe form of shock that may occur with spinal cord injuries at or above T6. The autonomic dysfunction produces an increased vagal

tone, which results in severe bradycardia, decreased cardiac output, peripheral dilatation. and decreased SVR.

61. **Correct answer: C**
AVMs are the most common cause of stroke in children younger than 12 years of age. AVMs are a complex tangle of misshapen blood vessels. The AVMs lack the normal blood pathway from arterial to venous flow without going through a capillary bed. The resulting high-pressure flow makes them more likely to bleed. While AVMs are not common, they occur slightly more often in men than in women. The other family members should be assessed for the presence of an AVM, as this condition is associated with an inherited trait.

62. **Correct answer: D**
Spinal reflexes indicate functional lower motor neurons. For example, the knee jerk, also known as the patellar reflex, demonstrates a functional lower motor neuron. Such reflexes are also known as deep tendon reflexes. The nerve impulse makes an arc from the tendon to the sensory portion of the spinal cord to the motor root and back to the patella, causing extension of the lower leg.

63. **Correct answer: A**
A sympathetic response to a stimulus results in heightened awareness, increased blood pressure, bronchial constriction, and increased glucogenosis. There are many responses to sympathetic stimuli as the body prepares for "flight, fright, or fight." Additional responses are dilated pupils (for increased visual acuity), increased heart rate, increased myocardial contractility, increased blood pressure, increased respiratory rate, decreased gastric motility, and decreased gastric secretion. Decreased urine output, decreased insulin production, and decreased renal blood flow also occur.

64. **Correct answer: B**
Approximately 85% of cerebral aneurysms are located at the anterior bifurcations of the Circle of Willis, and 15% at the posterior bifurcations. Cerebral aneurysms are often caused by a familial trait. Any family members who have severe headaches or visual disturbances should be evaluated for aneurysms.

65. **Correct answer: D**
An explosive headache is the most common symptom of a ruptured cerebral aneurysm. Frequently, the last thing patients say before losing consciousness is how bad the headache feels, describing it as "the worst headache of my life." It is the sudden onset and severity of the headache that is the clue to this emergent problem.

66. **Correct answer: B**
Glasgow Coma Scale assessment is imperative in monitoring for vascular spasm, a potentially life-threatening problem for a patient with a cerebral aneurysm. Vascular spasm occurs secondary to meningeal irritation from the blood in the subarachnoid space. The earliest sign of vasospasm is a change in the level of consciousness in the patient.

67. **Correct answer: A**
Clinical signs of ataxia include refusal to walk, nystagmus, and the patient is afebrile. Acute cerebral ataxia in children often occurs after an infection, including influenza and chickenpox. This form of ataxia rarely attacks children older than 10 years of age

and is more common in children in the 18 month to 7 year range. Immunizations do not cause acute cerebral ataxia, as they contain mostly dead viruses. A CT scan of the head is imperative to rule out other causes, such as cerebral tumor or hemorrhage.

68. **Correct answer: B**
The symptoms of Tourette syndrome often fade as the child ages. Tourette syndrome is often managed with antipsychotic medications such as Pimozide if the tics are disabling or interfere with learning. This condition is often seen in conjunction with attention-deficit disorder (ADD) or attention-deficit/hyperactivity disorder (ADHD).

69. **Correct answer: C**
A CT scan or MRI should be done early in Dasan's evaluation to rule out a mass such as a tumor. This child most likely has a brain abscess as a result of his untreated otitis media. The focal neurologic deficits make it dangerous to start diagnostic testing with a lumbar puncture. If Dasan's ICP is elevated, a lumbar puncture could result in herniation and death. Brain abscesses may be seen following infections involving the ears or sinuses, including the mastoid area. In older children, the abscess may be caused by snorting drugs such as cocaine. If left untreated, a brain abscess often leads to death either from the infection itself or from herniation of the brain tissue. Surgical removal of brain abscesses has a low overall mortality rate.

70. **Correct answer: B**
Astrocytoma is the most common form of pediatric brain tumor, followed by medulloblastoma. Lymphoma is not a form of brain tumor. While metastatic bone cancer can certainly lead to a mass in the brain, it is not a primary site.

71. **Correct answer: A**
Communicating hydrocephalus is the most common sequela after a subarachnoid hemorrhage (SAH). This type of hemorrhage moves through the subarachnoid space, where it may clog the arachnoid villi, preventing absorption of cerebrospinal fluid. This condition may be permanent, requiring placement of a ventriculo-peritoneal shunt.

72. **Correct answer: D**
Cranial nerve I (olfactory) is most commonly injured with a basilar skull fracture, causing the patient to lose his or her sense of smell. Cranial nerve VII (facial) may also be injured, causing ipsilateral facial paralysis. If cranial nerve VIII (vestibulocochlear) is injured, hearing and equilibrium may be impaired.

73. **Correct answer: B**
Ipsilateral (same-side) pupil dilation is evidence of increasing ICP in the lateral middle fossa of the brain, creating a shift in the temporal lobe. This area contains the uncus, which is forced through the dura mater that supports the temporal lobe. The herniation catches cranial nerve III (oculomotor) and the posterior cerebral artery on the same side as the lesion.

74. **Correct answer: B**
The Tensilon test is the "gold standard" for diagnosing myasthenia gravis. Tensilon is a rapid-acting cholinesterase inhibitor that improves motor impulses. In this case, the ptosis would resolve briefly. Myasthenia gravis in children has a high remission rate when a thymectomy is performed.

75. **Correct answer: A**
Purple glove syndrome is a potential complication of phenytoin administration that can lead to fasciotomy or amputation of a limb.

76. **Correct answer: C**
Topiramate (Topamax) is used to treat partial seizures. Partial seizures are localized seizures that may last anywhere from a few seconds to minutes, during which the patient is conscious. The symptoms may be motor or sensory in nature. In the Jacksonian march, the seizure progresses to another part of the body in a predictable progression. In complex partial seizures, the patient loses consciousness.

77. **Correct answer: C**
The patient who experiences a partial seizure does not lose consciousness, nor does he or she go into a postictal state. In some other types of partial seizures, such as complex partial seizeure, the patient loses consciousness for a short period of time.

78. **Correct answer: B**
Febrile seizures are the type of seizure most likely to occur in children between 6 months and 6 years of age. They are usually seen in children with no prior history of febrile seizures, central nervous system infection, or inflammation. The seizures may last 15 minutes or longer.

79. **Correct answer: D**
Triptans are not recommended in children younger than 18 years of age. Nonsteroidal anti-inflammatory drugs are most commonly used to treat childhood migraines.

80. **Correct answer: C**
All of the medications in this class, such as Adderall, (amphetamines) are contraindicated in this situation. Amphetamine use can lead to increased blood pressure, tachyarrhythmias, and even sudden cardiac death.

81. **Correct answer: C**
Mannitol is a powerful osmotic diuretic. It can induce cardiovascular collapse if given too quickly. Mannitol is always given via the in-line 5-micron filter over 20–30 minutes or a time appropriate for the patient's age.

82. **Correct answer: A**
Phenobarbital should be given as a slow intravenous push at a rate less than 30 milligrams per minute. Rapid infusion may lead to extravasation and tissue destruction.

83. **Correct answer: D**
Airway protection is the highest priority in teaching and in practice. Nothing should ever be placed in the mouth of a patient who is experiencing a seizure. While it may be necessary to call 911 during a seizure, 911 operators do not need to be notified each time Tess has a seizure. Birth control pills are contraindicated with antiepileptic drugs, as they may lower the seizure threshold.

84. **Correct answer: B**
You should explain that the term coup-contra-coup brain injury is a complicated brain injury that may have lasting effects. A coup-contra-coup brain injury is a complex injury that may have lasting effects such as chronic headaches, seizures, and memory

or personality difficulties. The brain is injured in two or more areas, with secondary injury resulting from the ensuing cerebral edema.

85. **Correct answer: D**
Ataxia is not a symptom of a cerebellar tumor. Cerebellar tumors do cause nystagmus, truncal ataxia, and impaired coordination and balance.

86. **Correct answer: A**
Deep cerebral hemispheric tumors cause hemiplegia and visual field defects.

87. **Correct answer: C**
The type of supratentorial tumor that causes metabolic dysfunctions, eating dysfunctions, and autonomic seizures is known as a sella-turcica area tumor.

88. **Correct answer: C**
The type of hydrocephalus that results from a loss of brain parenchyma is known as hydrocephalus ex vacuo.

89. **Correct answer: D**
Separation of cranial sutures may occur in infants and children and is known as diastasis. If this type of fracture is accompanied by a dural tear, the separation may progress to a larger fracture.

90. **Correct answer: B**
Blood collection behind the tympanic membrane in a patient post head injury indicates a temporal bone fracture. If the dura mater is also torn, CSF may leak out of the patient's ear.

91. **Correct answer: B**
Anosmia is a loss of the sense of smell because of damage to the olfactory nerve.

92. **Correct answer: C**
Inequality of pupils greater than a 1-mm difference is known as anisocoria. Some people normally have unequal pupils, however, they usually demonstrate less than a 1-mm difference.

93. **Correct answer: D**
An injury to the sacral cord and lumbar nerve roots resulting in areflexia of the lower limbs, bowel, and bladder is known as conus medullaris.

94. **Correct answer: A**
Depressed skull fractures in infants may result in indentation or pliable skull bone(s) without loss of bone integrity, a phenomenon known as a "Ping-Pong" depression.

95. **Correct answer: D**
A mycotic aneurysm results from a bacterial embolic arteritis. A fusiform aneurysm is the result of atherosclerotic changes. A saccular aneurysm is a berry aneurysm.

96. **Correct answer: B**
An epidural catheter is the type of ICP monitoring device that is inserted below the skull and above the dura mater.

97. **Correct answer: C**
The P_2 wave on a normal ICP waveform represents decreased intracranial compliance.

98. **Correct answer: D**
B waves on an abnormal ICP waveform are related to respirations. B waves may occur during a headache, when there is a decreased level of consciousness, or posturing. B waves may actually precede A waves if the patient is seizing.

99. **Correct answer: D**
Sustained, rapid, and moderately deep hyperpnea is known as central neurogenic hyperventilation. It is unknown exactly how this mechanism functions.

100. **Correct answer: D**
Pyrogenic respirations are a completely irregular breathing pattern with deep and shallow breaths.

101. **Correct answer: B**
Normal ICP in children is 3–7.5 mmHg. Normal ICP in newborns is 0.7–1.5 mmHg. In infants, the normal ICP is 1.5–6 mmHg. In an adult, the ICP should be less than 10 mmHg.

102. **Correct answer: D**
Approximately 20% of cardiac output is delivered to the brain of an older child.

103. **Correct answer: A**
A moderate reduction in alertness, increased sleeping, and decreased interest in the environment is called obtundation.

104. **Correct answer: C**
A child who is unresponsive except to repeated stimuli is stuporous.

105. **Correct answer: C**
Jugular venous oxygen saturation (SjO_2) is used to measure the balance between cerebral oxygen delivery and cerebral oxygen consumption.

106. **Correct answer: A**
The normal range for SjO_2 is between 60% and 75%.

107. **Correct answer: A**
SjO_2 monitoring should be used for patients who are older than age 8 or who weigh at least 30 kg. SjO_2 monitoring is used in conjunction with ICP or CPP monitoring. SjO_2 values may be abnormally high in patients with nonviable brain tissue, because nonviable brain tissue does not abstract oxygen. The SjO_2 catheter should be calibrated at regular intervals with venous blood gas analysis.

108. **Correct answer: C**
The intravenous fluid of choice to help lower cerebral hypertension is 3% saline. The 3% saline is usually administered as a continuous infusion at a rate between 0.1 mL and 1 mL/kg of body weight per hour. You should use the lowest dose necessary to maintain the ICP below 20 mmHg.

109. **Correct answer: D**
The long-term effects of anticonvulsive therapy with phenytoin include gingival hyperplasia, in addition to ataxia, nystagmus, lymphadenopathy, rickets, and folate deficiency.

110. **Correct answer: C**
An arteriovenous malformation is an abnormal connection between arteries and veins with no common capillary bed.

111. **Correct answer: B**
A grade III periventricular intraventricular hemorrhage is an intraventricular hemorrhage with ventricular dilation. This classification of bleeding is used to assess both the amount of bleeding and the location of the bleeding.

112. **Correct answer: D**
A salutatory syndrome is a very subtle deterioration that may occur over a period of hours to days. The patient may exhibit a decrease in the hematocrit, a decrease in the level of consciousness, hypotonia, abnormal eye movements, and altered spontaneous movements.

113. **Correct answer: A**
A patient with stage II Reye syndrome will present with stupor, agitation, and delirium.

114. **Correct answer: C**
Patients who sustain spinal injuries above T1 are at risk for impaired temperature regulation. With this type of injury, the connection between the hypothalamus and the sympathetic outflow of the spinal cord is lost.

115. **Correct answer: A**
Incontinence occurs only very rarely with syncope. A sense of an impending loss of consciousness, an actual loss of consciousness, and a headache can be associated with both conditions. Additional signs and symptoms of a prodromal period, including nausea, diaphoresis, and pallor, are common to both conditions. Recovery is usually rapid with syncope, and the child often feels fatigued.

116. **Correct answer: A**
Cerebral spinal fluid (CSF) is primarily produced by the choroid plexus of the lateral ventricles. The CSF flows through the foramen of Monroe, into the third ventricle, through the aqueduct of Sylvius. It next flows into the fourth ventricle, then through the foramen of Luschka and Magendie. The fluid bathes the spinal cord and brain before returning to the ventricular cisterns and subarachnoid space before being reabsorbed by the arachnoid villi.

117. **Correct answer: B**
Ascending, descending, Miller-Fischer variant, and pure motor are the four types of Guillain-Barré syndrome. Ascending GBS is the classic form, consisting of weakness and numbness that starts in the legs and moves up the trunk to involve the cranial nerves in some patients. The weakness is symmetrical. The descending type affects the cranial nerves first and the weakness progresses caudally. Respiratory failure is a major problem for these patients. The Miller-Fischer variant is a very rare form of GBS characterized by a triad of symptoms—ophthalmoplegia, areflexia, and pronounced ataxia. The pure motor form of Guillain-Barré is identical to ascending GBS, except there is limited sensory involvement and, therefore, no pain.

118. Correct answer: C

Brain tumors, including those arising from the glial cells, do not metastasize to other organs. Conversely, lung, breast, stomach, pancreas, lower GI tract, and kidney tumors easily metastasize to the brain.

119. Correct answer: B

Downward deviation of both eyes post head injury likely means the midbrain is being compressed.

120. Correct answer: C

An infratentorial herniation that produces decerebrate posturing and small, reactive pupils is known as a pontine compression.

121. Correct answer: C

When a nerve is not conducting an impulse, the phase is known as the resting membrane potential. During this phase, the intracellular fluid contained in a neuron is more negatively charged than the extracellular fluid. The intracellular fluid contains high levels of K^+, and the intracellular fluid contains high levels of Na^+ and Cl^-.

122. Correct answer: A

The action potential represents the response of a neuron to depolarization.

123. Correct answer: B

Arterial circulation to the skin and muscle of the face and scalp (the extracerebral structures) is provided by the external carotid arteries.

124. Correct answer: D

The basal ganglia and the lateral portion of the cerebral hemispheres are supplied with blood by the middle cerebral artery.

125. Correct answer: B

The primary respiratory and cardiac centers, along with the vasomotor centers, are controlled by the medulla oblongata.

126. Correct answer: D

The specific membrane that attaches directly to the roots of the spinal cord and brain is the pia mater. The pia mater is vascular, unlike the arachnoid and dura mater.

127. Correct answer: A

Normal cerebral spinal fluid (CSF) flow should be approximately 3–5 mL/hr in a toddler and 10–15 mL/hr in an adolescent.

128. Correct answer: A

The type of edema that usually occurs in gray matter due to water quickly shifting into cells is known as cytotoxic edema.

129. Correct answer: B

When a child suffers an arteriovenous malformation (AVM), the most common presenting symptom is spontaneous hemorrhage.

130. Correct answer: C

Elliot should be stable enough for surgery if he attains the following physiological parameters: CPP < 70 mmHg, MAP > 70 mmHg, and ICP < 20 mmHg.

131. **Correct answer: D**
CSF results for bacterial meningitis will show a decreased glucose level.

132. **Correct answer: C**
In BMD, children lose the ability to walk by the time they reach 20 years of age or older. In DMD, children lose the ability to walk by about 10 years of age. Both types of dystrophy are X-linked. Pseudohypertrophy of the calves is more prevalent in DMD. This condition occurs when excess lipids replace degenerating muscle fibers.

133. **Correct answer: B**
Uttering obscenities is known as coprolalia. Sydenham chorea is another term for St. Vitus's dance. The other terms are not medical conditions.

134. **Correct answer: A**
Primary causes of an intracranial headache include tension, a cluster headache, and migraine (muscle or dysfunctional neurons). Secondary causes of headaches include meningeal irritation and increased ICP.

135. **Correct answer: A**
Absence seizures are characterized by the lack of a postictal state. The seizures last less than 15 seconds and there is no loss of posture. A discharge of neurons in one hemisphere causes focal (partial) seizures.

136. **Correct answer: D**
Bilateral cortical injury results in decorticate posturing. This condition is manifested by the patient extending the legs and flexing the arms.

137. **Correct answer: C**
A decrease in facial strength indicates a lesion in cranial nerve VII.

138. **Correct answer: B**
Bell's palsy is a viral inflammatory disease that causes demyelination of cranial nerve VII. This condition also causes loss of the ability to chew and unilateral loss of facial expression.

139. **Correct answer: D**
The neurologist is assessing the patient for stereognosis—the ability to recognize objects by touching and manipulating them. Graphesthesia is the ability of a patient to identify letters or numbers written on each palm with a blunt object. Kinesthetic sensation is the ability to recognize which position one or more parts of the body are in when the eyes are closed.

140. **Correct answer: B**
Hallucinations would not be an extrapyramidal side effect of an antipsychotic medication. Dystonia is a spasm or involuntary muscle movement, most often involving the arms, legs, face, and neck. Akathisia means that the patient is restless or fidgets.

141. **Correct answer: D**
The ability to discriminate between sweet, sour, salt, and bitter tastes is known as ageusia. Agnosia is the ability to discriminate sensory stimuli. Anosmia is the term for a patient's inability to smell. Hyposmia means a diminished sense of smell.

142. Correct answer: A

Ella has pain in her hands and feet as well as paresthesias. These symptoms are most likely due to a vitamin B_{12} deficiency.

143. Correct answer: D

Jeffrey will undergo a rhizotomy, in which the nerve root of the trigeminal nerve will be severed.

144. Correct answer: A

The Salter-Harris classification system is used to classify growth plate fractures in children. Nine types of fractures are addressed within this classification system.

NEUROLOGY REFERENCES

Aehlert, B. (Ed.). (2005). *Comprehensive pediatric emergency care*. St. Louis, MO: Mosby.

Afi, S., Diaz-Arrastia, R., Madden, C., et al. (2008). Intracranial pressure monitoring in brain-injured patients is associated with worsening of survival. *Journal of Trauma, 64,* 335–340.

Akbar, M., Bresch, B., Seyler, T. M., Wenz, W., Bruckner, T., Abel, R., & Carstens, C. (2009). Management of orthopaedic sequelae of congenital spinal disorders. *Journal of Bone & Joint Surgery, 91*(suppl 6), 87–100.

Akopian, G., Gaspard, D. J., & Alexander, M. (2007). Outcomes of blunt head trauma without intracranial pressure monitoring. *American Surgeon, 73*(5), 447–450.

Ali, M., Khan, A., Khan, H., & Khwanzada, K. (2009). Short-term complications of ventriculo-peritoeal shunt in children suffering from hydrocephalus. *Journal of Pediatric Neurology, 7*(2), 165–169.

Alspach, J. G. (2006). *American Association of Critical-Care Nurses: Core curriculum for critical care nursing* (6th ed.). Philadelphia: W. B. Saunders.

American Association of Neurological Nurses. (2006). Guide to the care of the patient with craniotomy post-brain tumor resection. AANN reference series for clinical practice. Retrieved September 12, 2010, from http://www.aacn.org

American Heart Association. (2010). Guidelines 2010 for cardiopulmonary resuscitation and emergency cardiovascular care. Retrieved from www.americanheart.org

Arts, M. P., & de Jong, T. H. R. (2004). Thoracic meningocele, meningomyelocele or myelocystocele? Diagnostic difficulties, consequent implications and treatment. *Pediatric Neurosurgery, 40*(2), 75–79.

Bader, M. K., & Littlejohns, L. R. (2004). *AANN core curriculum for neuroscience nursing* (4th ed.). St. Louis, MO: Saunders.

Barker, E. (Ed.) (2002). *Neuroscience nursing: A spectrum of care* (2nd ed.). St. Louis, MO: Mosby.

Bergqvist, A. G. (2008). Encephalitis. In M. W. Schwartz (Ed.), *The 5-minute pediatric consult* (5th ed., pp. 296–297). Philadelphia: Wolters Kluwer Health/Lippincott Williams & Wilkins.

Betz, R. R., Ranade, A., Samdani, A. F., Chafetz, R., D'Andrea, L. P., Gaughan, J. P., . . . Mulcahey, M. J. (2010). Vertebral body stapling: A fusionless treatment option for a growing child with moderate idiopathic scoliosis. *Spine, 35*(2), 169–176.

Bickley, L. S., & Szilagyi, P. G. (2003). *Bates' guide to physical examination and history taking* (8th ed.). Philadelphia: Lippincott, Williams & Wilkins.

Blom, H. J., Shaw, J. M., den Heijer, M., & Finnell, R. H. (2006). Neural tube defects and folate: Case far from closed. Nature reviews. *Neuroscience, 7*(9), 724–731.

Bowen, K. A., & Chung, D. H. (2009). Recent advances in neuroblastoma. *Current Opinion in Pediatrics, 21*(3), 350–356.

Braunwald, E., Fauci, A. S., Kasper, D. L., Hauser, S. L., Longo, D. L., & Jameson, J. L. (Eds.). (2008). *Harrison's principles of internal medicine* (17th ed.). New York: McGraw-Hill.

Burns, S. M. (Ed.). (2007). *American Association of Critical-Care Nurses (AACN): AACN protocols for practice: Healing environments* (2nd ed.). Sudbury, MA: Jones and Bartlett.

Centers for Disease Control and Prevention. (2008). Spinal cord injuries: Acute injury care. Retrieved March 23, 2008, from http://www.cdc.gov/ncipc/dir/AcuteInjuryCare.htm

Chambers, M. A., & Jones, S. (Eds.). (2007). *Surgical nursing of children*. Philadelphia: Elsevier.

Chan, E., Ong, C., & Hsu, L. (2008). Corticosteroids for bacterial meningitis. *New England Journal of Medicine, 358*(13).

Chernecky, C., & Berger, B. (2004). *Laboratory tests and diagnostic procedures* (4th ed.). Philadelphia: Saunders.

Crocoli, A., Madafferi, S., Jenkner, A., Zaccara, A., & Inserra, A. (2008). Elevated serum alpha-fetoprotein in Wilms tumor may follow the same pattern of other fetal neoplasms after treatment: Evidence from three cases. *Pediatric Surgery International, 24*(4), 499–502.

Crowe, L., Babl, F., Anderson, V., & Catroppa, C. (2009). The epidemiology of paediatric head injuries: Data from a referral centre in Victoria, Australia. *Journal of Pediatric and Child Health, 45,* 346–350.

Cultrera, F., D'Andrea, M., Battaglia, R., & Chieregato, A. (2009). Unilateral oculomotor nerve palsy: Unusual sign of hydrocephalus. *Journal of Neurosurgical Sciences, 53*(2), 67–70.

Dekker, C., & Arvin, A. (2009). One step closer to a CMV vaccine. *New England Journal of Medicine, 360*(12), 1250–1252.

Dicianno, B. E., Bellin, M. H., & Zabel, A. T. (2009). Spina bifida and mobility in the transition years. *American Journal of Physical Medicine & Rehabilitation, 88*(12), 1002–1006.

Drake Melander, S. (Ed.). (2004). *Case studies in critical care nursing: A guide for application and review* (3rd ed.). Philadelphia: Saunders.

Eide, P. K., Egge, A., Due-Tennesses, B. J., & Helseth, E. (2007). Is intracranial pressure waveform analysis useful in the management of pediatric neurosurgical patients. *Pediatric Neurosurgery, 43,* 472–481. Retrieved June 28, 2010, from Pro Quest database.

Eide, P., & Sorteberg, W. (2008). Changes in intracranial pulse pressure amplitudes after shunt implantation and adjustment of shunt valve opening pressure in normal pressure hydrocephalus. *Acta Neurochirurgica, 150*(11), 1141–1147; discussion 1147.

Emergency Nurses Association & Newberry, L. (2005). *Sheehy's emergency nursing: Principles and practice,* 65th ed. St. Louis, MO: Mosby/Elsevier.

Figaji, A., & Adelson, P. (2009). Does ICP monitoring in children with severe head injuries make a difference? *American Surgeon, 75*(5), 441–442.

Fisher, M. J. (2008). Brain tumor. In M. W. Schwartz (Ed.), *The 5-minute pediatric consult* (5th ed.). Philadelphia: Wolters Kluwer Health/Lippincott Williams & Wilkins.

Fitzgerald Macksey, L. (2009). *Pediatric anesthetic and emergency drug guide.* Sudbury, MA: Jones & Bartlett.

Frazier, J. L., Ahn, E. S., & Jallo, G. I. (2008). Management of brain abscesses in children. *Neurosurgical Focus, 24*(6), E8.

Gilman, S., & Newman, S. W. (2003). *Manter and Gatz's essentials of clinical neuroanatomy and neurophysiology* (10th ed.). Philadelphia: F. A. Davis.

Gora-Harper, M. (1998). *The injectable drug reference.* Princeton, NJ: Bioscientific Resources.

Hardin, S. R., & Kaplow, R. (Eds.). (2004). *Synergy for clinical excellence: The AACN Synergy Model for Patient Care.* Sudbury, MA: Jones and Bartlett.

Hartfield, D. S., Tan, J., Yager, J. Y., Rosychuk, R. J., Spady, D., Haines, C., & Craig, W. R. (2009). The association between iron deficiency and febrile seizures in childhood. *Clinical Pediatrics, 48*(4), 420–426.

Hassanein, S., Moharram, H., & Monib, A. (2008). Perinatal ventriculomegaly. *Journal of Pediatric Neurology, 6*(4), 293–307.

Hay, W. W. Jr., Levin, M. J., Sondheimer, J. M., & Deterding, R. R. (Eds.). (2007). *Current diagnosis and treatment in pediatrics* (18th ed.). New York: McGraw-Hill.

Hickey, J. V. (2008). *The clinical practice of neurological and neurosurgical nursing* (6th ed.). Philadelphia: Lippincott Williams & Wilkins.

Jones & Bartlett Learning. (2011). *2011 nurse's drug handbook* (10th ed.). Sudbury, MA: Jones & Bartlett Learning.

Jones, K. L. (2006). Smith's recognizable patterns of human malformation (6th ed.). Philadelphia: Elsevier.

Kim, D-K., Yoo, S. K., Park, I-C., Choa, M., Bae, K. Y., Kim, Y-D., & Heo, J-H. (2009). A mobile telemedicine system for remote consultation in cases of acute stroke. *Journal of Telemedicine and Telecare, 15*(2), 102–107.

Kuriyama, N., Tokuda, T., Kondo, M., Miyamoto, A., Yamada, K., Ushijima, Y., . . . Nakagawa, M. (2008). Evaluation of autonomic malfunction in idiopathic normal pressure hydrocephalus. *Clinical Autonomic Research, 18*(4), 213–220.

Laskowitz, D. T., Kasner, S. E., Saver, J., Remmel, K. S., & Jauch, E. C.; BRAIN Study Group. (2009). Clinical usefulness of a biomarker-based diagnostic test for acute stroke: The Biomarker Rapid Assessment in Ischemic Injury (BRAIN) study. *Stroke, 40*(1), 77–85.

Littlejohns, L. R., & Bader, M. K. (Eds.). (2009). *AACN-AANN protocols for practice: Monitoring technologies in critically ill neuroscience patients*. Sudbury, MA: Jones & Bartlett.

Lückhoff, C., & Starr, M. (2010). Minor head injuries in children: An approach to management. *Australian Family Physician, 39*(5), 284–287.

Majed, M., Nejat, F., El Khashab, M., Tajik, P., Gharagozloo, M., Baghban, M., & Sajjadnia, A. (2009). Risk factors for latex sensitization in young children with myelomeningocele. *Journal of Neurosurgery: Pediatrics, 4*(3), 285–288.

Martin, B. (2010). Family presence during resuscitation and invasive procedures: AACN practice alert. Retrieved from http://www.aacn.org

McCance, K. L., & Huether, S. E. (2002). *Pathophysiology: The biologic basis for disease in adults and children* (4th ed.). St. Louis, MO: Mosby.

Medina, J., & Puntillo, K. (2006). *AACN protocols for practice: Palliative care and end-of-life issues in critical care*. Sudbury, MA: Jones and Bartlett.

Merck Manuals Online Library. (2008). *Intracranial and spinal tumors*. Retrieved July 1, 2009, from http://www.merck.com/mmpe/print/sec16/ch225/ch225a.htmL

Moe, P. G., Benke, T. A., Bernard, T. J., & Levisohn, P. (2009). Neurologic and muscular disorders. In W. W. Hay, M. J. Levin, J. M. Sondheimer, & R. R. Deterding (Eds.), *Current diagnosis and treatment in pediatrics* (19th ed., pp. 673–697). New York: McGraw-Hill Medical.

Montañana, A. P., Palacios, I. E., & Cariñena, L. S. (2008). Dexamethasone therapy for bacterial meningitis in children and newborns. *Acta Pediatrica Espanola, 66*(8), 390–395.

Montefiore Medical Center. (2009). Birth injuries. Retrieved July 2, 2009, from http://www.montefiore.org/healthlibrary/centers/pregnancy/birthinj

Nabavi, A., Goebel, S., Doerner, L., Warneke, N., Ulmer, S., & Mehdorn, M. (2009). Awake craniotomy and intraoperative magnetic resonance imaging: Patient selection, preparation, and technique. *Topics in Magnetic Resonance Imaging: TMRI, 19*(4), 191–196.

Ogilvie, J. (2010). Adolescent idiopathic scoliosis and genetic testing. *Current Opinion in Pediatrics, 22*(1), 67–70.

Park, J. R., Eggert, A., & Caron, H. (2008). Neuroblastoma: Biology, prognosis, and treatment. *Pediatric Clinics of North America, 55*(1), 97–120.

Partap, S., & Fisher, P. G. (2007). Update on new treatments and developments in childhood brain tumors. *Current Opinion in Pediatrics, 19*(6), 670–674.

Perry, S. E., Hockenberry, M. J., Lowdermilk, D. L., & Wilson, D. W. (2010). *Health problems of children: Maternal–child nursing care* (4th ed., pp. 1572–1574). Maryland Heights, MO: Mosby.

Prescribing reference. (2009, Summer). *NPPR: Nurse Practitioner's Prescribing Reference, 16*(2).

Rangel-Castillo, L., Gopinath, S., & Robertson, C. S. (2008, May). Management of intracranial hypertension. *Neurologic Clinics, 2*(26), 521–541. Retrieved July 2, 2009, from http://www.neurologic.theclinics.com/article/S0733-8619(08)00021-2/abstract

Riffaud, L., Moughty, C., Henaux, P., Haegelen, C., & Morandi, X. (2008). Acquired Chiari I malformation and syringomyelia after valveless lumboperitoneal shunt in infancy. *Pediatric Neurosurgery, 44*(3), 229–233.

Robertson, J., & Sholkofski, N. (2005). *The Harriet Lane handbook* (17th ed.). Philadelphia: Elsevier-Mosby.

Rogerson, S., Malenga, G., & Molyneux, E. M. (2004, June). Integrated pathways: A tool to improve infant monitoring in a neonatal unit. *Annals of Tropical Paediatrics, 24*(2), 171–174. Retrieved June 28, 2009, from Pro Quest database.

Rowe, D. E., & Jadhav, A. L. (2008). Care of the adolescent with spina bifida. *Pediatric Clinics of North America, 55*(6), 1359–1374, ix.

Salim, A., Hannon, M., Brown, C., et al. (2008). Intracranial pressure monitoring in severe isolated pediatric blunt head trauma. *American Surgeon, 74,* 1088–1093.

Santarius, T., Kirkpatrick, P. J., Ganesan, D., Chia, H. L., Jalloh, I., Smielewski, P., & Hutchinson, P. J. (2009). Use of drains versus no drains after burr-hole evacuation of chronic subdural haematoma: A randomised controlled trial. Lancet, 374(9695), 1067–1073.

Sawin, K. J., Bellin, M. H., Roux, G., Buran, C. F., & Brei, T. J. (2009). The experience of self-management in adolescent women with spina bifida. *Rehabilitation Nursing, 34*(1), 26–38.

Shaked, O., Peña, B. M., Linares, M. Y., & Baker, R. L (2009). Simple febrile seizures: Are the AAP guidelines regarding lumbar puncture being followed? *Pediatric Emergency Care, 25*(1), 8–11.

Shaw, S. (2009). Endocrine late effects in survivors of pediatric brain tumors. *Journal of Pediatric Oncology Nursing, 26*(5), 295–302.

Siedel, H. M., Ball, J. W., Dains, J. E., & Benedict, G. W. (2003). *Mosby's physical examination handbook* (3rd ed.). St. Louis, MO: Mosby.

Siegel, A., & Siegel, H. (2002). *Neuroscience: Pretest self-assessment and review* (5th ed.). New York: McGraw-Hill.

Singh, R. K., & Gaillard, W. D. (2009). Status epilepticus in children. *Current Neurology and Neuroscience Reports, 9*(2), 137–144.

Singh, R. K., Stephens, S., Berl, M. M., Chang, T., Brown, K., Vezina, L. G., & Gaillard, W. D. (2010). Prospective study of new-onset seizures presenting as status epilepticus in childhood. *Neurology, 74*(8), 636–642.

Slota, M. C. (Ed.). (2006). *Core curriculum for pediatric critical care nursing* (2nd ed.). St. Louis, MO: Saunders.

Smeltzer, S., & Bare, B. G. (2003). *Brunner and Suddarth's textbook of medical–surgical nursing* (10th ed.). Philadelphia: Lippincott Williams & Wilkins.

Spratto, G. R., & Woods, A. L. (2001). *PDR: Nurse's drug handbook.* Montvale, NJ: Delmar & Medical Economics.

Stemp-Morlock, G. (2007). Pesticides and anencephaly. *Environmental Health Perspectives, 115*(2), A78.

Strayer, D. A., & Pravikoff, D. (2010, September 17). Melanoma: Placental and fetal metastasis. *CINAHL Nursing Guide, Cinahl Information Systems,* 2.

Strengell, T., Uhari, M., Tarkka, R., Uusimaa, J., Alen, R., Lautala, P., & Rantala, H. (2009). Antipyretic agents for preventing recurrences of febrile seizures: Randomized controlled trial. *Archives of Pediatrics & Adolescent Medicine, 163*(9), 799–804.

Trivits Verger, J., & Lebet, R. M. (Eds.). (2008). *AACN procedure manual for pediatric acute and critical care.* St. Louis, MO: Saunders.

University of Maryland Medical Center. (2007). Increased intracranial pressure-treatment. Retrieved June 29, 2009, from http://www.umm.edu/ency/article/000793trt.htm

Valeo, T. (2007). How best to rule out bacterial meningitis? Neurologists weigh in on new guidelines. *Neurology Today, 7*(3), 4, 6–7.

Verboon-Maciolek, M. A., Groenendaal, F., Hahn, C. D., Hellmann, J., van Loon, A. M., Boivin, G., & de Vries, L. S. (2008). Human parechovirus causes encephalitis with white matter injury in neonates. *Annals of Neurology, 64*(3), 266–273.

Woodhouse, C. (2008). Myelomeningocele: Neglected aspects. *Pediatric Nephrology, 23*(8), 1223–1231. www.genetics.emory.edu/pdf/Emory_Human_Genetics_Cystic_Hygroma.PDF

Yadav, Y., Jaiswal, S., & Adam, N. (2006). Endoscopic third ventriculostomy in infants. *Neurology India, 54*(2), 161–163.

Yoong, M., Chin, R. F., & Scott, R. C. (2009). Management of convulsive status epilepticus in children. *Archives of Disease in Childhood: Education and Practice Edition, 94*(1), 1–9.

Zoair, A., El-Aziz, S., & Awny, M. (2008). Neonatal cerebrospinal fluid plasminogen and plasminogen activator inhibitor-1 assay as predictors of posthemorrhagic hydrocephalus. *Journal of Pediatric Neurology, 6*(3), 237–242.

SECTION 8

Gastrointestinal

1. **At what stage of fetal development does the GI tract begin to develop?**
   A. 2–4 weeks gestational age
   B. 4–8 weeks gestational age
   C. 6–10 weeks gestational age
   D. 12–16 weeks gestational age

2. **How do an omphalocele and gastroschisis differ?**
   A. An omphalocele is the herniation of some or all the abdominal contents into a sac at the umbilicus
   B. Gastroschisis is the herniation of all the abdominal contents into a sac at the umbilicus
   C. An omphalocele is the herniation of the small bowel into a sac outside the abdomen
   D. Gastroschisis is a herniation of the midgut contents into a sac around the umbilicus

3. **The parents of an infant born with gastroschisis are concerned about postoperative care. Which important facts will you teach them about the correction of this problem?**
   A. It is a minor surgical procedure done at the bedside
   B. It will take many days for their baby to recover
   C. This condition will require at least three correctional procedures
   D. Their baby will be monitored for fluid status, signs of infection, and NG suction will be in place

4. **Melena stools indicate bleeding from which area?**
   A. Mouth
   B. Upper gastrointestinal tract
   C. Descending colon
   D. Esophagus

5. **Which of the following preventive actions can reduce the risk of an infant developing necrotizing enterocolitis?**
   A. Breastfeeding is the only cause of this condition
   B. Adequate fluids, reduced stress, and careful feedings
   C. NG tube placement and surgery to repair the perforation
   D. Breastfeeding is the only prevention necessary

6. **Which of the following infants is at the greatest risk of developing necrotizing enterocolitis?**
   A. A 38 week gestational age, breastfed baby
   B. A 40 week gestational age baby whose mother had *Salmonella* food poisoning just prior to giving birth
   C. A 37 week gestational age baby who is currently stable
   D. A 38 week gestational age, formula fed baby

7. **Aside from lower gastrointestinal bleeding, what are some additional symptoms seen with necrotizing enterocolitis?**
   A. Lethargy, bradycardia, retractions
   B. Lethargy, apnea, bradycardia, abdominal distention
   C. Lethargy, tachypnea, fever
   D. Lethargy, tachycardia, jitteriness

8. **Your patient has a history of transphenoidal hypopysectomy. Which of the following procedures is absolutely contraindicated?**
   A. Nasal placement of a gastric tube
   B. Oral placement of a gastric tube
   C. Oral intubation with an endotracheal tube
   D. Tracheal intubation

9. **Infants born with diaphragmatic hernia are described as having a scaphoid abdomen on assessment. What does scaphoid mean?**
   A. A rounded appearance
   B. A sunken or convex appearance
   C. A concave or protruding appearance
   D. A sunken or concave appearance

10. **You have just assisted with the insertion of an esophageal and gastric balloon. Tamponade therapy duration should be carefully documented because**
    A. Hgb and Hct should drop after placement
    B. Comfort increases 24 hours after placement
    C. Prolonged inflation may lead to necrosis or ulceration
    D. Enteral feeding may be given via the tube after 36 hours

11. **Your 18 year old patient overdosed on Valium and Paxil. Gastric lavage is ordered. This is best accomplished**
    A. If done within 60 minutes of ingestion
    B. If 0.45% normal saline is used
    C. Lavage is not recommended for this type of overdose
    D. If the ingestion is liquefied first

12. **VATER association presents with which of the following anomalies?**
    A. Vertebral anomalies, anal anomalies, tracheoesophageal fistula, esophageal atresia, and renal anomalies
    B. Vertebral anomalies, anal anomalies, tracheoesophageal fistula, ear anomalies, and renal anomalies

C. Vertebral anomalies, anal anomalies, thoracic anomalies, esophageal atresia, and rectal anomalies
D. Ear anomalies, cranial vault anomalies, and multiple umbilical arteries

13. **Which of the following symptoms would be considered late signs of acute liver failure?**
A. Increased ICP, increased mean arterial pressure, and normal CPP
B. Decreased ICP, decreased mean arterial pressure, and elevated CPP
C. Increased ICP, decreased mean arterial pressure, and decreased CPP
D. Decreased ICP, increased mean arterial pressure, and normal CPP

14. **The most common cause of death related to acute hepatic failure is**
A. Pulmonary embolism
B. Anemia
C. Brain stem herniation
D. Pulmonary edema

15. **Hepatorenal syndrome is a complication of hepatic failure due to**
A. Vasodilation
B. Increased circulating plasma
C. Increased renal circulation
D. Release of mediators

16. **A 3 day old, 36 week gestational age male has suddenly started having bilious vomitus without abdominal distention. What could be the cause of his distress?**
A. Biliary atresia
B. Meconium plug
C. Malrotation of the midgut and volvulus
D. Duodenal atresia

17. **For an infant with malrotation of the midgut and volvulus, which treatments in addition to surgery would you expect?**
A. Feeding tube with basic soy formula
B. NG tube, antibiotics, NPO status
C. NG tube only
D. Only feeding with breastmilk

18. **A 3 week old infant was admitted to the PICU for pneumonia. She now has a diaper full of bloody stool. What are some common causes of lower gastrointestinal bleeding?**
A. Infection, meconium plug, maternal drug abuse
B. Maternal infection, lactose intolerance, necrotizing enterocolitis
C. Hirschsprung's disease
D. Hazelton's disease

19. **Cullen's sign is**
A. A marbled appearance to the abdomen
B. Bruising of the scrotum or labia
C. A bluish discoloration of the flanks
D. A bluish discoloration of the periumbilical area

20. **Bruce, a 15 year old student, came to the PICU with an acute appendix 4 days ago. Antibiotics and morphine have controlled his symptoms. As you are transferring him to a medical–surgical unit, Bruce asks if the pain will ever come back. You tell him**
    A. "No. You should not ever have this problem again"
    B. "Yes, but not for several years"
    C. "Yes, but the pain will not be as severe"
    D. "Possibly. About one third of patients are readmitted and require surgery within 1 year"

21. **Judy is a 17 year old student who weighs 85 pounds. She was found unconscious in the bathroom and was admitted for severe dehydration and starvation. Which of the following symptoms would you expect to observe with this patient?**
    A. Decreased serum lactate
    B. Normal urinary nitrogen excretion
    C. Conservation of body fluids with third spacing
    D. Decreased serum catecholamines, glucagon, and cortisol

22. **Sarah, a 13 year old, is a recovering anorexic. You are preparing to transfer her to a medical–surgical unit when you note that she has not touched her lunch. You would tell her**
    A. "It's okay. I know that hospital food is not gourmet, but the dinners are more appetizing"
    B. "If you don't eat, we will have to put a feeding tube in you"
    C. "You need to eat to regain strength and prevent complications. We will work with you to find foods that you like"
    D. "Food is not your enemy. Eating this is not going to make you fat"

23. **Joe, a 16 year old student with cirrhosis, was admitted to the PICU yesterday after a weekend party where he indulged in alcohol, drugs, and smoking. His morning lab results were as follows:**

    ALT 245 U/L   AST 147 U/L
    PT 24 sec   PLT 75 × 10^3/mm^3
    Hgb 8.4 g/dL   Hct 31%.
    Bilirubin 10 mg/dL

    These results indicate that Joe is at high risk for
    A. Variceal bleeding
    B. Peptic ulcer disease
    C. Gastritis
    D. Boerhaave's syndrome

24. **Which form of hepatitis originates as a DNA virus?**
    A. Hepatitis A
    B. Hepatitis B
    C. Hepatitis C
    D. Hepatitis D

25. **Which of the following forms of hepatitis is often misdiagnosed as gastroenteritis?**
    A. Hepatitis A
    B. Hepatitis B
    C. Hepatitis C
    D. Hepatitis E

26. **Meena, a 16 year old exchange student from Hungary, is brought in to the ED by her host family. Meena has been suffering for 2 weeks with flu-like symptoms, increasing bruising, headaches, pounding pulses, and fever. She was reluctant to seek treatment until this morning, when her headache became unbearable. Which diagnosis is the mostly likely cause of Meena's symptoms?**
    A. DIC related to bacterial infection
    B. Acute liver failure related to unintentional overdose of acetaminophen
    C. Vitamin K deficiency related to poor nutritional intake
    D. Anemia related to Gaucher's disease

27. **Ascites is a common finding in children with chronic liver failure. Which of the following statements about ascites is true?**
    A. Ascites is a result of an increase in albumin
    B. Ascites is the result of decreased hydrostatic pressure and increased oncotic pressures in the portal system
    C. Ascites occurs secondary to aldosteronism
    D. Ascites is due to an increased ventilation/perfusion (V/Q) ratio

28. **Tina is a 16 year old with severe Crohn's disease and perforation. She returns from surgery with an ileostomy. Tina is at greatest risk for which of the following complications?**
    A. Dehydration
    B. Hypernatremia
    C. Hemorrhage
    D. Prolapsed stoma due to vigorous exercise once discharged

29. **Nate had abdominal surgery for perforation yesterday. Today's abdominal X-rays show a double-bubble appearance. He is complaining of nausea and has stained emesis, abdominal distention, pain, and fever. The appropriate nursing intervention would be to**
    A. Contact the surgeon and prepare for immediate surgery
    B. Administer morphine and Tylenol, then call the physician if there is no improvement
    C. Position the patient flat and give him Tylenol
    D. Do nothing. This is normal. The physician should only be notified if the abdomen becomes discolored

30. **During a Whipple procedure, which of the following organs is removed?**
    A. Esophagus
    B. Gallbladder
    C. Ascending colon
    D. Jejunum

31. **Sue underwent the Whipple procedure 10 days ago for pancreatic cancer. She was started on clear liquids and then advanced to a soft diet. Two hours after lunch, you enter her room to find her sweating profusely, shaking, and confused. On the monitor, you note tachypnea and tachycardia. You suspect Sue is experiencing**
    A. An anxiety or panic attack
    B. Gastroesophageal reflux disease (GERD)
    C. Dumping syndrome
    D. Hypoglycemia

32. **Your patient had abdominal surgery 2 hours ago. Now you note a decrease in urine output, an increased CVP, increased PAP, increased SVR, and decreased cardiac output. In addition, the ventilator continuously alarms low volume despite intact circuits. Based on these findings, you would expect which of the following intra-abdominal pressure values?**
    A. 5 mmHg
    B. 15 mmHg
    C. 25 mmHg
    D. 50 mmHg

33. **Which of the following lab results would contraindicate administration of peritoneal lavage?**
    A. RBC 5.2 million/mm^3
    B. PLT 79,000 mm^3/mL
    C. PT 12.5 sec and PTT 75 sec
    D. Hgb 14.7 g/dL and Hct 46%

34. **You are preparing Bobby for a paracentesis. Which of the following actions is the first step in assisting with a paracentesis?**
    A. Have Bobby void or insert a Foley catheter
    B. Examine the abdomen for dullness
    C. Order an upright X-ray of the abdomen
    D. Position Bobby with the affected side up

35. **Brendon is a 15 year old student who was hospitalized for a myocardial infarction with an emergency cardiopulmonary artery bypass graft surgery yesterday. He has been having recurrent uncontrolled atrial fibrillation intermittently for the last 6 hours. This evening Brendon complains of abdominal pain with distention, intolerance for his soft diet, nausea, vomiting, and fever. The physician orders a plain film of the abdomen. Which of the following results would you expect to see on Brendon's X-ray?**
    A. Air in the biliary tree with signs of small bowel obstruction and calculus in the pelvis
    B. Dilated small bowel loops and air–fluid levels
    C. Dilation of the entire bowel including the stomach, "thumb printing," and pneumatosis intestinalis
    D. Air under the diaphragm on the right upper chest or over the right lobe of the liver

36. Mary is being treated in the PICU for burns sustained to 55% of her body after she was trapped in her house during a fire. She is at high risk for developing which of the following conditions?

A. Peptic ulcer
B. Pancreatitis
C. Cholecystitis
D. SRES

37. During gastric lavage for stress-related erosion syndrome (SRES), your patient becomes hyperthermic and tachycardic, and she complains of sudden abdominal pain and abdominal rigidity. As a PICU nurse, you should

A. Continue with the lavage—these symptoms are normal
B. Stop the infusion and contact the physician
C. Stop the infusion and rewarm the fluid
D. Slow the infusion and change the fluid

38. Your 14 year old patient with severe acute pancreatitis now has a blood pressure of 68/40. She has a heart rate of 138 and a respiratory rate of 32. You suspect hypovolemic shock, which is probably due to

A. Blood loss from a ruptured gallbladder
B. Third spacing related to capillary leaking
C. Insufficient volume intake related to vomiting
D. Excessive fluid loss due to diarrhea

39. Your patient was diagnosed with Barrett's esophagus. Which of the following conditions is your patient at greatest risk for developing?

A. Esophageal varices
B. Gastritis
C. Esophageal cancer
D. GERD

40. Patients and their parents considering gastric bypass for weight management control should begin bariatric education

A. Prior to the decision being made
B. When the decision to have surgery is made
C. Just prior to surgery
D. After the surgery is complete

41. Martha was admitted to the PICU prior to undergoing bariatric surgery. Which of the following assessments is the most important when caring for a patient considering bariatric surgery?

A. Nutritional assessment
B. Psychological evaluation
C. Activity or muscular/skeletal assessment
D. Physiological assessment

42. Which of the following is the most common complication of gastric banding?

A. Band slippage
B. Stoma obstruction
C. GERD
D. Stomach erosion

43. Your patient underwent the Roux-en-Y gastric bypass procedure 2 days ago. Which nutritional complication is your patient most at risk of developing?

A. Hypercalcemia
B. Vitamin C deficiency
C. Vitamin B_{12} deficiency
D. Hyperalbuminism

44. Anastomotic leaks are common with bariatric surgeries. Symptoms can be subtle and may include hyperthermia, tachycardia, tachypnea, abdominal pain, and anxiety. If an anastomotic leak goes undiagnosed, all of the following complications may result except

A. Hyperoxyia
B. Sepsis
C. MODS
D. Death

45. Barbara was admitted to the pediatric intensive care unit for abdominal pain. She recently had knee surgery, for which she received Tylenol #3 for pain control. She has no bowel sounds, her abdomen is firmly distended, and she is diffusely tender across the abdomen. What is probably wrong with Barbara?

A. Appendicitis from the pain medication
B. Paralytic ileus from the codeine
C. Gastroenteritis after eating undercooked chicken
D. Pancreatitis from lack of exercise

46. What is the optimal postfeeding position for an infant with gastroesophageal reflux?

A. Supine or right lateral position with the head of the crib at 30°
B. Right lateral position with the head of the crib at 20°
C. Prone or left lateral position with the head of the crib at 30°
D. Prone with the head of the crib at 20°

47. Prolonged TPN administration can lead to which of the following conditions?

A. Hypoglycemia
B. Cholestasis
C. Pleural effusion
D. Hemorrhagic cystitis

48. Hyperbilirubinemia is diagnosed based on the elevation of which of the following lab values?

A. Total serum bilirubin
B. Alanine transferase

C. Hepatic transferase
D. Polycythemia

49. **What is the most common presentation of gastroesophageal reflux (GER) in children and infants?**
A. Sandifer syndrome
B. Flatulence
C. Abdominal distention
D. Emesis

50. **The mother of a 2 week old infant is concerned about the frequency of the baby's bowel movements. The mother had not seen the baby since they were traveling home with the baby after discharge from the hospital. On the way home, their car was struck by another car. The baby was admitted to the PICU and the mother to the orthopedic unit. The mother states, "You always seem to be changing diapers and I have been here only four hours." Which of the following statements is the most therapeutic?**
A. "This is nothing; you should see the baby in the next bassinet"
B. "He is having a lot of stools. I will call the physician"
C. "Your baby should actually be stooling at least every 2 hours"
D. "It is normal for a newborn to have stools four to five times a day"

51. **Jeremy has been diagnosed with α_1-antitrypsin deficiency liver disease. Which lab findings or symptoms would you expect with Jeremy's condition?**
A. Elevated gamma-glutamyl transpeptidase, clay-colored stools
B. Jaundice, decreased GGTP
C. Increased LDH, jaundice
D. Flat abdomen, decreased LDH

52. **Common adverse reactions to cimetidine include**
A. Elevated BUN and creatinine
B. Rash, nausea, and agitation
C. Decreased liver enzymes, and anorexia
D. Jitteriness, and mottled skin

53. **Cimetidine, famotidine, and ranitidine belong to which class of medications?**
A. Proton pump inhibitors (PPIs)
B. Antacids
C. H_2 blockers
D. Antiemetics

54. **How do proton pump inhibitors (PPIs) work?**
A. PPIs inhibit the release of cytokines
B. PPIs antagonize the H_2 histamine receptors
C. PPIs increase gastric emptying, thereby reducing acid production
D. PPIs inhibit the release of hydrochloric acid by gastric parietal cells

55. **You are transporting an infant with severe abdominal distention and tenderness to your facility for a higher level of care. Which of the following consent forms should the team ensure is signed prior to departure from the tertiary facility?**
   A. Consent for morphine administration
   B. Consent for blood transfusion
   C. Consent for pictures
   D. Consent for an IV

56. **Francine is 15 years old and delivered a 29 week gestation neonate 5 days ago. Francine was taken to the PICU for hypovolemic shock, post uterine rupture, and a hysterectomy. She still wants to breastfeed her baby and has begun pumping. What effect will the delay have on her total breastmilk supply?**
   A. Francine will produce exactly the same total amount of breastmilk regardless of her complications
   B. Francine will likely produce less milk than the expected total if she had not developed complications
   C. Francine will likely produce more milk than the expected total if she had not developed complications
   D. Francine will probably not be able to breastfeed at all because her milk supply is dwindling

57. **Vitamin E is considered to be**
   A. An antagonist for vitamin K
   B. An effective oxidant
   C. Absorbed readily when given in formula
   D. A treatment for anemia

58. **Which treatments would you expect for an infant with neonatal hepatitis?**
   A. No treatment is necessary; this is a self-limiting disorder
   B. Breast milk, corticosteroids, broad-spectrum antibiotics
   C. Adequate nutrition, fluids, fat-soluble vitamins
   D. Water-soluble vitamins, corticosteroids

59. **Which symptoms would you expect in a child with neonatal hepatitis?**
   A. Jaundice, fever, tarry stools
   B. Jaundice, hepatomegaly, lethargy
   C. Jaundice, petechiae, hyperactivity
   D. Jaundice, hypothermia, hyperactivity

60. **Similac PM 60/40 is frequently given for**
   A. Fatty acid metabolism defect
   B. Renal insufficiency
   C. Neurologic disease
   D. Abdominal distention

61. **Soy-based formulas are indicated for which of the following conditions?**
   A. Low birth weight
   B. Bloody stools
   C. Lactase deficiency
   D. Hepatitis C

62. Portagen is frequently used for infants with which of the following conditions?

A. Hepatic disorder
B. Fatty acid metabolism
C. Feeding intolerance
D. Amino acid deficiency

63. Medications that are bound to protein may have which of the following effects?

A. Increased availability
B. Rapid distribution
C. Less available drug to produce the desired effect
D. Idiosyncrasy

64. A long-term complication of congenital diaphragmatic hernia repair is

A. Gastroesophageal reflux
B. Chylothorax
C. Cor pulmonale
D. Diarrhea

65. Assessment of the abdomen should occur in which order?

A. Inspection, palpation, auscultation, percussion
B. Auscultation, inspection, palpation, percussion
C. Percussion, inspection, palpation, auscultation
D. Inspection, auscultation, percussion, palpation

66. Your patient has been diagnosed with chronic liver disease. In addition to a venous hum or murmur, which of the following findings should you hear during abdominal auscultation?

A. Aortic bruit
B. Hepatic bruit
C. Iliac artery bruit
D. Renal artery bruit

67. Normal portal pressures are

A. 5–10 mmHg
B. 10–20 mmHg
C. 5 mmHg less than the inferior vena cava pressure
D. 10 mmHg greater than the inferior vena cava pressure

68. Your patient has acute esophageal and gastric varices. Which esophagogastric tamponade tube is the best choice for differentiating bleeding from the esophagus and bleeding from the stomach?

A. Minnesota tube
B. Sengstaken-Blakemore tube
C. Linton-Nachlas tube
D. Standard nasogastric tube

69. The 10 year old brother of your patient with severe biliary obstruction notices that his sister has multiple scratches and excoriations over her skin. He is concerned that his sister is being abused. You explain

A. "Do not panic—we are not abusing her"
B. "I understand you are concerned. Because of her high bilirubin levels, she scratches herself unconsciously"
C. "She must have gotten out of the restraints"
D. "She did it to herself as a result of PICU psychosis"

70. Hepatic encephalopathy has ____ grades based on ____ clinical findings

A. 3; 4
B. 4; 4
C. 4; 5
D. 5; 5

71. The family of your 7 year old patient with chronic liver failure would like to know what they can do to make him more comfortable. You tell them that they can

A. Provide deep tissue massage every 2 hours
B. Apply a moisturizing lotion when visiting
C. Assist with rapid range of motion every 4 hours
D. Limit visitation to once a day

72. Your 15 year old patient was involved in a motor vehicle accident and suffered blunt abdominal trauma related to the seat belt placement. He begins complaining of severe abdominal pain around the epigastric area that is knife-like and twisting. You also note that he has a low-grade fever with diaphoresis, abdominal distention, decreased bowel tones, and rebound tenderness. You suspect

A. Pancreatitis
B. Acute liver failure
C. Gastrointestinal bleeding
D. Abdominal bruising

73. A patient with acute pancreatitis had labs drawn this morning. A result you would expect to see is

A. Elevated serum amylase
B. Decreased serum lipase
C. Elevated albumin
D. Decreased trypsin level

74. Dorothy has been in the PICU for 11 days and has developed a stress ulcer. Family members ask why she has developed an ulcer. You acknowledge their concern and explain that

A. Ulcers are caused by a decrease in mucosal blood flow
B. Ulcers are caused by an increase in mucus production
C. Ulcers are caused by fungal infections
D. Dorothy had the ulcer before she was admitted to the hospital

75. Luke is 12 years old and a nonalcohol abusing patient. He was diagnosed with portal hypertension with direct variceal bleeding. His wedge hepatic venous pressure is less than his portal pressure due to portal vein thrombosis. This effect may be due to

A. Chronic active hepatitis
B. Umbilical vein catheterization as a neonate
C. Metastatic carcinoma
D. Congestive heart failure

76. Joel, despite being only 12 years old, is frequently admitted to your unit for alcohol-induced comas. Just prior to his transfer to a step-down unit, he begins projectile vomiting bright red blood. Your first action should be to

A. Position the patient flat
B. Obtain and insert a Linton-Nachlas tube
C. Make the patient NPO and verify IV access
D. Start dopamine at 5 mcg/kg/min

77. Jake, a 16 year old student, had an appendectomy a week ago in another state while on spring break. He is admitted to the PICU with fever, nausea and vomiting, and abdominal pain, with a red, swollen surgical incision. You anticipate his next treatment to include

A. Immediate surgery with IV antibiotics
B. Hydration and antibiotics
C. Bedside excision of an abscess
D. Bedside wound debridement

78. Penny just had surgery for peritonitis related to diverticulitis. During drug reconciliation, which of the following medications should Penny continue?

A. Advil for headaches
B. Prednisone for bronchitis
C. Morphine for surgical pain
D. Verapamil for atrial fibrillation

79. Eric has chronic pancreatitis and develops respiratory distress with dyspnea and pulmonary edema. These symptoms are due to

A. Pulmonary capillary endothelial damage related to phospholipase
B. Bronchospasm related to stress
C. Aspiration
D. Atelectasis

80. Nicolai was admitted to the PICU with vague epigastric discomfort, vomiting times one week, inability to eat more than a few bites of solid foods, weight loss, weakness, and postprandial fullness. Labs showed a Hgb 10.8 g/dL and a positive stool guiac. Based on these findings, which result you would expect to see on the upper gastrointestinal studies?

A. "Unitis plastia"—leather bottle stomach
B. Localized ulcer
C. Esophageal varices
D. Pyloric stenosis

81. **Jerry is 11 years old. He was admitted to the PICU for dehydration and malnutrition after collapsing in his bedroom. His mother reports that Jerry has been eating very bland, soft foods for 3 weeks due to reflux and difficulty swallowing. You suspect that this patient has**
    A. Partial tongue paralysis
    B. Gastric cancer
    C. Tracheal neoplasm
    D. Esophageal neoplasm

82. **Robert is visiting his sister after she underwent surgery for colorectal cancer. Their familial history includes polyposis and inflammatory bowel disease. Robert is worried about his own risk of developing cancer. Which of the following statements is true regarding colorectal cancers?**
    A. Adenocarcinomas are the least common cancer
    B. Right colon lesions are rare
    C. Left colon tumors spread, ulcerate, and erode blood vessels
    D. Rectal tumors are associated with localized metastasis

83. **Diane just got a tattoo and a lip ring last week. Now she complains of flu-like symptoms. She has increasing lethargy and decreased appetite with weight loss of 10 pounds. Generally a cheerful and active person, she reports overwhelming malaise with a sense of foreboding. Nursing interventions include**
    A. Weight-bearing physical therapy every 6 hours
    B. Extended teaching sessions regarding her disease process
    C. An order for a low-fat, high-carbohydrate diet
    D. Allowing visitors 24-hour visitation to cheer Diane up

84. **Which of the following patients with acute liver failure has the best prognosis if liver transplantation does not occur?**
    A. A 17 year old candy striper with hepatitis C
    B. A 13 year old with *Galerina autommars* poisoning
    C. A 7 year old with accidental overdose of acetaminophen
    D. A 14 year old bone marrow transplant recipient with graft-versus-host disease

85. **Sandra's mother is concerned that her daughter, who has cirrhosis, is not urinating. You tell her that this is a common complication of the disease process, because cirrhosis is associated with**
    A. An increased glomerular filtration ratio
    B. Increased renal blood flow
    C. Decreased sodium reabsorption
    D. Increased renin and aldosterone levels

86. **You are admitting an emergency room patient in the PICU after a head injury. As you perform your assessment, you note a stoma to the right iliac fossa in the lower abdomen. There are soft, scattered bowel tones. Output is loose, brownish tinged, and without form. You would document your findings as a(n)**
    A. Sigmoid colostomy
    B. Ileostomy
    C. Loop colostomy
    D. Ascending colostomy

87. **Which of the following methods for measuring intra-abdominal pressures is most commonly utilized in the pediatric critical care setting?**
    A. Intraperitoneal measuring with a peritoneal dialysis catheter
    B. Measurement of the bladder pressures via indwelling urinary catheter
    C. Intragastric measurement with a nasogastric tube
    D. Rectally with a rectal tube

88. **Marie was diagnosed with pancreatic cancer 2 weeks ago. A Whipple procedure is recommended. Which of the following health issues might worsen after she undergoes this procedure?**
    A. Diabetes
    B. Crohn's disease
    C. Hyperbilirubinemia
    D. Obesity

89. **Renee is experiencing dumping syndrome post gastric bypass surgery after eating any meal. Which of the following medications should Renee stop immediately?**
    A. Nitroglycerin
    B. Insulin
    C. Pepcid
    D. Reglan

90. **Ella is 7 months pregnant and was admitted to your unit for severe HELLP syndrome. She is also at risk for which of the following conditions?**
    A. Intra-abdominal hypertension (IAH) and abdominal compartment syndrome (ACS)
    B. Decreased intracranial pressure (ICP)
    C. Hypocarbia
    D. Increased platelets

91. **When patients have liver failure, fatty nodules may develop subcutaneously due to cholesterol accumulation. These nodules are called**
    A. Asterixis
    B. Factor hepaticus
    C. Xanthomas
    D. Telangiectasis

92. **Which of the following types of bowel obstructions leads to infarction or strangulation?**
    A. Acute
    B. Subacute
    C. Chronic
    D. Intermittent

93. **Jacob is a 17 year old Orthodox Jew who presents with an unintentional weight loss of 20 pounds. Jacob also suffers from fatigue, anorexia, and chronic, watery diarrhea with bloody mucus. He is tachycardic, tachypneic, hyperthermic, with a Hgb of 7 g/dL and Hct of 21%. You suspect Jacob is suffering from**
    A. Colonic diverticulitis
    B. Ulcerative colitis
    C. Pancreatitis
    D. Cholecystitis

94. When checking nasogastric tube placement on your burn patient, you note frank blood returning from the tube. Which of the following therapies would be most effective in managing gastric bleeding in this patient?

A. Vasopressin infusion
B. Endoscopic thermal therapy
C. Endoscopic injection therapy
D. Variceal ligation

95. The physician orders a gastric lavage to aid in controlling gastric bleeding in your burn patient. The best fluid choice for gastric lavage is

A. Hot tap water
B. Iced 3% saline
C. Iced sterile water
D. Room-temperature normal saline

96. Matteo has recurrent gallstones and has been treated medically at home for the last 6 months. He was brought into the ICU for severe dehydration, vomiting, and fever. On admission, your assessment reveals abdominal distention, guarding, tympany, absent bowel tones, jaundice, Grey-Turner's sign, and Cullen's sign. Matteo's blood pressure is 75/50, his heart rate is 140, and his respiratory rate is 40 and shallow. You suspect Matteo has

A. Cholecystitis
B. Pancreatitis
C. Cirrhosis
D. Gastritis

97. Ethan has been medically treated for GERD for the past 3 years. He has been admitted to your unit for aspiration pneumonia due to increasing difficulty swallowing and vomiting. He admits to noncompliance with his GERD medication regimen, and was diagnosed with Barrett's esophagus 6 months ago. During his stay in the PICU, Ethan is diagnosed with esophageal cancer. Which surgical procedure would Ethan likely have to remove his cancer?

A. Whipple procedure
B. Modified Whipple procedure
C. Esophagectomy
D. Esophagastrectomy

98. Which of the following bariatric surgical methods does not result in the suturing or removal of gastrointestinal tissue or organs?

A. Vertical banding
B. Gastric banding
C. Biliopancreatic diversion
D. Roux-en-Y proximal gastric bypass

99. Which bariatric surgery method allows for a larger usable stomach pouch?

A. Vertical banding
B. Gastric banding
C. Biliopancreatic diversion
D. Roux-en-Y proximal gastric bypass

100. The TIPS (transjugular intrahepatic portosystemic shunt) is used in which of the following patients?

A. Patients who experience portal hypertension once bleeding has stopped
B. Patients with a portal pressure gradient of <10 mmHg
C. Transplant patients
D. Patients with HITS

101. Sandostatin is ordered for your patient with portal hypertension. Which of the following nursing actions is most important to perform when first starting this drug?

A. Carefully monitor input and output
B. Check nerve stimulation
C. Perform blood glucose checks
D. Check blood pressure every 5 minutes

102. The baby you are caring for was born 2 days ago at home. She has been feeding poorly. While you are attempting to feed the baby, she begins coughing and choking. She has large amounts of oral secretions as well. Her color is poor and she is in respiratory distress. What is the most likely cause of these symptoms?

A. Esophageal atresia
B. Diaphragmatic hernia
C. BPD
D. Trisomy 21

103. Which of the following is the most common cause of intestinal obstruction in the newborn?

A. Intussusception
B. Meconium ileus
C. Intestinal atresia
D. Volvulus

104. The infant you are caring for had meconium plug syndrome at birth. The mother reports the baby has a salty taste when kissed. What could be wrong with this infant?

A. Hirschsprung's disease
B. Cystic fibrosis
C. Malrotation with volvulus
D. Hypernatremia

105. While resuscitating an infant with a diaphragmatic hernia, which oxygen delivery method is best?

A. Bag-valve-mask device
B. Intubation and mechanical ventilation
C. Simple oxygen mask or blow-by oxygen
D. Nasal cannula

106. Your patient, who is 1 month old and has Down syndrome, has started vomiting. You notice his abdomen is becoming distended. Which of the following conditions may be the cause of this problem?

A. High meconium plug
B. Malrotation and volvulus
C. Duodenal atresia
D. NEC

107. Ductal atresia is often seen with trisomy 13. Which other conditions are associated with trisomy 13?

A. Congenital heart defects, malrotation of the gut, and tracheoesophageal abnormalities
B. Congenital heart disease, limb abnormalities, and tracheoesophageal abnormalities
C. Congenital heart disease, anorectal defects, and neural tube defects
D. Neural tube defects, choanal atresia, and limb abnormalities

108. The infant you are caring for is suspected of having Hirschsprung's disease. Which diagnostic procedures do you anticipate the infant to undergo for this disease?

A. Plain abdominal films and blood work, including amylase and lipase
B. Rectal biopsy, plain abdominal X-rays, and barium enema
C. Rectal biopsy and MRI
D. MRI and barium enema

109. The parents of the infant you are caring for are very concerned about their baby's ability to have a normal life with Hirschsprung's disease. What can you tell them?

A. Nothing; all information has to come from the physician
B. There will be no residual problems
C. Surgery may help, but their child may still have some long-term issues
D. Surgery is the only cure

110. Which of the following problems is often associated with meconium plug and Hirschsprung's disease?

A. Down syndrome
B. Cystic fibrosis
C. VATER association
D. Trisomy 13

111. Aside from lower gastrointestinal bleeding, what are some additional symptoms seen with necrotizing enterocolitis?

A. Lethargy, tachycardia, jitteriness
B. Lethargy, apnea, bradycardia, abdominal distention
C. Lethargy, tachypnea, fever
D. Hyperactivity, decreased gastric residuals

112. Short bowel syndrome puts neonates at increased risk for which of the following deficiencies?

A. Vitamins A, D, E, and K deficiency
B. Vitamin B complex and vitamin K deficiency
C. Vitamin C, vitamin B complex, and vitamin D deficiency
D. Vitamin C, vitamin B complex, and vitamin K deficiency

113. What is the drug of choice for treating gastroesophageal reflux?

A. Metoclopramide
B. Questran
C. Regitine
D. Procan

114. Which of the following conditions can cause early upper gastrointestinal bleeding in the neonate?

A. Swallowed maternal blood
B. Necrotic enterocolitis
C. Infectious colitis
D. Volvulus

115. Lower gastrointestinal bleeding is often caused by which of the following conditions?

A. Necrotizing enterocolitis
B. Gastroesophageal reflux disease
C. Intestinal polyps
D. Esophageal varices

116. Three or more episodes of acute, midline abdominal pain lasting from 2 hours to several days, with periods without symptoms, is known as

A. An abdominal migraine
B. Chronic appendicitis
C. Functional dyspepsia
D. Esophagitis

117. Hirschsprung's disease is classified as a(n)

A. Neurologic disorder
B. Metabolic disorder
C. Intrinsic motor disorder
D. Functional disorder

118. Your patient has been diagnosed with gastroenteritis. The primary causative agent for this condition is

A. *Clostridium difficile*
B. *Salmonella typhi*
C. *Cryptosporidium*
D. A rotavirus

119. Diana was admitted to the PICU after a motor vehicle accident that left her bruised and with a fractured leg. She is now complaining of diffuse abdominal pain. Which symptom probably indicates an early sign of appendicitis?

A. Flank pain
B. Pain while resting
C. Night waking
D. Pain after vomiting

120. Steven frequently eats at fast-food restaurants. He was admitted to the PICU with severe abdominal pain and diarrhea. The probable causative organism for his condition is

A. *Giardia lambia*
B. *E. coli*
C. *Staphylococcus aureus*
D. Norwalk virus

121. The most frequent cause of parasitic gastroenteritis in the United States is

A. *Giardia lambia*
B. *Clostridium difficile*
C. *Entamoeba hostolytica*
D. *Cryptosporidium*

122. Administration of an antimicrobial drug should improve diarrhea caused by

A. *E. coli*
B. *Staphylococcus aureus*
C. *Shigella*
D. A rotavirus

123. As a PICU nurse, you know that there is an increased risk for development of pyloric stenosis if an infant is exposed to ________ during the first few months of life

A. Omeprazole
B. Famotidine
C. Gentamycin
D. Erythromycin

124. A glycoprotein produced in the stomach that is required for vitamin B_{12} absorption is

A. Hydrochloric acid
B. Pepsinogen
C. Secretin
D. Intrinsic factor

125. Which of the following statements about splanchnic circulation is true?

A. The splanchnic circulation supplies blood to the kidneys
B. The splanchnic circulation receives one-fourth of the body's total cardiac output
C. The splanchnic circulation empties via the hepatic vein to the liver
D. The splanchnic circulation is the flow from the liver to the duodenum

126. **Which of the following medications inhibits gastrin synthesis and gastric acid output, and decreases splanchnic circulation?**
   A. Vasopressin
   B. Famotidine
   C. Octreotide acetate
   D. Ranitidine

127. **Which of the following drugs is classified as an ammonia detoxicant and a hyperosmotic laxative?**
   A. Lactulose
   B. Cyclosporine
   C. Tacrolimus
   D. Muromonab

128. **One side effect associated with erythromycin is**
   A. Tachycardia
   B. Headache
   C. Eosinophilia
   D. Anemia

129. **A contraindication for use of magnesium hydroxide (milk of magnesia) would be**
   A. Intestinal obstruction
   B. Hyperacidity
   C. Bowel evacuation
   D. A depressed immune system

130. **On the splenic injury scale, a capsular tear that is not bleeding and is less than 1 cm of parenchymal depth is classified as**
   A. Grade I
   B. Grade II
   C. Grade III
   D. Grade IV

131. **On the pancreatic injury severity scale, a proximal transaction or parenchymal injury with probable duet injury would be classified as a**
   A. Class I injury
   B. Class II injury
   C. Class III injury
   D. Class IV injury

132. **Which of the following terms describes bleeding that consists of bright or dark red blood and is passed from the rectum?**
   A. Melena
   B. Occult
   C. Hematemesis
   D. Hematochezia

133. The current treatment of choice for esophageal varices in children is

A. Ligation

B. Endoscopic variceal sclerosis

C. TIPS

D. Barium reduction

134. Jasmine was admitted to the PICU with recurrent pneumonia and severe dysphagia. You are unable to pass either an OG or a NG tube. You suspect Jasmine is suffering from

A. Tracheoesophageal fistula

B. Varices

C. Intestinal atresia

D. A diaphragmatic hernia

135. The type of jaundice that results from failed biliary excretion and includes increased direct bilirubin is known as

A. Cholestatic bilirubinemia

B. Hepatocellular bilirubinemia

C. Physiologic jaundice

D. Kernicterus

136. The stage of hepatitis characterized by jaundice, pallor, pale stool, dark urine, and pruritis is called the _______ stage

A. Preicteric

B. Fulminant

C. Toxic

D. Icteric

SECTION 8

Gastrointestinal Answers

1. **Correct answer: B**
   The organs of the GI system begin developing at 4 weeks gestation and are generally well defined by 8 weeks. At 10 weeks, the midgut moves to the abdomen. It is during this time that a problem may occur with herniation of some or all of the GI contents. At 12 weeks gestation, the GI tract begins peristalsis.

2. **Correct answer: A**
   An omphalocele is the herniation at the umbilicus of abdominal contents, contained in a sac, that may include the large and small bowel, liver, pancreas, and spleen. An omphalocele is often seen with other congenital abnormalities such as other GI disorders, congenital cardiac anomalies, and chromosomal disorders. Gastroschisis is the herniation of the intestines only through an abdominal wall defect. There is no sac covering the intestines in gastroschisis.

3. **Correct answer: D**
   Postoperative care for an infant with gastroschisis includes monitoring fluid status for signs of infection and an NG to suction. Gastroschisis is the herniation of the intestines through a defect in the abdominal wall and is usually found to the right of the umbilicus. Unlike an omphalocele, gastroschisis does not involve other GI organs, nor are the intestines contained in a sac. The surgery to correct this defect may be difficult, as the bowel may be friable and there is a chance of perforation. Infants with gastroschisis rarely have any other congenital anomalies.

4. **Correct answer: B**
   Melena is black, tarry stool containing blood from the upper gastrointestinal area or ascending colon. Oral bleeding may result in hematemesis. Descending colon bleeding may lead to bright red stools. Consumption of iron, bismuth, and other foods may produce stools that are sometimes mistaken for melena, but an occult blood test of the stool will rule out these sources.

5. **Correct answer: B**
   Prevention of necrotizing enterocolitis can be maximized by keeping an infant's stress to a minimum, maintaining adequate fluids, and starting feedings slowly. Prebiotics and probiotics such as *Bifidobacterium* species have been administered in some hospitals, but there is no long-term study demonstrating either the safety or the efficacy of this approach.

6. **Correct answer: B**
   A maternal infection such as *Salmonella* can lead to necrotizing enterocolitis in an infant. This infant should be carefully monitored for abdominal distention, hypotension, lethargy, and bloody stools.

7. **Correct answer: B**
   In addition to abdominal distention, symptoms seen with necrotizing enterocolitis include increased gastric residuals, lethargy, apnea, bradycardia, temperature instability, decreased urine output, hypotension, and bilious vomitus.

8. **Correct answer: A**
   Nasal placement of a gastric tube is contraindicated. This surgical procedure allows for easier access into the cranial vault. Oral gastric tube placement is safe. Oral intubation carries no increase in complications. Tracheal intubations carry no increase in complications related to this history.

9. **Correct answer: D**
   Scaphoid means "hollowed out" or "boat shaped." The abdomen of an infant with a diaphragmatic hernia is sunken or concave in shape because the abdominal contents are displaced into the thoracic cavity.

10. **Correct answer: C**
    Maximum therapy time is 24 to 36 hours for esophageal balloons and 48 to 72 hours for gastric balloons. Time of therapy exceeding these limits is associated with increased risk for necrosis, ulceration, erosion of skin around the nares, airway obstruction, and aspiration of gastric or oropharyngeal contents. Comfort decreases over time, and the risk of erosion to mucosal lining increases. Hgb and Hct levels should increase or stabilize with cessation of bleeding and blood replacement. The gastrointestinal lining may be inflamed related to blood in the system and feedings should be held until the bleeding is stopped.

11. **Correct answer: A**
    Unless they were taken enterically or in sustained-release form, materials are best lavaged within 60 minutes of ingestion. Normal saline or tap water should be used for gastric lavage. Lavage is contraindicated only if the overdose involves corrosive or hydrocarbon materials. Liquid ingestion would have a faster absorption rate than pills, needing faster treatment.

12. **Correct answer: A**
    VATER also encompasses the VATERR, VACTRL, and VACTERL associations. VATER includes vertebral anomalies, anal anomalies, tracheoesophageal fistula, esophageal atresia, and renal anomalies. The other forms of this condition may include cardiac defects, radial dysplasia, limb anomalies, and a single umbilical artery. The causes of these anomalies are unknown but it is believed that the defects begin to form as early as 4–6 weeks of gestational age. VATER association may require numerous surgeries to correct the anomalies as the child grows.

13. **Correct answer: C**
    In acute hepatic failure, late signs include increased ICP, normal or decreased mean arterial pressures, and decreased CPP. Increased ICP, increased mean arterial pressures, and normal CPP are early indicators of acute hepatic failure.

14. **Correct answer: C**
    Brain stem herniation is the most common cause of death related to increased coagulation times, intracranial hemorrhaging, and hypoxia leading to cerebral edema. Anemia is a complication of prolonged bleeding times, but is not the primary cause of death. Pulmonary impairment is the result of hemorrhaging, not embolism or edema.

15. **Correct answer: D**
Hepatorenal syndrome is a complication of hepatic failure due to release of mediators. The release of mediators results in vasoconstriction, which diverts blood flow to the kidneys. A decrease in circulating plasma occurs as the patient develops ascites. Vasoconstriction—not vasodilation—occurs in end-stage liver failure. A decrease in renal circulation occurs due to plasma shifting and vasoconstriction.

16. **Correct answer: C**
Bilious vomitus is the hallmark of malrotation and volvulus. This surgical emergency requires immediate treatment to prevent necrotic bowel. Duodenal atresia may also be associated with bilious vomitus, but a dilated abdomen and duodenum are seen on abdominal X-rays. For meconium plug and Hirschsprung's disease, abdominal distention and delayed stooling are the hallmark symptoms.

17. **Correct answer: B**
For an infant with malrotation of the midgut and volvulus, it is important to decompress the stomach and decrease the risk of aspiration. Most infants have a return to normal bowel function within 10 days. The NPO status is maintained until bowel motility has resumed. Feedings are then slowly resumed. The infant may be maintained on TPN to allow for gut rest. Antibiotics are routinely given in these cases.

18. **Correct answer: B**
Lower gastrointestinal bleeding in the neonate is often due to maternal infection such as *Salmonella* or lactose intolerance. Lower GI bleeding is also common in infants who are under stress, such as an infant with pneumonia. The stress of prematurity can lead to necrotizing enterocolitis.

19. **Correct answer: D**
Cullen's sign refers to the bluish discoloration of the periumbilical area seen in conjunction with pancreatitis and/ or abdominal trauma. A marbled appearance is common with abdominal trauma. Coopernail's sign is bruising of the scrotum or labia. Turner's sign is bruising of the flanks.

20. **Correct answer: D**
This question requires honest communication with the patient and family regarding possible recurrence of symptoms. Approximately one-third of patients with appendicitis who are treated with antibiotics and pain management are readmitted and require appendectomies within one year. The remaining answers are stated as absolutes and are inappropriate responses by the nurse. Because the appendix was not removed, the patient may have a recurrence of symptoms at a later date. There is no way to predict if and when an appendix may become infected or diseased. There is also no way to predict the pain level of appendicitis, as pain is perceived differently by each patient.

21. **Correct answer: C**
Prolonged starvation and protein loss result in fluid shifting and third spacing. Muscle wasting results in an increase in serum lactate levels, not a decrease. Initially, there is an increased urinary nitrogen excretion, which is then followed by a decrease in the excretion rate. Increases in serum catecholamine, glucagons, and cortical levels occur as the body releases elements to maintain energy and make glucose available to the cells.

22. **Correct answer: C**
The goal when working with bulimic and anorexic patients and their families is to support positive nutritional changes while acknowledging and supporting the psychological changes in body and food perception. By acknowledging the difficulties the patient has with food perception and willingness to provide support and counseling with a nutritionist, dietician, and psychologist, the patient will find foods that are both appealing and provide needed nutrition. The remaining answers are abrasive or do not address the patient's physiological or psychological struggle with eating.

23. **Correct answer: A**
Fifty percent of deaths of patients with cirrhosis are from variceal bleeding. These lab tests are used to differentiate causes of bleeding. The history and lab values both lean toward a diagnosis of varices. Although the Hgb and Hct levels would be decreased in peptic ulcer disease and gastritis, the other changes in the lab results would not be occurring. Boerhaave's syndrome is a full-thickness rupture or perforation of the esophageal wall due to prolonged and frequent vomiting related to eating disorders.

24. **Correct answer: B**
Hepatitis B is the only DNA virus listed. The other forms of hepatitis are RNA viruses.

25. **Correct answer: A**
Hepatitis A is often misdiagnosed initially as gastroenteritis, as its symptoms are usually self-limiting. Fecal–oral transmission may also be mistaken as food poisoning.

26. **Correct answer: B**
Acute liver failure related to acetaminophen overdose would be consistent with this patient's presentation. Individuals without full command of the English language are at risk for overdose when self-medicating if the medication label is not read and understood correctly. The symptomology is inconsistent with the DIC and vitamin K deficiency. Gaucher's disease is a genetic enzyme-deficiency disease that is typically diagnosed in childhood. Symptoms are progressive, as the glucocerebroside is collected in the spleen and liver. This patient would also present with skeletal weakness, neurological complications, swollen lymph nodes, and pain not related to just the last 2 weeks.

27. **Correct answer: C**
Aldosteronism initiates sodium retention, thereby increasing portal hypertension. Low albumin levels with increased hydrostatic pressure and decreased oncotic pressures result in ascites. Due to fluid shifting, there would be a decrease in the ventilation/perfusion (V/Q) ratio.

28. **Correct answer: A**
Dehydration is a severe complication in patients with ileostomies. Water reabsorption is normally accomplished by the colon. This patient may have had a large portion or all of the large intestine removed related to the Crohn's disease process. Fluids should be encouraged and IV support maintained to prevent hypovolemic shock. Postoperative teaching should include signs and symptoms of shock and preventive home management. Although a stoma prolapse may occur after discharge home, the stoma can be reopened without major complications. Hyponatremia—not hypernatremia—is a serious complication, as sodium uptake also occurs in the colon. Hemorrhage is not a

concern unless the stoma is scratched or damaged during care. Light pressure should be applied until bleeding stops, but bleeding is not a life-threatening complication.

29. **Correct answer: A**
The patient is exhibiting signs and symptoms of malrotation and duodenal obstruction related to a volvulus. The nurse should contact the physician immediately and prepare for surgery before necrosis of the bowel occurs. Tylenol and morphine will mask these serious symptoms. Pain is related to ischemia experienced by the intestines as their blood supply is prevented by the malrotation. The fever may indicate perforation or necrosis of the areas of the intestines impacted by the volvulus. The patient will need to sit upright to prevent aspiration post vomiting. These symptoms are not normal, and discoloration of the abdomen indicates greater ischemia and a higher risk of perforation.

30. **Correct answer: B**
The Whipple procedure removes the tip or head of the pancreas, the gallbladder, the duodenum, and part of the bile duct. Occasionally, part of the stomach may also be removed. The extent of the cancerous pancreatic tumor will indicate the extent of removal.

31. **Correct answer: C**
Sue's symptoms are consistent with late dumping syndrome related to the partial gastrectomy during the Whipple procedure. With late dumping syndrome, symptoms occur 1 to 3 hours after meals. Additional symptoms include weakness, fatigue, dizziness, anxiety, palpitations, and fainting. Patients may also exhibit early signs of dumping syndrome approximately 15 to 30 minutes after a meal with nausea, vomiting, cramps or abdominal pain, diarrhea, bloating, tachycardia, dysrhythmias, and dizziness. Although anxiety may be exhibited with dumping syndrome, an alteration in mental status in relation to food consumption and the patient's history support a dumping syndrome diagnosis. Hypoglycemia is a greater risk for patients who have undergone just gastrectomy or bypass. GERD presents with heartburn and epigastric pain.

32. **Correct answer: C**
Intra-abdominal pressures of 5 to 15 mmHg indicate a low to moderate pressure problem. When respiratory function is impaired, the values will range to about 25 mmHg, and you would expect to see more extensive respiratory distress and compromise. Severe compromise is seen with pressures exceeding 40 mmHg. Thoracic pressures increase as intra-abdominal pressures increase, which inhibits lung expansion and diaphragm movement, resulting in hypoventilation and hypoxia.

33. **Correct answer: B**
A patient with a platelet count of 79 mm^3/mL is thrombocytopenic and at risk for coagulation complications. Heparin is normally added to the solution to prevent clotting and can lead to further complications of bleeding. The other lab values are within the normal range for either males or females.

34. **Correct answer: A**
The correct order for interventions when assisting with a paracentesis is (1) have the patient void or insert a Foley catheter, (2) order an upright X-ray of the abdomen, (3) position the patient with the affected side up, and (4) examine the abdomen for dullness.

35. **Correct answer: B**
Brendon is exhibiting signs of an early ischemic bowel. At this time, there will be some dilation of the bowel with loops behind the ischemic bowel, because the ischemic bowel is not performing peristaltic actions. Late signs, if this condition is not diagnosed and treated early, include dilation of the entire bowel, including the stomach. "Thumb printing" is seen on an X-ray when edema of the bowel wall shows the convex indentations of the lumen and pneumatosis intestinalis is evident as a mottled gas pattern in the bowel wall. Air in the biliary tree is indicative of a gallbladder emergency, and air under the diaphragm is a pneumoperitoneum.

36. **Correct answer: D**
Mary is at risk for developing SRES. The diagnosis of SRES or Stress-Related Erosive Syndrome, was once used to explain gastric complications related to critical care illnesses. The stress response within the patient may lead to rapid erosion of the mucosal lining and result in ulcerations. Patients suffering from severe physiological illnesses are at high risk of SRES and, if this condition goes untreated, gastric bleeding.

37. **Correct answer: B**
The patient is exhibiting signs and symptoms of gastric perforation. This is a surgical emergency and the lavage should be stopped, fluid aspirated, and the physician notified immediately. Additional actions should include the placement of at least two large-bore IVs, preparing to administer IV fluid replacement if hypovolemic shock occurs, and preparing the patient for immediate surgery.

38. **Correct answer: B**
Patients with pancreatitis undergo massive fluid shifts as part of the inflammatory response to pancreatic self-digestion. Mediators released during the inflammatory response lead to vasodilation and increased capillary permeability. Fluid may shift into the bowel, into the mucosal lining, and within the lungs leading to acute lung injury (ALI). The drop in blood pressure may lead to acute kidney injury (AKI) and renal failure. Immediate fluid replacement with crystalloids and colloids is required to maintain intravascular volume. A history of poor volume intake worsens the hypovolemia, but is not the primary and most severe cause of the hypovolemic shock.

39. **Correct answer: C**
Barrett's esophagus is a result of mucosal changes in the esophagus after repeated and prolonged exposure to gastric secretions seen in untreated GERD (gastroesophageal reflux disease). Due to cellular changes in the esophageal lining, the patient is at increased risk for esophageal cancer.

40. **Correct answer: A**
Gastric bypass surgery can lead to permanent gastric changes and places the obese patient at risk for both surgical and anesthesia-related complications. For many patients undergoing bariatric procedures, the initial gastric bypass surgery is not necessarily the only surgery required. Often cosmetic surgery to remove loose skin around the stomach, back, thighs, arms, and chest is required to improve self-image. Each surgery carries additional risk. Therefore, complete bariatric education should be provided to any patient and his or her parents if they are considering bariatric surgery. Education should include preoperative changes in diet, nutritional consultation, psychological evaluation, and full medical evaluation including lab work and cardiovascular

testing. Education and support for the patient undergoing bariatric surgery should continue throughout the surgical process, with ongoing education, nutritional support, and physiological support for years after surgery.

41. **Correct answer: B**
Although each of these assessments is vital prior to bariatric surgery, psychological evaluation assesses the patient's psychological health regarding weight management, food, diet, nutrition, activity, exercise, health, and surgery. In addition, evaluation of the patient's coping mechanisms, self-image, and self-esteem needs may help estimate the surgery's chance of long-term success. Obesity has many different causes, and an assessment of psychological health may reveal dangerous beliefs and behaviors related to food and nutrition that will need to be addressed prior to surgery.

42. **Correct answer: C**
GERD or gastroesophageal reflux disease is a common complication of gastric banding. Due to the smaller gastric size and the close proximity of the band to the sphincter, the patient experiences reflux, and possibly nausea and vomiting, after eating. Deflation of the band with slower reinflation adjustments every 2 weeks will ease these symptoms. Stoma obstruction may occur if the patient fails to chew food properly and thoroughly. Band slippage may lead to erosion and perforation of the stomach or a folding of the larger portion of the stomach over the smaller portion.

43. **Correct answer: C**
Because the gastric size is greatly reduced, there is less intrinsic factor to facilitate vitamin B_{12} absorption—a condition that is needed to prevent pernicious anemia. Oral supplements are not recommended, as they may not be absorbed quickly enough. Instead, sublingual or injected vitamin B_{12} may be required. Iron, thiamin, and calcium are all absorbed in the duodenum. In gastric bypass, the duodenum is also bypassed, which greatly limits the absorption of these vitamins and minerals. Careful supplementation is mandatory to prevent malnutrition. Protein deficiencies are also common and supplementation is necessary, especially in early postoperative recovery, to prevent muscle wasting during the rapid weight loss period.

44. **Correct answer: A**
This patient would suffer a shortage of oxygen to the tissues, not an excessive amount of oxygen.

45. **Correct answer: B**
Barbara is probably suffering from a paralytic ileus caused by the codeine. Codeine slows gastric motility throughout the GI tract. This patient needs a nasogastric tube and motility medications such as metoclopramide.

46. **Correct answer: C**
The optimal postfeeding position for an infant with gastroesophageal reflux is the prone or left lateral position, which facilitates gastric emptying. Keeping the head of the crib elevated to 30° also helps reduce reflux.

47. **Correct answer: B**
Prolonged TPN administration can lead to cholestasis. Cholestasis is the impaired flow of bile. This condition may be seen with other conditions as well, such as cystic fibrosis, biliary atresia, and infection. Cholestasis can also occur as a result of cholelithiasis.

48. **Correct answer: A**
Total serum bilirubin is the measure of hyperbilirubinemia. The condition may be mild to severe. A patient with hyperbilirubinemia presents with jaundice in a cephalocaudal (head-to-toe) pattern, and the condition resolves in the reverse order. If hyperbilirubinemia occurs acutely and if it is severe enough, it can cause severe neurologic damage and death.

49. **Correct answer: D**
Emesis is the most common symptom of GER, and it may be dramatic. Infants with gastroesophageal reflux are sometimes called "happy spitters." More than 50% of all infants have episodes of spitting up that are not pathologic, and for most infants, this condition resolves in the first year of life.

50. **Correct answer: D**
Newborns typically stool 4–5 times per day. This number decreases to 1–2 per day by age 1 year.

51. **Correct answer: A**
An infant with α_1-antitrypsin (α_1-AT) deficiency liver disease has increased gamma-glutamyl transpeptidase (GGTP) levels, jaundice, clay-colored stools, and malabsorption. Small for gestational age, hepatosplenomegaly, and a family history of emphysema or cirrhosis will also be seen with this condition. Jeremy will probably need a liver transplant at some time. He is also very susceptible to developing emphysema or cirrhosis at a young age.

52. **Correct answer: B**
Adverse reactions to cimetidine may include rash, nausea, agitation, vomiting, diarrhea, flushing, neutropenia, elevated liver enzymes, and drowsiness.

53. **Correct answer: C**
Cimetidine, famotidine, and ranitidine are H_2 blockers. They inhibit gastric acid production by antagonism of the histamine H_2 receptors. These medications are used for prevention of ulcers and in the treatment of GI bleeding.

54. **Correct answer: D**
Proton pump inhibitors inhibit an enzyme that triggers the gastric parietal cells to release hydrochloric acid. This reduction in acid production can reduce the effectiveness of many oral medications such as antifungal agents. It may increase the absorption of drugs such as digoxin and furosemide.

55. **Correct answer: B**
During transportation of a critically ill infant, it is important to obtain consent for blood and blood products in addition to consent for transport and treatment. This patient presents with severe gastrointestinal distress. If the cause is related to perforation or megacolon, sepsis and hypovolemic shock may result, threatening life. Proactive staff will anticipate potential administration of blood and blood products and prevent any delay in treatment if the patient becomes critical.

56. **Correct answer: B**
Francine will likely produce less milk than the amount that would have been expected if she had not had complications of hypovolemic shock with delayed pumping.

57. **Correct answer: D**
Vitamin E is a fat-soluble vitamin that is used concurrently with iron and erythropoietin to treat anemia. It is also an antioxidant and has been used in the healing of damaged tissues.

58. **Correct answer: C**
Treatments you would expect for an infant with neonatal hepatitis include adequate nutrition, fluids, and fat-soluble vitamins. The infant may not be able to tolerate PO nutrition, and may need IV fluids or TPN and fat-soluble vitamins. Corticosteroids would be contraindicated in this case. Antibiotics or antivirals should be given only if the diagnosis warrants their use.

59. **Correct answer: B**
Infants with neonatal hepatitis may present with jaundice, hepatomegaly, vomiting, poor sucking, anorexia, lethargy, fever, and petechiae. The causes of neonatal hepatitis can range from idiopathic to inborn metabolic errors and infection.

60. **Correct answer: B**
Similac PM 60/40 is frequently given to neonates with renal insufficiency. This formula has a low mineral content, low iron content, and optimal electrolyte balance.

61. **Correct answer: C**
Soy-based formulas are indicated for lactase deficiency, as their carbohydrate content is plant based, rather than lactose based. Lactase is the enzyme that breaks down lactose.

62. **Correct answer: B**
Portagen is frequently used for infants with fatty acid metabolism deficiency. These patients are unable to digest and utilize the long-chain fatty acids from foods.

63. **Correct answer: C**
Medications that are bound to protein may have less drug available to produce the desired effect.

64. **Correct answer: A**
Gastroesophageal reflux is a long-term complication of congenital diaphragmatic hernia repair. Parent teaching should include management and prevention of reflux and aspiration with resulting respiratory distress.

65. **Correct answer: D**
This is another of those deceptively easy questions. Make absolutely certain you know the correct order for assessment: (1) inspection to determine landmarks and appearance, (2) auscultation to establish location and quality of bowel tones, (3) identification of percussion notes or tones, which are different for various internal organs, and (4) palpation to establish wall tone, tenderness, and size of organs. Performing percussion and palpation prior to inspection or auscultation could affect the assessment findings.

66. **Correct answer: B**
Hepatic bruits are heard over the liver and may indicate primary liver cancer, alcoholic hepatitis, or vascular liver metastases. An aortic bruit over the epigastric area indicates a partial aortic occlusion. Iliac artery bruits are heard over the left and right inguinal areas. Renal artery bruits indicate renal artery stenosis.

67. **Correct answer:** A
Normal portal pressures are 5 to 10 mmHg (7 to 14 cm H_2O). This would indicate portal hypertension. Portal pressures should be 4 to 5 mmHg higher than the inferior vena cava pressures. Pressures this high above the inferior vena cava pressures indicate severe portal hypertension.

68. **Correct answer:** A
The Minnesota tube contains separate suction and balloons that can function independently. The Sengstaken-Blakemore tube has three lumens, but only one suction port. The Linton-Nachlas tube is used only for gastric varices. The Standard nasogastric tube has no balloon function, so it cannot be used to tamponade bleeding.

69. **Correct answer:** B
This answer acknowledges the brother's concerns and provides education. Elevated bilirubin levels deposited in the skin result in unconscious scratching and excoriations. With the presence of increased PT, PTT, and INR levels, hematomas may also be present. Denying abuse provides no explanation for the scratches and decreases communication with the brother. Restraints are inappropriate for this patient. PICU psychosis can lead to abnormal behavior, but is not the reason for this patient's behavior.

70. **Correct answer:** C
Four grades of hepatic encephalopathy are distinguished based on five clinical findings: level of consciousness, orientation, intellectual functions, behavior, mood, and neuromuscular function.

71. **Correct answer:** B
In patients with chronic liver failure, the skin becomes very dryentle. Application of a moisturizer may relieve their discomfort. Deep tissue massage is contraindicated due to the decreased platelet count and increased tendency toward bruising. Development of orthostatic hypertension prohibits any rapid movement, as it is associated with dizziness and greater risk of fall. Patients and family members are at risk for depression, but visits may decrease this risk and will provide staff with an opportunity to assess for and intervene if depression is observed.

72. **Correct answer:** A
Acute pancreatitis may occur as a result of seat belt trauma to the pancreatic duct or abdominal ischemia. Acute liver failure is characterized by flu-like symptoms, jaundice, confusion, and enlarged liver. Gastrointestinal bleeding is often associated with a history of ulcers and/or esophageal varices with hemodynamic changes, narrowing pulse pressures, hematemesis, and hyperactive bowel tones. Abdominal trauma does not produce the knife-like and twisting pain, and tenderness and a marbled appearance would be noted.

73. **Correct answer:** A
You would see elevated serum amylase. Serum lipase would be increased, not decreased. Albumin levels would drop, not rise. Trypsin levels would also increase, not decrease, with the buildup of pancreatic enzymes.

74. **Correct answer:** A
Severe illnesses result in blood shunting to protect cardiac, respiratory, and neurological function. Any mucosal ischemia may lead to a loss of protective functions within

the gastrointestinal system. Mucus acts to protect function within the gastrointestinal system, so a decrease in its production would be harmful. Fungal infections are rare within the gastrointestinal system; bacteria are more common causes of gastric ulcers. Although it is possible to have ulcers on admission to the PICU, the diagnosis in this case is a new-onset illness.

75. **Correct answer: B**
Prehepatic (presinusoidal) factors lead to hepatic venous pressures that are less than portal pressures. Umbilical vein catheterizations in a neonate (within the first month of life) due to neonatal illness or prematurity may cause damage to the vessel. Chronic active hepatitis is an intrahepatic (sinusoidal) factor. Wedge hepatic venous pressures are increased or equal to portal pressures. Metastatic carcinoma and cardiac diseases such as CHF can cause portal hypertension and may indirectly cause variceal bleeding.

76. **Correct answer: C**
This patient has likely ruptured a varix (the singular form of "varices"). Priorities are to maintain the airway, stop bleeding, and verify venous access for blood replacement, fluid management, and homeostasis. Placing the patient NPO and obtaining IV access is the first correct answer listed. You would want to position the patient upright (not flat) to prevent aspiration. You would anticipate the placement of a Minnesota tube, not a Linton-Nachlas tube. Dopamine at 5 mcg/kg/min would better support renal function—not blood pressure, as is needed in this patient.

77. **Correct answer: A**
This patient is exhibiting signs and symptoms of an abscess post surgical intervention for appendicitis, which occurs in 5–33% of patients. Surgical debridement of the incision and IV antibiotics are appropriate immediate treatment to prevent sepsis. Hydration and antibiotics alone will not treat the abscess. Bedside excision of the abscess alone may reduce the amount of infected fluid and tissue at the site, but will not prevent further infection. Bedside wound debridement carries a high risk of further contamination of the site. In approximately 2% of cases, the abscess may be intra-abdominal and may require surgical intervention under anesthesia as well as continued antibiotic treatment.

78. **Correct answer: D**
This patient may safely continue verapamil for atrial fibrillation. Calcium channel blockers have been found to provide some protection against complications of diverticulae. Nonsteroidal anti-inflammatory agents, corticosteroids, and opiate analgesics have been noted to increase risk of perforation of diverticulae.

79. **Correct answer: A**
Chronic pancreatitis results in the release of digestive enzymes into the body. Phospholipase A_2 breaks down the cellular structure of the capillary beds, resulting in tissue injury throughout the body. In the lungs, capillary damage is manifested by pulmonary edema and dyspnea, leading to respiratory distress. Although stress may lead to bronchospasm in patients with existing respiratory diseases such as asthma, that finding is not part of the information given in this question. Aspiration and atelectasis are occasional complications in PICU patients, but do not explain both symptoms as related to the ongoing disease process.

80. **Correct answer: A**
This patient is exhibiting subjective and objective signs and symptoms of stomach cancer. A higher incidence of stomach cancer is noted in males from cultures farthest from the equator. With this diagnosis, an upper gastrointestinal series would show a "leather bottle" stomach. The symptoms do not support a diagnosis of an ulcer. Radiological studies would show ulceration or free air with perforation. Radiological studies for varices would not show any distinct changes. Pyloric stenosis is typically seen in infants and would be evident as a distended abdomen, accompanied by nonbilious, projectile vomiting.

81. **Correct answer: D**
This patient is exhibiting classic progression of a developing esophageal neoplasm. Complications that coincide with this disease process are related to changes in nutritional intake. Narrowing of the esophageal lumen results in increasing difficulties and pain when swallowing, leading to a softer diet until the patient can swallow only liquids. Partial tongue paralysis would be supported if the patient also had difficulty speaking, but that symptom is not included in the information given in this question. Gastric cancer is indicated with indigestion and fullness, not difficulty swallowing. A tracheal neoplasm would be associated with more respiratory distress.

82. **Correct answer: C**
Left colon (descending) lesions typically spread, ulcerate, and erode blood vessels within the colon. Obstruction is a very common complication with this type of lesion. Adenocarcinomas are the most common of these neoplasms. Right colon (ascending) lesions are typically polypoid lesions and are associated with a familial history of polyps. Rectal lesions may spread to the vagina or prostate, but are known for systemic metastasis.

83. **Correct answer: C**
This patient's history and symptomology are consistent with new-onset hepatitis C. Hepatitis C results in a hypermetabolic state. Nursing interventions should focus on minimizing symptoms and reducing stress on the body. A low-fat, high-carbohydrate diet supports the body's increased caloric demand and helps prevent weight loss. The greater the liver compromise related to infection, the lower the fat and protein intake, because the liver may not be able to assist with effective digestion. This patient should remain on strict bed rest to allow for energy conservation while she is in the acute phase of her illness. Light ambulation is permitted as long as the patient does not become fatigued with the activity. Although teaching is vital for this patient and her family, extended teaching sessions may tax the patient's ability to concentrate. Teaching should be available in multiple forms that can be referred to at the patient's and family's leisure. Family may be supportive, but planned rest periods should be maintained and supported as patient tolerance allows.

84. **Correct answer: C**
The patient with the acetaminophen overdose has the best prognosis even in the absence of a liver transplant. The patients with viral hepatitis, *Galerina autumnaas* (mushroom) poisoning, and bone marrow transplant all have very poor prognoses if liver transplants are not available. Management goals include stabilizing hemodynamics, preventing infection, maintaining stable glucose levels, protecting the airway, and supporting adequate tissue perfusion.

85. **Correct answer: D**
Due to the cirrhosis, renal function may be impaired, resulting in poor urine output. Common complications that lead to poor urine output are an increased secretion of renin and aldosterone levels leading to sodium retention. There is a decrease in glomerular filtration rate, along with a decrease in renal blood flow.

86. **Correct answer: B**
An ileostomy is located at the right ileac fossa just prior to the colon. Given that the majority of water absorption occurs in the colon, stool from the small intestines is loose and unformed. Sigmoid colostomy stools more closely resemble normal stools, as most of the water has been absorbed. Loop (transverse) and ascending colostomies will yield loose stools with more formation.

87. **Correct answer: B**
The most commonly used method for measuring intra-abdominal pressure is via the bladder. A specialized catheter with a transducer allows for direct measurement of pressures with equipment that is usually found in the pediatric critical care unit.

88. **Correct answer: A**
If a patient has been diagnosed with diabetes or has uncontrolled blood glucose levels, then removal of the pancreatic head may result in diabetes or worsening symptoms. It is imperative that the patient's blood glucose levels be monitored closely. With removal of part of the pancreas, the pancreas may not produce and release insulin at previous levels. Consequently, insulin injections may be required to make up for the shortfalls. The Whipple procedure removes part of the bile duct, which may improve bilirubin levels. With removal of part of the stomach and pancreas, patients are at risk of long-term malnutrition and weight loss.

89. **Correct answer: D**
Renee is experiencing dumping syndrome post gastric bypass surgery and should stop taking reglan. Reglan increases gastric emptying by increasing peristalsis, thus increasing the effects of dumping syndrome. Reglan may be used post gastrectomy when gastroparesis is present, but once peristalsis has resumed, it should be stopped.

90. **Correct answer: A**
Due to the pregnancy and resulting HELLP syndrome, there is an increased risk for fluid to collect in the abdominal cavity and for development of tissue edema. Signs and symptoms of IAH and ACS include an increased ICP, hypercarbia, decreased platelet values, decreased cardiac output, poor or absent urinary output, and abdominal wall rigidity.

91. **Correct answer: C**
When patients have liver failure, fatty nodules called xanthomas may develop subcutaneously due to cholesterol accumulation.

92. **Correct answer: A**
Acute bowel obstruction is the only type of obstruction that leads to infarction or strangulation. Obstruction occurs rapidly and may inhibit delivery of blood to a portion of the bowel. The other types of obstructions permit limited or intermittent blood flow that sustains tissue function, albeit at a compromised level.

93. **Correct answer: B**
Based on the presenting symptoms and his ethnicity, Jacob has ulcerative colitis. He may also have leukocytosis and cachexia. Colonic diverticulitis presents with left upper quadrant pain, hyperthermia, vomiting, chills, diarrhea, and tenderness over the descending colon. Pancreatitis presents with left upper quadrant pain that radiates to the back or chest, hyperthermia, rigidity, rebound abdominal tenderness, nausea and vomiting, jaundice, Cullen's sign, Grey-Turner's sign, abdominal distention, and diminished bowel sounds. Cholecystitis presents with right upper quadrant or epigastric pain, pain that lasts for as long as 6 hours after a fatty meal, vomiting, and increased white blood cell counts.

94. **Correct answer: A**
This patient is likely having gastric bleeding related to stress-related erosion syndrome. Due to the generalized bleeding associated with this condition, endoscopic therapies are not as effective as arginine vasopressin infusion into the gastric artery, which causes splanchnic vasoconstriction. There is no indication that this patient has varices that would require ligation.

95. **Correct answer: D**
The best fluid choice for gastric lavage is room temperature normal saline. In the past, iced solutions were used in controlling gastric bleeding. More recently, research has shown that the iced solutions may cause additional bleeding by irritating healthy and compromised mucosal lining. Their low temperature may also produce core hypothermia and a shift in the oxyhemoglobin dissociation curve, resulting in decreased oxygen delivery to the tissues. A 3% saline solution would cause a fluid shift. Tap water should be avoided, as it may increase the risk of systemic infection if the water is contaminated.

96. **Correct answer: B**
Although Matteo's initial symptoms and family history may indicate cholecystitis, his symptoms are the classic presentation for pancreatitis. Abdominal rigidity, Grey-Turner's sign, and Cullen's sign are late indicators of pancreatitis. In addition, Matteo is presenting with severe hypovolemic shock. Fluid resuscitation should be initiated immediately to support his cardiovascular function.

97. **Correct answer: C**
The correct name for this procedure is an esophagectomy. It involves removal of the damaged esophagus to the proximal portion of the stomach. The stomach is then resectioned to form a new esophagus. If the stomach is also cancerous, the stomach is removed and the small bowel is resectioned to create a new esophagus.

98. **Correct answer: B**
Gastric banding uses an adjustable band placed around the upper portion of the stomach to create a small, 1- to 2-ounce area to act as the stomach. Because the size is restricted without suturing off the stomach or removal of any tissue, this procedure may be reversed for medical reasons such as pregnancy. Vertical banding, biliopancreatic diversion, and Roux-en-Y proximal gastric bypass all inflict some permanent change on the normal gastric pathway.

99. **Correct answer: C**
Biliopancreatic diversion uses a 5-ounce stomach pouch and wide anastomosis. The biliary branch or limb connects a portion of the small bowel to the biliary tract to allow for normal biliary excretion. To prevent further preoperative or postoperative complications associated with cholecystitis, the gallbladder may be removed during the procedure.

100. **Correct answer: C**
In transplant patients, TIPS serves as a bridge between the two livers in a hemodynamically unstable patient, so as to increase his or her stability. TIPS can be used when patients are experiencing active bleeding via varices. Patients must have a directly measured portal pressure gradient of more than 10 mmHg. If bleeding is due to HITS (heparin-induced thrombocytopenia) this procedure should be postponed until the patient is stabilized.

101. **Correct answer: C**
Glycemic emergencies may occur with administration of sandostatin, especially in the diabetic patient. It is important to monitor blood glucose to prevent hyperglycemia or hypoglycemia. Blood pressure and urinary function may also be affected, but these dysfunctions do not become life-threatening as quickly as unstable glucose levels.

102. **Correct answer: A**
This collection of symptoms is classic for esophageal atresia and often occurs with a tracheoesophageal fistula—a condition that affects 1 in every 25,000 infants. Esophageal atresia is a failure of the esophagus to complete the connection between the throat and stomach, forming a blind pouch. Often a fistula forms between the esophagus and the trachea, called a tracheoesophageal fistula. Assessment of these infants involves insertion of a nasogastric tube into the blind pouch, followed by a chest X-ray. Depending on the severity of the atresia, it may be possible to close the fistula. It is important to close the fistula as soon as possible to reduce the risk of aspiration pneumonia. A G-tube may be inserted for feedings, and the nasogastric tube placed on low suction. Nursing care includes elevating the head of the bassinet, giving IV fluids, providing oxygen, and maintaining the NG tube. Approximately half of all infants born with esophageal atresia have other congenital problems, such as VATER association, other GI abnormalities of the anus and rectum, renal malformations, cardiac abnormalities, and skeletal deformities.

103. **Correct answer: C**
Intestinal atresia is the most common cause of intestinal obstruction in the newborn. Bile-colored vomitus is the hallmark of intestinal atresia. The site of the obstruction may occur anywhere in the small or large bowel. Symptoms depend on the obstruction's location. Duodenal atresia is often seen with Down syndrome. Malrotation with volvulus usually occurs at the duodenal–jejunal junction and is a surgical emergency. Jejunal atresia, often seen with meconium ileus, presents with bile vomitus at birth. Meconium plug syndrome is often seen with Hirschsprung's disease and cystic fibrosis and causes diffuse distention of the bowel.

104. Correct answer: B

Cystic fibrosis is often seen with meconium plug syndrome. Symptoms include abdominal distention, a salty taste, no meconium plug passage, and vomiting. X-rays of the abdomen will show distention with fine bubbles in the bowel. Most states require infant testing for cystic fibrosis as a part of the national newborn screening requirements. GI abnormalities that occur with cystic fibrosis in addition to meconium plug syndrome include rectal prolapse, pancreatic disorders, chronic liver disease, failure to thrive, low protein levels with edema, fat-soluble vitamin deficiencies, sodium depletion, electrolyte imbalances, and alkalosis.

105. Correct answer: B

Immediate intubation and mechanical ventilation with 100% oxygen is the only approved oxygenation method for this infant. A bag-valve-mask device can cause distention of the bowel, which is already impeding breathing. The simple oxygen mask and blow-by are inappropriate in this case.

106. Correct answer: C

Duodenal atresia is seen in about approximately 30% of infants born with Down syndrome. On X-ray, a "double bubble" of gas is often seen. Treatment will include placement of an NG tube, NPO status, and IV fluids. The infant may also receive antibiotics.

107. Correct answer: A

Approximately 30% of infants with ductal atresia also have congenital heart defects, malrotation of the gut, tracheoesophageal abnormalities, and anorectal defects. Generally, patients with ductal atresia have an excellent prognosis.

108. Correct answer: B

After plain films are taken, a barium enema may be performed. The rectal biopsy is the best diagnostic tool for Hirschsprung's disease. In patients with this disease, a biopsy shows a lack of parasympathetic ganglions in the distal bowel and rectum. This problem usually develops around the 12th week of gestation. Hirschsprung's disease is seen in males four to five times more often than in females, and it may also run in families.

109. Correct answer: C

With Hirschsprung's disease, surgery may help, but the child may still have some long-term issues. Surgery is performed to move the innervated bowel to the anus. There may be some delay in bowel training. In some cases, a child with Hirschsprung's disease may have fecal incontinence or chronic constipation.

110. Correct answer: B

Cystic fibrosis is associated with meconium plug and Hirschsprung's disease in approximately 10% of cases. All 50 states require chloride sweat testing on all newborns as an assessment for cystic fibrosis.

111. Correct answer: B

In addition to abdominal distention, symptoms seen with necrotizing enterocolitis include increased gastric residuals, lethargy, apnea, bradycardia, temperature instability, decreased urine output, hypotension, and bilious vomitus.

112. Correct answer: A
Neonates are at risk for deficiencies of vitamins A, D, E, and K. These fat-soluble vitamins are absorbed in the ileum. The ileum is responsible for the absorption of the majority of the nutrition consumed, vitamin B_{12}, and bile salts, in addition to the fat-soluble vitamins. In the neonate, the two most common causes of short bowel syndrome are volvulus and necrotizing enterocolitis.

113. Correct answer: A
Metoclopramide increases gastric emptying and motility, thereby reducing reflux symptoms. The infant should be monitored for diarrhea and neurologic signs such as tremors or muscle twitching.

114. Correct answer: A
Early upper gastrointestinal bleeding in the neonate may be caused by swallowing maternal blood during birth. Blood from fissured nipples may also be swallowed and later vomited.

115. Correct answer: A
Necrotizing enterocolitis is the primary cause of lower gastrointestinal bleeding in neonates. Other causes include swallowed maternal blood, allergic colitis, Hirschsprung's disease, and volvulus. Gastroesophageal reflux disease, intestinal polyps, and Mallory-Weiss tear are seen in older children.

116. Correct answer: A
An abdominal migraine is characterized by three or more episodes of acute, midline abdominal pain lasting from 2 hours to several days, with periods without symptoms.

117. Correct answer: C
Hirschsprung's disease is classified as an intrinsic motor disorder.

118. Correct answer: D
The primary causative agent for gastroenteritis is a rotavirus.

119. Correct answer: C
Night waking is an early sign of appendicitis. An affected patient has nonspecific discomfort and wakes frequently.

120. Correct answer: B
E. coli infection is linked with abdominal pain and diarrhea caused by consumption of fast foods.

121. Correct answer: A
Giardia lambia infection is the most frequent cause of parasitic gastroenteritis in the United States.

122. Correct answer: C
An antimicrobial drug should improve diarrhea caused by *Shigella* infection.

123. Correct answer: D
As a PICU nurse, you know that there is an increased risk for development of pyloric stenosis if an infant is exposed to erythromycin during the first few months of life.

124. **Correct answer: D**
Intrinsic factor is a glycoprotein produced in the stomach that is required for vitamin B_{12} absorption.

125. **Correct answer: B**
The splanchnic circulation receives one-fourth of the cardiac output to the body.

126. **Correct answer: C**
Octreotide acetate inhibits gastrin synthesis, gastric acid output, and decreases splanchnic circulation.

127. **Correct answer: A**
Lactulose is classified as an ammonia detoxicant and a hyperosmotic laxative.

128. **Correct answer: C**
Eosinophilia is a side effect of erythromycin. Other side effects of this medication include bradycardia, abdominal pain, nausea, ventricular arrhythmia, and cholestatic jaundice.

129. **Correct answer: A**
Intestinal obstruction is a contraindication for use of magnesium hydroxide (milk of magnesia). Additional contraindications would include ileostomy, colostomy, and appendicitis.

130. **Correct answer: A**
If the patient at this grade had a laceration: capsular tear, nonbleeding, and less than 1 cm of parenchymal depth is classified as a grade I on the splenic injury scale.

131. **Correct answer: C**
On the pancreatic injury severity scale, a proximal transaction or parenchymal injury with probable duet injury would be known as a Class III injury.

132. **Correct answer: D**
Hematochezia is the term used to describe bleeding that consists of bright or dark red blood that is passed from the rectum.

133. **Correct answer: B**
The current treatment of choice for esophageal varices in children is endoscopic variceal sclerosis. The sclerosing agent is administered through a flexible fiber-optic endoscope. This agent may be placed near the varices or injected directly into the varix.

134. **Correct answer: A**
With a tracheoesophageal fistula, the nurse will be unable to pass either an OG tube or a NG tube in a patient presenting with recurrent pneumonia and severe dysphagia.

135. **Correct answer: A**
Cholestatic bilirubinemia is the type of jaundice that results from failed biliary excretion and includes increased direct bilirubin.

136. **Correct answer: D**
The stage of hepatitis characterized by jaundice, pallor, pale stool, dark urine, and pruritis is called the icteric stage.

GASTROINTESTINAL REFERENCES

Aehlert, B. (Ed.). (2005). *Comprehensive pediatric emergency care.* St. Louis, MO: Mosby.

Ahmed, I., & Beckingham, I. J. (2007). Liver trauma. *Trauma, 9*(3), 171–180.

American Heart Association. (2010). Guidelines 2010 for cardiopulmonary resuscitation and emergency cardiovascular care. Retrieved from www.americanheart.org

Applegate, K. (2009). Evidence-based diagnosis of malrotation and volvulus. *Pediatric Radiology: Supplement, 39,* 161–163.

Babl, F. E., Goldfinch, C., Mandrawa, C., Crellin, D., O'Sullivan, R., & Donath, S. (2009). Does nebulized lidocaine reduce the pain and distress of nasogastric tube insertion in young children? A randomized, double-blind, placebo-controlled trial. *Pediatrics, 123*(6), 1548–1555.

Betz, T. G., Lee, P., & Victor, J. C. (2008). Hepatitis A vaccine versus immune globulin for post-exposure prophylaxis. *New England Journal of Medicine,* 358(5), 531–532.

Birmingham Children's Hospital. (2008, December). Pierre-Robin syndrome: Research from Birmingham Children's Hospital NHS Trust in the area of Pierre-Robin syndrome in children published. *Health & Medicine Week,* 2903.

Burns, S. M. (Ed.). (2007). *American Association of Critical-Care Nurses (AACN): AACN protocols for practice: Healing environments* (2nd ed.). Sudbury, MA: Jones and Bartlett.

Carlotti, A. P., & Carvalho, W. B. (2009). Abdominal compartment syndrome: A review. *Pediatric Critical Care Medicine, 10*(1), 115–120.

Chambers, M. A., & Jones, S. (Eds.). (2007). *Surgical nursing of children.* Philadelphia: Elsevier.

Chernecky, C., & Berger, B. (2004). *Laboratory tests and diagnostic procedures* (4th ed.). Philadelphia: Saunders.

Columbus Children's Hospital. (2009, July). Pediatric surgery: Research from Columbus Children's Hospital yields new data on pediatric surgery. *Pediatrics Week,* 115.

Dartmouth Hitchcock Medical Center. (2009). Polyhydramnios. Retrieved August 21, 2009, from http://www.dhmc.org/webpage.cfm?site_id=2&org_id=828&morg_id=0&sec_id=0&gsec_id=47098&item_id=47108

Drake Melander, S. (Ed.). (2004). *Case studies in critical care nursing: A guide for application and review* (3rd ed.). Philadelphia: Saunders.

Eghbalian, F., Monsef, A., & Mousavi-Bahar, S. (2009, April). Urinary tract and other associated anomalies in newborns with esophageal atresia. *Urology Journal, 6*(2), 123–126.

Emergency Nurses Association & Newberry, L. (2005). *Sheehy's emergency nursing: Principles and practice* (6th ed.). St. Louis, MO: Mosby/Elsevier.

George Washington University. (2009, August). Pediatrics: Findings in pediatrics reported from George Washington University. *Pediatrics Week,* 199.

Gora-Harper, M. (1998). *The injectable drug reference.* Princeton, NJ: Bioscientific Resources.

Hardin, S. R., & Kaplow, R. (Eds.). (2004). *Synergy for clinical excellence: The AACN Synergy Model for Patient Care.* Sudbury, MA: Jones and Bartlett.

Harvard University. (2008, September). Pediatric gastroenterology and nutrition: New pediatric gastroenterology and nutrition research from Harvard University discussed. *Pediatrics Week,* 25.

Hay, W. W. Jr., Levin, M. J., Sondheimer, J. M., & Deterding, R. R. (Eds.). (2007). *Current diagnosis and treatment in pediatrics* (18th ed.). New York: McGraw-Hill.

Heinlein, C. R. (2009). Dumping syndrome in Roux-en-Y bariatric surgery patients: Are they prepared? *Bariatric Nursing & Surgical Patient Care, 4*(1), 39–47.

Hickey, J. V. (2008). *The clinical practice of neurological and neurosurgical nursing* (6th ed.). Philadelphia: Lippincott Williams & Wilkins.

Jiang, D., Xu, C., Wu, B., Li, Z. Z., Zhang, Y. B., & Han, F. Y. (2009). Effects of botulinum toxin injection on anal achalasia after pull-through operations for Hirschsprung's disease: A 1-year follow-up study. *International Journal of Colorectal Disease, 24*(5), 597–598.

Jones & Bartlett Learning (2011). *2011 nurse's drug handbook.* (10th ed.). Sudbury, MA: Jones & Bartlett Learning.

Koch, T. R., & Finelli, F. C. (2010). Postoperative metabolic and nutritional complications of bariatric surgery. *Gastroenterology Clinics of North America, 39*(1), 109–124.

Kulick, D., Hark, L., & Deen, D. (2010). The bariatric surgery patient: A growing role of registered dietitians. *Journal of the American Dietetic Association, 110*(4), 593–599.

Lee, C. W., Kelly, J. J., & Wassef, W. Y. (2007). Complications of bariatric surgery. *Current Opinion in Gastroenterology, 23*(6), 636–643.

Lillehei, C., & Hansen, A. (2009). *SIX: Respiratory disorders: Part 1: Esophageal atresia and tracheoesophageal fistula* (pp. 159–168). Beijing, China: People's Medical Publishing House USA.

Macksey, L. F. (2009). *Pediatric anesthetic and emergency drug guide.* Sudbury, MA: Jones and Bartlett.

Martin, B. (2010). Family presence during resuscitation and invasive procedures: AACN practice alert. Retrieved from http://www.aacn.org

McNiel, M. E., Labbok, M. H., & Abrahams, S. W. (2010). What are the risks associated with formula feeding? A re-analysis and review. *Birth: Issues in Perinatal Care, 37*(1), 50–58.

Medina, J., & Puntillo, K. (2006). *AACN protocols for practice: Palliative care and end-of-life issues in critical care.* Sudbury, MA: Jones and Bartlett.

National Craniofacial Association. (2006). Pierre Robin sequence. Retrieved September 6, 2009, from http://www.faces-cranio.org/Disord/PierreRobin.htm

Oestreicher-Kedem, Y., DeRowe, A., Nagar, H., et al. (2008, December). Vocal fold paralysis in infants with tracheoesophageal fistula. *Annals of Otology, Rhinology, and Laryngology, 117*(12), 896–901.

Olgun, H. (2009, May). Gastroenterology: New gastroenterology study findings recently were reported by H. Olgun and co-researchers. *Cardiovascular Week,* 166.

Rizoli, S., Mamtani, A., Scarpelini, S., & Kirkpatrick, A. W. (2010). Abdominal compartment syndrome in trauma resuscitation. *Current Opinion in Anaesthesiology, 23*(2), 251–257.

Root, E. (2009). *The ecology of birth defects: Socio-economic and environmental determinants of gastroschisis in North Carolina.* PhD dissertation, University of North Carolina at Chapel Hill, NC. Retrieved September 6, 2009, from Dissertations & Theses: Full Text.

Sanjay Gandhi Postgraduate Institute of Medical Sciences. (2009, February). Biliary atresia epidemiology: Studies from Sanjay Gandhi Postgraduate Institute of Medical Sciences, Department of Pathology in the area of biliary atresia epidemiology described. *Hepatitis Weekly,* 31.

Shew, S. (2009). Surgical concerns in malrotation and midgut volvulus. *Pediatric Radiology: Supplement, 39,* 167–171.

Slota, M. C. (Ed.). (2006). *Core curriculum for pediatric critical care nursing* (2nd ed.). St. Louis, MO: Saunders.

Spratto, G. R., & Woods, A. L. (2001). *PDR: Nurse's drug handbook.* Montvale, NJ: Delmar & Medical Economics.

Stanford School of Medicine. (2009). Bilirubin screening and management of hyperbilirubinemia. Retrieved August 21, 2009, from http://newborns.stanford.edu/BiliSummary.htmL# PhototxGuide

Thaisetthawatkul, P. (2008). Neuromuscular complications of bariatric surgery. *Physical Medicine & Rehabilitation Clinics of North America, 19*(1), 111–124, vii.

Trivits Verger, J., & Lebet, R. M. (Eds.). (2008). *AACN procedure manual for pediatric acute and critical care.* St. Louis, MO: Saunders.

University of Heidelberg. (2009, February). Diaphragmatic hernia: Research from University of Heidelberg provides new insights into diaphragmatic hernia. *Gastroenterology Week,* 196.

University of Washington. (2009, August). Hirschsprung disease: Research in the area of Hirschsprung disease reported from University of Washington. *Gastroenterology Week,* 105.

von Drygalski, A., & Andris, D. A. (2009). Anemia after bariatric surgery: More than just iron deficiency. *Nutrition in Clinical Practice: Official Publication of the American Society for Parenteral and Enteral Nutrition, 24*(2), 217–226.

Wu, Y., Yan, Z., Hong, L., Hu, M., & Chen, S. (2009, June). Thoracoscopic repair of congenital esophageal atresia in infants. *Journal of Laparoendoscopic & Advanced Surgical Techniques, 19*(3), 461–463.

Yale University Medical Department. (2008, November). Cleft lip: Studies from Yale University, Medical Department further understanding of cleft lip. *Genomics & Genetics Weekly*, 52.

SECTION 9

Renal

1. **Your patient is 14 years old. A normal value for intracellular potassium (K^+) in this patient would be**
   A. 4.5 mEq/L
   B. 140 mEq/L
   C. 45 mEq/L
   D. 104 mEq/L

2. **Juan is a renal patient who needs to have a radiologic procedure that requires contrast dye. He has no known allergies. Which of the following medications administered prior to the test would be effective and safe for this patient?**
   A. Bicarbonate
   B. Mucomyst
   C. BNP
   D. NSAIDs

3. **Foster will be receiving Nesiritide as part of his treatment for heart failure. Effects of Nesiritide include**
   A. Vasoconstriction
   B. Decreased wedge pressure
   C. Anemia
   D. Decreased cardiac output

4. **Mannitol would be classified as which type of diuretic?**
   A. Loop
   B. Thiazide
   C. Osmotic
   D. Potassium sparing

5. **It is incumbent upon the PICU nurse to know the adverse effects of any medication his or her patient receives. Potential complications of loop diuretics would include**
   A. Hypokalemia
   B. Increase in BUN
   C. Hypercalcemia
   D. Hypertension

6. **Diuretics that are classified as carbonic anhydrase inhibitors would include**
   A. Methazolamide
   B. Mannitol
   C. Urea
   D. Metolazone

7. **Ethacrynic acid works on the body by**
   A. Inhibiting the aldosterone mechanism
   B. Inhibiting reabsorption of Na and Cl
   C. Increasing osmotic pressure
   D. Blocking carbonic anhydrase

8. **A normal value for bicarbonate (HCO_3) in the intravascular space would be**
   A. 11 mEq/L
   B. 45 mEq/L
   C. 80 mEq/L
   D. 24 mEq/L

9. **Which hormone would be released if your patient's CVP suddenly rose from 5 to 18 mmHg?**
   A. BNP
   B. Aldosterone
   C. ANP
   D. ADH

10. **Which of the following solutions would be used to expand the intravascular volume?**
    A. Hypertonic saline
    B. D_5W
    C. 0.45 NS
    D. 0.9% NS

11. **If your patient has a decreased extracellular fluid volume, which of the following hemodynamic profiles would be indicative of this condition?**
    A. Decreased CO, CVP, and SVR
    B. Decreased CVP, PAP, MAP, and CO; increased SVR
    C. Decreased SVR, MAP, and CVP; increased CO
    D. Increased CVP, CO, and PAP; decreased SVR

12. **Myra was aggressively treated with 0.3% hypertonic saline for profound hyponatremia. Now she is having tremors, LOC changes, and paresthesias. Myra is probably developing**
    A. ICU psychosis
    B. Hyponatremia veridans
    C. Osmotic demyelinization syndrome
    D. Red cell sequestration

13. **Joey is an 8 year old boy who was hit in the lower back while playing football with friends. His X-ray shows T11 and T12 transverse process fractures. Which of Joey's symptoms probably indicates renal injury?**
   A. Flank pain
   B. 2 mL/kg/hr of urinary output
   C. Urinary incontinence
   D. Urine osmolarity of 300 mOsm/L

14. **You are caring for Hector, a 16 year old patient who weighs 205 pounds. Hector was admitted to the PICU for arrhythmias after drinking several energy drinks during rugby practice. You need to calculate his urine output for the 12-hour shift. Hector's minimum urinary output should be**
   A. 360 mL
   B. 558 mL
   C. 1116 mL
   D. 1227.6 mL

15. **Which of the following statements is true regarding kidney function in the pediatric population?**
   A. Nephrons continue to develop until age 8
   B. Kidney location is fixed at L1–L3
   C. Infant kidneys are less susceptible to fluid changes
   D. Approximately 20% to 25% of cardiac output is directed to the kidneys

16. **Which of the following statements is true regarding kidney structure in the pediatric population?**
   A. Cortical nephrons account for 99% of all nephrons
   B. Cortical nephrons have long Loops of Henle for water conservation
   C. The tubular components of the nephron include the proximal tubule, Loop of Henle, and distal tubule
   D. Afferent arterioles take blood from the glomerulus to the second capillary bed

17. **The function of the proximal tubule is**
   A. Secretion and reabsorption of sodium
   B. Secretion of H^+
   C. Reabsorption of water when ADH is present
   D. Secretion of potassium

18. **During your morning assessment, you note that your 4 year old patient has a sallow complexion with a slight yellow cast that was not mentioned by the previous nurse. You should**
   A. Open the curtains so that the child can be exposed to indirect sunlight
   B. Not be concerned, as the patient's normal skin tone is slightly yellow
   C. Complete your assessment and report your findings to the physician
   D. Call the doctor immediately to report your finding

19. **Which of the following substances can be passively transported between membranes located within the nephron?**
    A. Potassium
    B. Glucose
    C. Bicarbonate
    D. Water

20. **A decrease in urine output may occur with**
    A. Afferent arteriole vasoconstriction
    B. Efferent arteriole vasoconstriction
    C. A serum albumin of 1.8 g/dL
    D. A heart rate of 160

21. **Sympathetic nerve stimulation affects kidney function by**
    A. Dilation of the Loop of Henle
    B. Vasoconstriction of the afferent and efferent arterioles
    C. Dilation of the Bowman's capsule
    D. Constriction of the distal tubule

22. **Which of the following statements best describes the definition or function of creatinine?**
    A. Creatinine is the endogenous waste product of muscle tissue that is excreted by the kidneys
    B. Creatinine is the volume of a specific substance filtered from plasma over a designated time
    C. The creatinine level represents constant filtration pressures by renal blood flow and GFR
    D. The creatinine level represents all the substances filtered from plasma

23. **The normal glomerular filtration rate for a 1 year old child is**
    A. 35 to 40 mL/min
    B. 60 mL/min
    C. 80 to 120 mL/min
    D. 140 to 180 mL/min

24. **Which of the following statements is true regarding antidiuretic hormone?**
    A. ADH is released from the thalamus
    B. ADH increases urine concentration
    C. ADH causes changes in permeability of the proximal tubule
    D. ADH is solely responsible for sodium retention

25. **Sodium retention in the kidneys is not affected by**
    A. Aldosterone secretion
    B. ADH
    C. Insulin
    D. Estrogen

26. **Harry is an 8 year old with acute renal failure. Which of the following lab results should be immediately reported to his physician?**
    A. An inorganic phosphate level of 6.1 mg/dL
    B. A sodium level of 144 mEq/L
    C. A potassium level of 4.8 mEq/L
    D. A calcium level of 10 mg/dL

27. **Missy is a 10 year old gymnast who has been suffering repetitive ankle injuries during practices. She has been taking ibuprofen 800 mg every 6 hours. Missy was admitted to the PICU following a tibial fracture and concussion after falling from the parallel bars. Her blood pressure is 110/85, her heart rate is 120, and her urinary output is 0.5 mL/kg/hr. Which of the following explanations may be the cause of Missy's poor renal function?**
    A. Missy is in prerenal failure due to her leg cast impeding return blood flow
    B. Missy is in intrinsic renal failure due to impaired autoregulation
    C. Missy is in postrenal failure due to poor intake
    D. Missy is in prerenal failure due to ibuprofen use

28. **Which of the following complications is associated with acute tubular necrosis?**
    A. Hypernatremia
    B. Metabolic acidosis
    C. High thyroxine levels
    D. Decreased parathyroid levels

29. **Urea is the waste product of ________ metabolism**
    A. Protein
    B. Blood
    C. Amino acid
    D. Nucleic acid

30. **Carter is 3 years old. Last night he did not eat dinner, and he fell asleep on the couch by 6 p.m. Today he complains of pain in the lower abdomen and cannot pass urine. Carter's anuria may be due to**
    A. Congestive heart failure
    B. An embolic event
    C. Prostate enlargement
    D. Azotemia

31. **Dexter has been diagnosed with acute renal failure. A general definition of acute renal failure would be**
    A. Trauma to one or both kidneys
    B. A decrease in renal perfusion from shock or anaphylaxis
    C. A sudden or rapid decline in renal filtration function
    D. An obstruction to passage of urine

32. **Intrinsic AKI is most commonly caused by**
    A. Arteriolar vasoconstriction
    B. Acute ischemic or cytotoxic injury
    C. Amphotericin
    D. Hypercalcemia

33. **Matthew is scheduled for his first apheresis treatment in an hour. Apheresis is best defined as**
    A. The removal of plasma and/or proteins from the blood
    B. The removal of an antigen from the blood
    C. The selective removal of cellular components from the blood
    D. The selective removal of cells, plasma, and substances from the blood

34. **Postrenal acute renal injury may be caused by**
    A. DIC and preeclampsia
    B. Transplant rejection
    C. A neurogenic bladder
    D. Malignant hypertension

35. **In the polyuric phase of acute kidney injury, it is important for the PICU nurse to carefully monitor**
    A. Potassium and phosphorus levels
    B. Nitrogen balance
    C. Dopamine and mannitol levels
    D. Desmopressin levels

36. **In a 15 year old patient, anuria is usually defined as a urine output of**
    A. Less than 30 mL/hr
    B. 200 mL/day
    C. 300 mL/day
    D. Less than 100 mL/day

37. **Mannitol and loop diuretics may be used in the treatment of AKI. Mannitol is nontoxic but must be used with caution because**
    A. Mannitol may damage the eighth cranial nerve
    B. Mannitol may cause vestibular impairment
    C. Mannitol may bind with proteins in the renal tubule
    D. Mannitol may produce a hyperosmolar state

38. **It is important for the PICU nurse to be aware that acute kidney injury may result from nephrotoxicity. Nephrotoxicity may be caused by**
    A. Furosemide
    B. Acyclovir
    C. Thioguanine
    D. Aspirin

39. The popularity of NSAIDs has increased among parents partly because of the availability of generic forms and their low prices. As a pediatric nurse, you are aware NSAIDs may cause

A. Prerenal AKI

B. Intrinsic AKI

C. Postrenal AKI

D. Increased urine osmolality

40. The primary site for urea synthesis in the body is the

A. Kidneys

B. Lungs

C. Liver

D. Pancreas

41. Increased production of urea may be due to

A. Hypothermia

B. A low-protein diet

C. Congenital kidney disease

D. GI bleeding

42. Jeffrey was admitted to your PICU after severely cutting his right arm on a piece of glass. You notice Jeffrey's hand spasming when the automatic blood pressure cuff inflates. When you attempt to take a manual blood pressure measurement, the same thing happens when you inflate the cuff just past the systolic pressure and maintain that pressure for several seconds up to approximately a minute. This carpopedal spasm is indicative of

A. Hypokalemia

B. Hyperphosphatemia

C. Hypocalcemia

D. Hypernatremia

43. Your patient is 4 years old and was admitted with CHF. While assessing the patient, you notice significant pretibial and pedal edema. When the patient is weighed, you note that the patient has gained 1 kg of weight in 24 hours. This would be equal to at least __________ of excess fluid

A. 2000 mL

B. 1000 mL

C. 2200 mL

D. 500 mL

44. Your patient has a calcium level of 7.8 mEq/L. You would expect which of the following changes to occur on the EKG tracing?

A. Tall, peaked T waves

B. A prominent U wave

C. A prolonged QT interval

D. A first-degree AV block

45. One way to check a patient for low calcium is to tap your finger over a branch of the individual's facial nerve. If the patient is hypocalcemic, the upper lip on the same side (ipsilateral) will twitch. This sign is known as

A. Trousseau's sign
B. Chvostek's sign
C. Grey-Turner's sign
D. Homan's sign

46. Aldosterone is secreted when the extracellular sodium level is _____ or when extracellular potassium is _____

A. Low, low
B. High, low
C. Low, high
D. High, high

47. __________ is the major extracellular cation, and ________ is the major intracellular cation

A. Calcium, magnesium
B. Sodium, calcium
C. Potassium, sodium
D. Sodium, potassium

48. Potassium is reabsorbed in the

A. Proximal tubules
B. Distal tubules
C. Ascending colon
D. Descending colon

49. Gavin is 14 years old and is an alcoholic. Chronic use of alcohol will have which of the following effects on Gavin's potassium levels?

A. Potassium moves out of the vascular circulation and into the cells
B. Potassium moves out of the cells and into the vascular circulation
C. Potassium moves out of the cells and into the interstitium
D. Potassium moves out of the vascular circulation and into the interstitium

50. Tara is hypokalemic because she had a huge diuresis from a dose of furosemide. Which of the following EKG changes would you expect to see with her condition?

A. Peaked T waves
B. A U wave
C. A shortened QT interval
D. An absent P wave

51. Bobby has problems regulating his potassium level. You and a new PICU nurse are discussing methods of cooking vegetables with this patient's parents. Which of the following cooking techniques leaches potassium out of the food?

A. Boiling
B. Baking
C. Steaming
D. Microwaving

52. In Addison's disease, the patient's potassium level results in

A. Hyperkalemia related to the decrease in aldosterone secretion
B. Hyperkalemia related to the increase in aldosterone secretion
C. Hypokalemia related to the decrease in aldosterone secretion
D. Hypocalcemia related to the increase in aldosterone secretion

53. Bronwyn has congestive heart failure and was given Lasix for water retention. Her feet and legs continued to swell, so she took extra Lasix this morning. Now she has been admitted to the PICU with profound muscle weakness and flat T waves. You would expect her potassium level this morning to be

A. 4.2 mEq/L
B. 3.8 mEq/L
C. 1.8 mEq/L
D. 6.1 mEq/L

54. Normal serum magnesium levels for a 16 to 17 year old patient are

A. 0.5–1.5 mg/dL
B. 1.5–2 mg/dL
C. 2–3 mg/dL
D. 4–5 mg/dL

55. Cora is receiving a magnesium drip to control premature contractions. As a pediatric nurse, you know magnesium alters intracellular calcium by influencing

A. Parathyroid function
B. Aldosterone secretion
C. Cortisol secretion
D. Glycosol production

56. Meredith had gastric bypass surgery two days ago. Gastric bypass surgery can dramatically affect which of the following electrolytes?

A. Sodium
B. Calcium
C. Magnesium
D. Potassium

57. Elaine eats a diet high in calcium because her family has a history of osteoporosis. She was admitted status post fractured pelvis and pulmonary embolism sustained when she fell off her horse. Elaine has been experiencing increasing weakness and muscle tremors. She has noted an increased number of "skipped" beats. Elaine stated that she was very dizzy and disoriented just before she fell. Based on her symptoms, which of the following labs should you assess immediately?

A. Calcium level
B. Sodium level
C. Hemoglobin and hematocrit levels
D. Magnesium level

58. Your patient was admitted for treatment of her ketoacidosis. Her magnesium level is 0.5 mEq/L. Which symptoms would you expect to see when a patient has this result for her magnesium level?

A. Lethargy

B. Convulsions

C. Negative Babinski sign

D. Decreased reflexes

59. What percentage of calcium is stored in the bone?

A. 65%

B. 85%

C. 80%

D. 99%

60. Which of the following statements about calcium is true?

A. Calcium is approximately 40% ionized in the serum

B. Calcium levels cannot be correlated with albumin levels

C. Calcium that is bonded to protein cannot pass through capillary walls

D. Calcium is not necessary for coagulation

61. Which of the following statements about calcium is not true?

A. Calcium increases vitamin D levels

B. Renal tubular excretion is affected by calcium

C. Calcium aids in gastrointestinal excretion

D. Bone demineralization is affected by calcium

62. As calcium levels __________, the parathyroid gland __________ its secretions

A. Increase, decreases

B. Increase, increases

C. Decrease, decreases

D. Decrease, increases

63. You are testing for hypocalcemia, using Trousseau's sign to aid in your assessment. You elicit this reaction by

A. Tapping the patient's cheek

B. Lifting the patient's left leg up and looking for the patient's knee to move toward the chest

C. Inflating a BP cuff to greater than the systolic pressure for 3 minutes and waiting for a carpal spasm

D. Taking a sharp object up from the heel to the toes and watching for the toes to spread

64. Rebecca is scheduled to undergo continuous renal replacement therapy (CRRT) this week. Which of the following drugs should be stopped 2–3 days prior to the beginning of this therapy?

A. Beta blockers

B. ACE inhibitors

C. Heparin

D. Calcium channel blockers

65. **For nonpumped continuous renal replacement therapy (CRRT) to function appropriately, the minimal mean arterial blood pressure must be**
    A. 40 mmHg
    B. 50 mmHg
    C. 60 mmHg
    D. 80 mmHg

66. **Which of the following continuous renal replacement therapies (CRRT) require only venous access and pumping function?**
    A. CVVHDF, SCUF
    B. CVVH, CAVH
    C. CAVH, CAVHD
    D. CVVH, CVVHD

67. **You are assessing your patient's vascular access prior to initiating hemodialysis. You note that there is no thrill or bruit. Your next nursing action would be to**
    A. Call the surgeon to do a new graft
    B. Administer a bolus of heparin
    C. Use a Doppler to determine graft patency
    D. Continue with the hemodialysis, there is nothing wrong

68. **Communication among all staff is vital. When transferring your patient with a graft, which of the following facts is a priority to communicate to all staff who may come in contact with this patient?**
    A. Last dialysis date
    B. Location of the graft
    C. Type of dialysis machine used
    D. Total fluid removed with last dialysis

69. **Hemodialysis is used to treat many metabolic abnormalities as well as renal failure. One possible treatment is to provide**
    A. Vitamin C and calcium carbonate for patients with osteoporosis
    B. Erythropoietin for patients with excessive iron
    C. Glucose for patients with hyperglycemia
    D. Phosphate binders for patients with hyperphosphatemia

70. **The usual amount of dialysate used in peritoneal dialysis is**
    A. 0.5–1 L
    B. 1–2 L
    C. 2–3 L
    D. 3–4 L

71. **Which of the following is the correct fluid exchange sequence in peritoneal dialysis?**
    A. Dump, dwell, drain
    B. Instillation, dwell, drain
    C. Drain, instillation, dwell
    D. Instillation, drain, dwell

72. **Peritoneal dialysis functions by using which two of the following principles?**
   A. Diffusion and osmosis
   B. Osmotic pressure and osmosis
   C. Ultrafiltration and oncotic pressure
   D. Diffusion and ultrafiltration

73. **For which of the following disease processes is immunoadsorption used as a treatment?**
   A. Multiple sclerosis
   B. Paraneoplastic neurologic syndromes
   C. Cutaneous T-cell lymphomas
   D. Heart transplant rejection

74. **Exchange plasma volume used in apheresis is usually delivered at a ratio of**
   A. 1.5:1
   B. 2:1
   C. 2.5:1
   D. 3:1

75. **Drew, age 14, has been diagnosed with hypertension. He states that to control his blood pressure he "will never eat another thing with salt. Now I can't even go to the movie and have popcorn." You should tell him**
   A. "That is not easy. Most fresh vegetables and fruit have tons of sodium"
   B. "Great. Sodium plays only a minor part in water balance and cellular activity, so your body won't know the difference"
   C. "You cannot completely eliminate sodium from your diet. Your body has an intricate system of safety measures to protect the level of sodium in your body"
   D. "Okay. Sodium is controlled by aldosterone that is released by the pituitary gland"

76. **Which of the following fruits has the lowest sodium content per 3.5-ounce serving?**
   A. Cantaloupe
   B. Blackberries
   C. Peaches
   D. Grapes

77. **Joseph is trying to limit his salt intake. Which of the following meat products would you recommend for Joseph to eat?**
   A. Chicken without the skin
   B. Canned beef hash
   C. Fresh fish
   D. Canned crab

78. **Cameron loves cheese, but must limit his sodium intake. Which of the following cheeses has the highest sodium per 3.5-ounce serving?**
   A. Swiss cheese
   B. Mozzarella cheese
   C. Cheddar cheese
   D. Parmesan cheese

79. **A common cause of hyponatremia is**
    A. Salt-water drowning
    B. Overhydration
    C. Administration of hypertonic solutions
    D. Hyperoxia

80. **The BUN may be elevated in patients who**
    A. Consume a low-protein diet
    B. Take streptomycin
    C. Take chloramphenicol
    D. Receive steroid treatments

81. **A renal transplant that results from humoral rejection or acute cellular rejection may be definitively diagnosed only via**
    A. The precise location of pain
    B. Nuclear scan
    C. Doppler scan
    D. Renal biopsy

82. **Betty was admitted to the PICU directly from her physician's office. She had been complaining of fatigue and generalized pain. Her lab work indicated a rapidly rising BUN, and she was admitted for further tests. While assessing Betty, you note that she has severe acne around her face and neck. You suspect that the increase in BUN may be due to her use of**
    A. Bumetanide
    B. HCTZ
    C. Tetracycline
    D. Mannitol

83. **Medications that can decrease BUN levels include**
    A. Neomycin and rifampin
    B. Chloral hydrate and furosemide
    C. Bacitracin and gentamycin
    D. Chloramphenicol and streptomycin

84. **Which of the following statements about creatinine is true?**
    A. A normal range for creatinine would be 0.8 to 1.4 mg/dL
    B. Creatinine levels are higher in females
    C. Lower than normal levels of creatinine may indicate pyelonephritis
    D. Low levels of creatinine are a precursor to eclampsia

85. **Allergic nephritis may be caused by**
    A. Inadequate protein consumption
    B. Cimetidine
    C. Weight loss
    D. Water intoxication

86. **Your patient is becoming confused, is lethargic, and has muscle weakness. A review of her lab reports shows a calcium level of 11.7. One way to treat this condition would be to use**
    A. Normal saline and a loop diuretic
    B. D_5W and a Kayexalate enema
    C. Glucose followed by insulin
    D. Nothing; this is a normal value

87. **What is the primary acid–base disturbance exhibited by patients with AKI?**
    A. Metabolic acidosis
    B. Respiratory acidosis
    C. Metabolic alkalosis
    D. Respiratory alkalosis

88. **Logan is 12 and was admitted to the pediatric intensive care unit for cocaine intoxication. He begins to complain of severe epigastric pain. His lab results are as follows: WBC 17.3 with 77% neutrophils, hematocrit 40%, LDH 341, platelets 226, BUN 7, creatinine 1.0. Urine analysis shows trace proteins, few RBCs, and a positive urine toxicology test for cocaine. What could cause Logan's pain?**
    A. Peptic ulcer disease
    B. Renal infarction
    C. Gastroenteritis
    D. Infarcted mesenteric artery

89. **Kenji is a 10 year old patient with cystic fibrosis. Kenji is at a high risk for**
    A. Hypernatremia
    B. Hypocalcemia
    C. Hyponatremia
    D. Hypercalcemia

90. **Sean has a J-tube post surgery for peritonitis. Which electrolyte deficit is he at risk for?**
    A. Sodium
    B. Magnesium
    C. Manganese
    D. Phosphorus

91. **Leila is a 9 year old diabetic with congestive heart failure. After 4 hours of no contact, her mother found Leila in her bed, unresponsive. Leila has a red, dry swollen tongue, a temperature of 102 ºF, and flushed, dry skin. She is tachycardic, hypotensive, and demonstrates decreased reflexes. Leila's urine specific gravity is 1.050. You suspect Leila has**
    A. Hypernatremia
    B. Hypocalcemia
    C. Hypermagnesemia
    D. Hypokalemia

92. Aldosterone secretions have what effect on potassium excretion?

A. Potassium excretion decreases

B. Potassium excretion increases

C. Potassium excretion remains the same

D. Aldosterone affects only sodium levels

93. Hypokalemia may cause

A. Respiratory alkalosis only

B. Metabolic alkalosis only

C. Both respiratory and metabolic alkalosis

D. Metabolic acidosis only

94. Which of the following conditions is not a potential cause of hypokalemia due to excessive urinary excretion?

A. Oliguria

B. Renal disease

C. Lasix

D. Increased adrenal cortical hormones

95. All of the following foods are high in potassium except

A. Avocados

B. Carrots

C. Potatoes

D. Raisins

96. All of the following are treatments for hyperkalemia except

A. Glucose and insulin

B. Kaon

C. Calcium glucanate

D. Bicarbonate administration

97. Your 4 year old patient's morning arterial blood gas indicates metabolic alkalosis. What is the expected effect on serum potassium?

A. Serum potassium will not be affected

B. Serum potassium will be higher than normal

C. Serum potassium will be lower than normal

D. Only the serum CO_2 level will be affected

98. Magnesium is not required for which one of the following functions?

A. To always act as an antagonist with calcium

B. For enzyme activation

C. Synthesis of nucleic acid and proteins

D. Sodium–potassium pump regulation

99. Magnesium is most prevalent in which of the following areas in the body?

A. Extracellular

B. In the liver

C. In the spleen

D. In the bone

100. Your patient was admitted and treated for torsades de pointes. You are teaching him about adding foods to his diet that are rich in magnesium. Your patient asks about each of the following foods. Which one is the poorest source of magnesium?

A. Almonds
B. Broccoli
C. Honey
D. Chocolate

101. Magnesium is ordered for your patient. During your assessment, however, you note flaccidity, absent patellar reflexes, shallow respirations, and a flushed face. You should

A. Give the magnesium—the patient is just sleeping
B. Hold the dose for 1 hour
C. Give the dose over 3 hours
D. Hold the dose, contact the physician, and obtain a magnesium level

102. One of the most common causes of hypermagnesemia is

A. Gastrointestinal bypass
B. Gastrointestinal fistulas
C. Renal failure
D. Overdose

103. The family of your patient with hypermagnesemia asks why the patient's face is flushed. You answer

A. "He has a temperature"
B. "His magnesium level is a little high and causes his face to look flushed"
C. "He is embarrassed because the hospital gown does not provide enough coverage"
D. "He just completed his physical therapy"

104. The physician has ordered the removal of the PICC line for your patient on full feeds and oral medications. Which of the following statements is true about this procedure?

A. Direct pressure should be held on the site for 30 seconds after removal of the PICC line
B. The PICC line length should be documented upon its removal
C. The PICC line should be pulled forcefully if any resistance is met
D. The PICC line must be pulled only by a physician

105. Acid–base regulation in the body occurs via the lungs and the kidneys. Which of the following statements is true regarding acid–base regulation?

A. Acids are hydrogen (H^+) receptors
B. Excess H_2O forms carbonic acid
C. Respiratory imbalances are determined by assessing HCO_3^-, and metabolic imbalances are determined by assessing PCO_2
D. HCO_3 is a buffer that binds with free hydrogen to form carbonic acid

106. Drake has renal failure and is preparing to have continuous renal replacement therapy (CRRT). He asks if he can have visitors during the procedure. You tell him

A. "Of course. There are no restrictions"
B. "No. They would be in the way of the equipment"
C. "No. The visitors will increase your risk of infection"
D. "Yes, but if they are sensitive to the sight of blood, they may want to wait until after the procedure is finished"

107. Lin is a patient in renal failure post multiple cardiac arrests and cardiogenic shock. He has continued cardiovascular instability. The best and safest method for removal of excess fluid in Lin's case is to use

A. Hemodialysis
B. Peritoneal dialysis
C. Continuous renal replacement therapy (CRRT)
D. Plasmapheresis

108. Alessio is undergoing hemodialysis for renal failure as a result of uncontrolled type 2 diabetes. His father asks you how you know the hemodialysis is effective. Adequacy of dialysis is measured by

A. Urine creatinine clearance
B. Sodium, chloride, and potassium levels
C. Urea clearance
D. Blood pressure

109. You are preparing Patricia for her first peritoneal dialysis session. It is important to tell her which of the following findings is a normal occurrence when undergoing this procedure?

A. "During the instillation phase, the insertion site may leak"
B. "During the dwell phase, you may feel abdominal fullness and have shortness of breath"
C. "During the dwell phase, subcutaneous fluid may be seen in the groin"
D. "During the drain phase, you will feel dizzy and have palpitations"

110. During the drain phase after peritoneal dialysis, you note only 50% return in the collection bag. What is the first action you should perform?

A. Position the patient prone
B. Double-check the amount instilled
C. Check for kinks, bends, or cracks in the tubing
D. Assess for subcutaneous fluid

111. You are providing discharge teaching to the family and the patient who will be undergoing peritoneal dialysis. As part of the discharge equipment, your patient will receive a home glucometer. The mother questions the necessity for this equipment because her daughter is not a diabetic. You should explain to the mother

A. "Peritoneal dialysis can cause diabetes"
B. "She didn't tell you? Your daughter was just diagnosed with diabetes"
C. "The dialysate contains glucose and can lead to hyperglycemia"
D. "Peritoneal dialysis may lead to pancreatitis"

112. Connie is undergoing lymphocytopheresis and plasma exchange as a treatment for progressive multiple sclerosis, with citrate as the anticoagulant. She begins to feel tingling. Which of the following lab results should you check first to determine the source of Connie's symptoms?

A. ABG, ionized calcium, and PT/PTT levels
B. ACT, ionized calcium level, and ABGs
C. INR, potassium, sodium, and chloride levels
D. Potassium, magnesium, and PT/PTT levels

113. What is the effect of acidosis on free ionized calcium levels in the serum?

A. There is no relationship between blood pH and free ionized calcium levels
B. Acidosis results in higher free ionized calcium levels
C. Acidosis results in lower free ionized calcium levels
D. Acidosis results in a lowered pH that decreases serum calcium

114. Bobby was put on a limited-sodium diet, and his family has been working with a nutritionist. He was admitted to your unit for chest pain (angina) and pulmonary edema. Bobby and his parents report that he has stopped all additional sodium intake, has been following his diet regimen closely, and has stopped eating out. Bobby is drinking 8–10 eight-ounce glasses of tap water every day, and is voiding well. His sodium level is 155 mEq/L. What is the likely cause of his hypernatremia?

A. Renal failure
B. Hypotonic fluids
C. Diabetes mellitus
D. Water softener system

115. You are receiving a report on James, who was injured when he had a seizure while working on his bicycle. His sodium level on admission was 120 mEq/L. Which symptoms of hyponatremia would you expect James to exhibit?

A. Lethargy
B. Tachypnea
C. Twitching
D. Flattened T waves

116. A normal range for serum potassium in a newborn would be

A. 3.5–4.2 mEq/L
B. 3.8–4.8 mEq/L
C. 4.5–6.8 mEq/L
D. 3.0–4.5 mEq/L

117. You just drew an arterial blood gas from your patient's radial arterial line. The pH is 7.23. What is the expected response from the kidneys to compensate for this acid–base deficit?

A. Increased secretion of hydrogen ions in the glomerulus
B. Reabsorption of bicarbonate in the distal tubules
C. Excretion of ammonia
D. Increased secretion of hydrogen ions in the distal tubules

118. The urine analysis for your patient indicates the presence of casts, tubular cells, and proteinuria. This result indicates

A. Prerenal failure
B. Intrinsic renal failure
C. Postrenal failure
D. Renal necrosis

119. Which of the following statements is true regarding renal failure?

A. A fluid challenge is used to rule out postrenal causes of renal failure
B. A urine output of less than 2 mL/kg/hr after furosemide administration indicates an intrinsic or postrenal cause of renal failure
C. Prerenal failure involves the ureters and bladder
D. Rapid and sustained diuresis within 1 to 2 hours of fluid bolus indicates a postrenal cause of renal failure

120. Hydronephrosis is best defined as

A. Dilation of the pelvis and calyces of one or both kidneys due to obstruction
B. An excess of urine production
C. Hypoperfusion of one or both kidneys, resulting in poor urine output
D. Dysplasia of one or both kidneys

121. Your 2 week old patient was diagnosed with mild unilateral hydronephrosis. Urine output is 1.5 mL/kg/hr. The parents ask you if surgery will be necessary. You should answer

A. "Surgery is always indicated and will occur at 3 months of life"
B. "Immediate surgery is indicated despite your baby having normal levels of amniotic fluid at birth"
C. "The need for surgery depends on the cause and severity of the hydronephrosis"
D. "This is not a case that requires surgery"

122. Ophelia is 3 months old and has congestive heart failure that is not responding to furosemide therapy. The physician orders bumetanide 0.05 g/kg, to be given every 6 hours via slow IVP. Which electrolyte imbalance would indicate an adverse effect of bumetanide administration?

A. Hypernatremia
B. Hyperkalemia
C. Hypercalcemia
D. Hypochloremia

123. Your patient with bronchopulmonary dysplasia (BPD) was started on Diuril 2 days ago for pulmonary edema. While drawing a capillary blood gas (CBG), you perform a bedside glucose check. The serum glucose is 180 mg/dL. The most likely cause for the hyperglycemia in this patient is

A. Suppression of the pancreatic release of insulin
B. The patient is under stress
C. Hypersecretion of bicarbonate
D. Stimulation of the adrenal glands

124. Which of the following statements is true regarding furosemide (Lasix) administration?

A. Oral Lasix should be taken with milk, not water

B. Lasix IV should be administered rapidly

C. Lasix solutions, whether oral or intravenous, should be protected from light

D. Oral Lasix should be administered with food

125. You are caring for a 2 year old child in chronic renal failure awaiting a renal transplant. Peritoneal dialysis is being started. Which of the following statements is true regarding nursing management during peritoneal dialysis?

A. Seizure precautions should be instituted at all times

B. If turbidity is noted, request a CBC with differential, Gram stain, and culture fluid

C. The best position for the infant is flat, supine, or prone

D. Maintain clean gauze dressings around the catheter insertion site

126. Which hormone is released by the pituitary when a hyperosmolar state is present?

A. Renin

B. Calcitonin

C. Prostaglandin

D. Antidiuretic hormone

127. The normal specific gravity of urine at 1.002–1.012 reflects the normal value of urine osmolality. Normal urine osmolarity for a 12 year old child is

A. 50–100 mOsm/L

B. 100–300 mOsm/L

C. 200–500 mOsm/L

D. 200–400 mOsm/L

128. You are preparing to admit a 6 day old term infant from home for dehydration. The infant has been vomiting and has had diarrhea for the past 2 days. Which of the following lab results would support the diagnosis of dehydration?

A. Low BUN and creatinine levels

B. A urine output of 2.2 mL/kg/hr

C. Depressed fontanelles

D. Metabolic acidosis obtained via capillary blood gas analysis

129. Which of the following statements regarding sodium is true?

A. Sodium is a major intracellular cation

B. Hypernatremia causes a fluid shift from the extracellular space to the intracellular space

C. Hyponatremia results in intravascular hypotonicity

D. Sodium is the major electrolyte responsible for cardiac muscle function

130. Today you are working in the capacity of charge nurse for your PICU. You are called to the nursery to evaluate a 2 day old term infant for suspected seizure activity. You note that this term infant has a high-pitched cry, irritability, dry mucous membranes, and sunken fontanelles. The mother reports that she is breastfeeding exclusively, but the baby "always seems to be sleepy and hard to wake up." While obtaining vital signs, you note a period of apnea and seizure

activity. You bring the infant to the PICU and notify the physician. Which order should be carried out first?

A. Obtain ABGs immediately

B. Obtain a chest X-ray

C. Draw a CBC, chemistry panel, and blood glucose

D. Set up seizure precautions

131. **Dakota is 1 year old and is to receive volume replacement for dehydration. She does not have any signs or symptoms of trauma. Which of the following is the most appropriate initial choice for immediate fluid replacement?**

A. 20 mL/kg of D_5W

B. Normal saline or lactated Ringer's solution

C. $D_{12.5}W$

D. Packed red blood cells

SECTION 9

Renal Answers

1. **Correct answer: B**
   A normal value of intracellular potassium would be 140 mEq/L. Intracellular fluid contains high concentrations of potassium, magnesium, proteins, phosphates, and sulfates.

2. **Correct answer: B**
   Mucomyst (*N*-acetylcysteine [NAC]) is used to help reduce renal failure or worsening of symptoms caused by contrast media. The contrast media can cause contrast-induced neuropathy. Mucomyst has antioxidant properties that may counteract the reactive oxygen species that occur when the contrast media causes tubular epithelial cell toxicity.

3. **Correct answer: B**
   Nesiritide is synthetic brain natriuretic peptide (BNP). It is used in the management of the heart failure associated with prerenal azotemia. The BNP causes vasodilation, decreased systemic resistance (SVR), decreased wedge pressure (PCWP or PAOP), increased cardiac output (or cardiac index), diuresis, and decreased renin–angiotensin activity.

4. **Correct answer: C**
   Mannitol and urea are osmotic diuretics. This type of diuretic acts by increasing the osmotic pressure of the filtrate, which in turn attracts water and electrolytes and prevents reabsorption. The problem is that osmotic diuretics can cause a rebound volume expansion, hyponatremia, and hypernatremia. Mannitol may be used in lieu of sodium bicarbonate to manage hemoglobinuria and myoglobinuria secondary to rhabdomyolysis or severe crush injury. The use of large volumes of fluid may also help reduce or prevent renal tubular obstruction.

5. **Correct answer: A**
   Potential complications of loop diuretics include hypokalemia. Because of the high volume of urine excreted, additional complications may include hypocalcemia, dilutional hyponatremia, hyperglycemia, and hypochloremic acidosis.

6. **Correct answer: A**
   Methazolamide is a diuretic that is classified as a carbonic anhydrase inhibitor. Other carbonic anhydrase inhibitors include dichlorphenamide and acetazolamide sodium. This type of diuretic blocks carbonic anhydrase and promotes excretion of water, Na^+, K^+, and bicarbonate. Potential complications include hypokalemia and hyperchloremic acidosis.

7. **Correct answer: B**
   Ethacrynic acid is a loop diuretic that prevents reabsorption of Na and Cl at the ascending loop of Henle (in the medulla of the kidney). Other loop diuretics include furosemide, torsemide, and bumetanide. As a group, they have vasodilatory effects on renal vasculature.

8. **Correct answer: D**
   A normal value for bicarbonate (HCO_3) in the intravascular space would be 24 mEq/L. Bicarbonate in the interstitial spaces contains approximately 3 mEq more than bicarbonate in the intravascular space, which averages 24 mEq/L.

9. **Correct answer: C**
   If your patient's CVP suddenly rose from 5 to 18, ANP would be released. ANP is atrial natriuretic peptide and is released by the atria as a response to fluid overload. ANP increases excretion of sodium and water from the kidneys. This action results in lowering the blood pressure. When the sodium and water are excreted, this decreases the release of antidiuretic hormone (ADH) and aldosterone.

10. **Correct answer: A**
    The hypertonic saline will expand the intravascular volume only. D_5W will be distributed equally between the intravascular and extravascular spaces. Other solutions used for volume replacement include Dextran (hetastarch) and Hextend, both of which are synthetic colloidal solutions.

11. **Correct answer: B**
    If your patient has a decreased extracellular fluid volume, they would exhibit the hemodynamic profile of decreased CVP, PAP, MAP, and CO, and an increased SVR. When all the fluid is in the extracellular space, systemic vascular resistance is increased. Because the fluid volume in the intravascular space is low, all the other parameters are decreased.

12. **Correct answer: C**
    Myra is probably developing osmotic demyelinization syndrome. Treatment should have occurred at a slower pace to prevent shrinkage and lysis of brain cells. If this condition is discovered early enough, fluid and electrolyte replacement can be slowed. If permanent damage is done, the patient may develop quadriparesis, flaccidity, and other neurological deficits. Seizure precautions should be in place.

13. **Correct answer: A**
    A report of flank pain indicates renal injury in pediatric patients who experience blunt trauma and transverse and vertebral body fractures to the T11–12 and L1–L4 levels. The kidneys in pediatric patients are proportionately larger than the kidneys in adults and move freely with respiration. As a result, the kidneys are more prone to injury in children. A urinary output of less than 0.5 to 1 mL/kg/hr and the presence of hematuria also would indicate renal impairment. Urinary incontinence may indicate spinal cord injury (not renal injury), so it should definitely be reported. A urine osmolarity of 300 mOsm/L is normal.

14. **Correct answer: A**
    A 205-pound 16 year old may be managed according to adult standards. To calculate the minimum urine output, multiply 30 mL/hr by 12 hours. The result equals 360 mL

per 12-hour shift. For pediatric patients weighing less than 60 kg, minimum urine output should be calculated based on a rate of 0.5–1 mL/kg/hr. This patient weighs 93 kg (204.6/2.2 = 93).

15. **Correct answer: D**
In pediatric patients, 20% to 25% of cardiac output is directed to the kidneys. Nephrons are completely formed at 28 weeks gestation. Kidney location is not fixed, but move easily with the diaphragm within the abdominal cavity between T11 and L4. Infant kidneys are more vulnerable to fluid changes, including dehydration and overhydration, due to their inability to concentrate urine effectively.

16. **Correct answer: C**
The tubular components of the nephron include the proximal tubule, Loop of Henle, and distal tubule. Cortical nephrons account for approximately 85% of all nephrons. The juxtaglomerular nephrons account for the other 15%. Cortical nephrons have long Loops of Henle—a factor that is important for water conservation. Afferent arterioles bring blood to the glomerulus, and efferent arterioles take blood from the glomerulus to the second capillary bed.

17. **Correct answer: B**
The proximal tubules are responsible for secretion of H^+. The distal tubules and collecting ducts may also secrete H^+ when an acidotic state exists. The Loop of Henle only secretes or reabsorbs Na^+ and water. Reabsorption of water when ADH is present occurs in the distal tubules and collecting ducts. The proximal tubules do not require ADH to reabsorb water. Secretion of potassium is controlled by the distal tubules and the collecting ducts.

18. **Correct answer: C**
Complete your assessment of this patient. A sallow complexion and yellowing or browning of the skin may indicate renal compromise. The color change may be due to deposits of urochrome under the skin. Prior to calling the doctor, assess the patient for other indicators of renal compromise, such as changes in LOC, respiratory and heart status, blood pressure, abdominal pain, urinary output quantity and quality, and the most recent chemistry and hematology reports.

19. **Correct answer: D**
Water is the only substance transported passively between membranes within the nephrons via osmosis. Potassium, glucose, sodium, calcium, amino acids, chloride, phosphate, and bicarbonate all require active transportation with adenosine triphosphate (ATP) to cross membranes.

20. **Correct answer: A**
Decreased urine output will occur when there is a decrease in glomerular filtration rate (GFR) with vasoconstriction of the afferent arterioles. The afferent arterioles bring blood to the glomerulus for filtration. Any drop in blood flow to or through the nephrons will result in a drop in GFR and urine output. Efferent arteriole vasoconstriction results in an increased hydrostatic pressure and GFR in the glomerulus. The blood is unable to move easily to the second capillary bed. A serum albumin of 1.8 g/dL will result in decreased plasma osmotic pressure and increased GFR. A heart rate of 160 increases blood flow to the kidneys, increasing the GFR. Less time is available for changes to occur in plasma osmotic pressures.

21. **Correct answer: B**
Sympathetic nerve stimulation affects kidney function by restricting blood flow through the afferent and efferent arterioles. Parasympathetic nerve stimulation causes vasodilation of the arterioles. Autoregulation in response to systemic arterial pressures may increase or decrease GFR, as the body attempts to stabilize blood pressure and circulating volume.

22. **Correct answer: A**
Creatinine is an endogenous waste product of muscle tissue that is excreted by the kidneys. Clearance refers to volume of a specific substance filtered from plasma over a designated time. Autoregulation represents the goal of constant filtration pressure by renal blood flow and glomerular filtration rate. Glomerular filtrate refers to all substances filtered from the plasma, such as electrolytes, blood, proteins, water, ketones, and white blood cells.

23. **Correct answer: C**
The normal glomerular filtration rate (GFR) for a 1 year old is 80 to 120 mL/min. The normal GFR for a newborn at the second week of life is 35 to 40 mL/min. A GFR of 60 mL/min is normal for a 6 month old child. GFR peaks in the 20s at 120 to 130 mL/min, then declines with age. A GFR of <60 mL/min indicates likely renal impairment and should be reported in any patient who is more than 1 year old.

24. **Correct answer: B**
Antidiuretic hormone causes urine to be more concentrated as water reabsorption is increased. ADH is released by the hypothalamus in response to high solute concentrations in the blood. Release of ADH results in active transportation of water in the distal tubules and collecting ducts, which increases the water content in the blood. Sodium retention is affected by aldosterone secretion by the adrenal cortex.

25. **Correct answer: B**
Sodium retention in the kidneys is not affected by ADH. ADH only affects water reabsorption in the kidneys. Sodium reabsorption is influenced by aldosterone excretion (which increases the absorption rate), insulin (which affects sodium retention), and estrogen release (which affects sodium retention).

26. **Correct answer: A**
An inorganic phosphate level of 6.1 mg/dL should be reported to the physician. The kidneys are the primary mechanism for controlling the phosphate concentration. Normal phosphate levels are 4.2 to 6.5 mg/dL in newborns, 3.5 to 6.5 mg/dL in children 1 to 5 years old, and 2.5 to 4.5 mg/dL in older children and adults. For this patient, the sodium, potassium, and calcium levels are within normal ranges.

27. **Correct answer: D**
Missy's poor urine output is due to prerenal failure from extensive ibuprofen use. NSAIDs impair renal autoregulation and inhibit the kidney's response to sympathetic stimulation, resulting in vasodilation and a drop in both renal blood flow and the glomerular filtration rate. Poor intake would lead to prerenal failure. Intrinsic failure refers to failure within the nephrons. There is no indication that Missy's cast is restrictive, and if it were too tight, it would impair blood flow to the limb, not blood flow to the kidneys.

28. Correct answer: B
Acute tubular necrosis (ATN) is associated with metabolic acidosis, as the kidneys are unable to excrete excess hydrogen ions or reabsorb bicarbonate. The bicarbonate binds with the hydrogen to form carbon dioxide and water, which can then be expelled by the lungs. Additional ATN complications include hyponatremia, low thyroxine levels, and increased parathyroid levels.

29. Correct answer: C
Urea, the waste product of amino acids in the liver, is excreted by the kidneys. Bilirubin, a blood waste product, is metabolized by the liver and excreted via the gastrointestinal tract. Creatinine is a waste product of protein metabolism. Uric acid is a waste product of nucleic acid metabolism.

30. Correct answer: C
Anuria is usually due to postrenal AKI, which is characterized by mechanical obstruction of the urinary collection system. The collection system consists of the renal pelvis, the ureters, the bladder, and the urethra.

31. Correct answer: C
An example of acute renal failure would be a sudden or rapid decline in renal filtration function. Acute renal failure is now known as acute renal injury or acute kidney injury (AKI) and can be classified as prerenal, intrinsic, or postrenal. Because material covered on the CCRN exam reflects practice up to two years ago, we thought that the new terminology should be added, as some item writers may use this new terminology on the exam.

32. Correct answer: B
Intrinsic AKI is most commonly caused by acute ischemic or cytotoxic injury. Other causes include cell detachment, dilation of the lumen, and injury to the distal nephrons. Arteriolar vasoconstriction, amphotericin, and hypercalcemia are causes of prerenal AKI.

33. Correct answer: D
Apheresis is the general term used for all pheresis techniques and encompasses any selective removal of cells, plasma, and substances from blood. Apheresis also includes the return of remaining components and volume to the patient. Plasmapheresis is the removal of plasma and/or proteins from the blood or as a plasma exchange. Cytopheresis is the selective removal of cellular components from the blood (e.g., WBCs). Leukocytopheresis is the removal of WBCs. Erythrocytopheresis is the removal of RBCs. Plateletpheresis is the removal of platelets.

34. Correct answer: C
Postrenal acute renal injury may be caused by a neurogenic bladder. Other causes of postrenal acute renal injury include tumor, tricyclic antidepressants, fibrosis, BPH, prostate cancer, urethral obstruction, stone disease, and ligation during surgery. DIC, preeclampsia, transplant rejection, and malignant hypertension are causes of intrinsic failure or injury.

35. Correct answer: A
In the polyuric phase of acute kidney injury, it is important for the PICU nurse to carefully monitor potassium and phosphorus levels because of the potential for dysrhythmias.

36. **Correct answer: D**
As a teenager approaches adulthood in terms of body weight, the criteria for anuria becomes that of an adult: less than 100 mL per day. It is doubtful such a question would be asked about younger children, because it would be impossible to memorize all of the different possible values based on age or weight.

37. **Correct answer: D**
Mannitol may produce a hyperosmolar state. Damage to the eighth cranial nerve, vestibular impairment, and binding with proteins in the renal tubules are characteristics of loop diuretics such as furosemide, bumetadine, and torsemide.

38. **Correct answer: B**
Acyclovir can crystallize in the kidney and cause AKI. It is important for the nurse to carefully monitor the infusion time and the amount of fluid used to dilute intravenous drugs. Other drugs that can crystallize in the kidney include sulfonamides, idinivir, and triamterine.

39. **Correct answer: A**
NSAIDs may cause prerenal AKI. These drugs block prostaglandin production, which in turn alters glomerular arteriolar perfusion.

40. **Correct answer: C**
More than 99% of urea synthesis occurs in the liver. Dietary protein is converted into amino acids and peptides. Approximately 90% of these molecules are absorbed and transferred to the liver. Any excess nitrogen is converted into urea.

41. **Correct answer: D**
Increased production of urea may be due to GI bleeding. Approximately 500 mL of whole blood equals 100 g of protein. The extra protein must be converted into urea.

42. **Correct answer: C**
A carpopedal spasm that occurs when a blood pressure cuff is inflated to just past the systolic pressure elicits Trousseau's sign, an indication of hypocalcemia. You can also elicit this response by having the patient hyperventilate. When the patient becomes alkalotic, the serum calcium level decreases and a carpopedal spasm occurs.

43. **Correct answer: B**
1 kilogram = 2.2 pounds = 1000 mL. Although you may think this is too basic a piece of information for a pediatric CCRN review, it is the little pieces of information like this that often trip people up on the exam.

44. **Correct answer: C**
This patient is hypocalcemic. Lack of calcium slows cardiac contractility (the prolonged QT interval) and the patient might develop torsades de pointes (polymorphic ventricular tachycardia). The torsades may also be caused by hyperkalemia.

45. **Correct answer: B**
If the patient is hypocalcemic, the upper lip on the same side (ipsilateral) will twitch—a response known as Chvostek's sign. With Trousseau's sign, a BP cuff is used to elicit a carpopedal spasm indicative of hypocalcemia. Grey-Turner's sign consists of ecchymosis around the umbilicus, indicating abdominal issues. Homan's sign may indicate DVT.

46. Correct answer: C
Aldosterone is secreted when the extracellular sodium level is low and/ or when extracellular potassium is high. Aldosterone is a hormone secreted by the adrenal glands. Aldosterone will also be secreted if the blood pressure is too low and when there is extreme physical stress.

47. Correct answer: D
Sodium is the major extracellular cation, and potassium is the major intracellular cation.

48. Correct answer: B
Potassium is reabsorbed in the distal tubules. Regulated excretion of potassium also occurs in the distal tubules.

49. Correct answer: A
Chronic alcohol use leads to an alkalotic state. Potassium has a positive charge and hydrogen moves in the opposite direction to potassium. Thus, when potassium moves into the cell, hydrogen moves out to correct the alkalosis.

50. Correct answer: B
A U wave is seen in conjunction with hypokalemia. A peaked T wave, a shortened QT interval, and an absent P wave are seen on EKG tracings for patients with hyperkalemia.

51. Correct answer: A
Boiling leaches out most of the vegetables' potassium and nutrients into the water. Baking is the best method of preparation, as it allows the vegetables to retain most of their potassium and other nutrients.

52. Correct answer: A
In Addison's disease, the patient's potassium level results in hyperkalemia related to the decrease in aldosterone secretion. This condition leads to hyperkalemia and hyponatremia, as sodium cannot be retained and potassium cannot be removed.

53. Correct answer: C
Bronwyn is exhibiting signs and symptoms of hypokalemia. Hypokalemia is defined as any potassium level less than 3.5 mEq/L.

54. Correct answer: C
The current recommended serum magnesium level is 2–3 mg/dL. This concentration may be higher in patients with cardiac disease or in their third trimester of pregnancy. Magnesium is also used to treat pregnancy-induced hypertension and to control premature contractions.

55. Correct answer: A
The parathyroid controls the calcium level within the body. Magnesium has been found to influence the secretion rate of the parathyroid and, therefore, influence calcium levels.

56. Correct answer: C
Because magnesium is absorbed in the small intestines, surgeries that remove or alter the small intestines, such as gastric bypass, place the patient at risk for developing

hypomagnesemia. Gastric surgeries also affect water reabsorption, processing time in the intestines, calcium levels, and the amount of lactose tolerated in the diet.

57. **Correct answer: D**
Elaine is exhibiting signs and symptoms of hypomagnesemia related to her high calcium intake. Calcium and magnesium are absorbed in the small intestines. Calcium in extremely high doses or intake competes with magnesium absorption. Elaine will need nutritional teaching to help her balance her diet.

58. **Correct answer: B**
A magnesium level of 0.5 mEq/L will result in convulsions. Ketoacidosis leads to excessive urinary secretion of magnesium as a result of osmotic diuresis caused by the elevated glucose concentration. In addition, the insulin therapy used to treat hyperglycemia forces magnesium into the cells, which causes a further drop in the extracellular concentration of magnesium. As magnesium levels drop, cellular irritability increases and the risk of convulsions increases. In this scenario, you would expect to see an increased overall irritability, positive Babinski sign, and increased reflexes.

59. **Correct answer: D**
Approximately 99% of the body's calcium is stored in the bone.

60. **Correct answer: C**
Calcium that is bonded to protein cannot pass through capillary walls. If calcium does bind to protein, the molecule is too large to pass from the extracellular fluid into the intracellular space due to the restrictive capillary permeability. Approximately 50% to 70% of serum calcium is ionized in the serum. Because of the protein-binding ability of calcium, albumin and calcium levels can be directly correlated. Calcium plays a major role in coagulation.

61. **Correct answer: A**
Vitamin D increases serum calcium. Calcium does not increase vitamin D levels.

62. **Correct answer: A**
As calcium levels increase, the parathyroid decreases secretions. The parathyroid hormone is the hormone most closely related to serum calcium management. In response to rising calcium levels, the parathyroid decreases its secretions to decrease or stabilize calcium levels.

63. **Correct answer: C**
The technique for eliciting a Trousseau's sign is to inflate a blood pressure cuff to greater than the systolic blood pressure for 3 minutes. A positive sign is observed when the carpal nerve spasms, causing the hand to curve inward with all fingers touching.

64. **Correct answer: A**
Beta blockers may cause an anaphylactic reaction with the membranes or the filter in the CRRT filter. Bradykinins are released as a result, which leads to systemic anaphylaxis.

65. **Correct answer: C**
The minimal mean arterial pressure must be 60 mmHg. The patient's blood pressure provides the gradient on which the system functions. If the blood pressure is too low, the system will not filter the blood appropriately.

66. **Correct answer: D**
CVVH and CVVHD require only venous access and pumping function. The "C" stands for continuous. The second two letters refer to the access and return sites, respectively. CVV types of filtration require a pump function, as the blood must be pumped throughout the system. CAV types of filtration use arterial pressures to drive the flow and the filtration. H, HD, and HDF refer to the type of filtration—hemofiltration, hemodialysis, and hemodiafiltration, respectively. SCUF or Slow continuous ultrafiltration is used to remove fluid from the patient and no replacement is given.

67. **Correct answer: C**
Lack of thrill and/or bruit may indicate that the graft has become occluded and dialysis is not possible. The nurse's best course of action is to use a Doppler to determine graft patency prior to making any calls or administering any medication. Although you may not hear or feel the thrill and bruit, the graft may still be patent.

68. **Correct answer: B**
It is imperative that all staff be made aware of the graft site location, including lab technicians, nursing assistants, student nurses, medical staff, physical therapists, and respiratory therapists. The goal is to avoid any lab or blood draws, blood pressures, or occlusions in the grafted limb.

69. **Correct answer: D**
Hemodialysis is used to administer phosphate binders to patients with hyperphosphatemia. In addition, it may be used to provide vitamin D and calcium carbonate for osteoporosis, erythropoietin for iron deficiencies (anemia), and glucose for hypoglycemia.

70. **Correct answer: C**
Approximately 2–3 L of dialysate is used in peritoneal dialysis. In small children, this amount is adjusted downward.

71. **Correct answer: B**
The correct sequence for fluid exchange in peritoneal dialysis is first to instill the dialysate, then to allow the fluid to dwell within the abdomen for a predetermined time, and finally to drain the fluid. The number of exchanges is determined by the physician and based on the desired outcome.

72. **Correct answer: A**
Peritoneal dialysis functions based on the principles of diffusion and osmosis. Diffusion is the passive movement of solutes across a membrane. The direction of diffusion is based on concentration (movement goes from areas of higher concentration to areas of lower concentration), heat, and pressure. The speed at which diffusion occurs depends on the grade or steepness of the differences in concentrations on each side of the membrane and the molecule moving across the membrane (i.e., its size and polarity). Osmosis is the passive movement of solvents (i.e., water) across a permeable membrane. Movement of the solvent depends on the permeability of the membrane: The more permeable the membrane, the more passive the movement of solutes and solvents. Permeability may affect the types of solutes that are able to unintentionally cross the membrane.

73. **Correct answer: B**
Each of these answers is a condition often treated with apheresis, but paraneoplastic neurologic syndromes are treated with immunadsorption. Multiple sclerosis is treated with plasma lymphocyte. Cutaneous T-cell lymphoma is treated using a combination of photopheresis and leukopheresis. Heart transplant rejections are treated with a combination of photopheresis and plasmapheresis.

74. **Correct answer: A**
Replacement of plasma volume in plasmapheresis is usually delivered at a 1:1 or 1.5:1 ratio. Replacement fluids include FFP, thawed plasma, albumin, and electrolytes and fluids based on the patient's condition.

75. **Correct answer: C**
Sodium cannot be completely eliminated from the diet. A major cation in the extracellular fluid within the body, sodium plays a role in driving the sodium–potassium pump and stabilizing polarization of cells and water balance. The body attempts to protect sodium levels by titrating aldosterone and antidiuretic hormone (ADH), and changing the filtration rate within the kidneys. Fresh fruits and vegetables contain minimal amounts of salt. Canned vegetables tend to utilize sodium to preserve flavor, so they will have the highest sodium levels.

76. **Correct answer: B**
Blackberries contain 1 mg of sodium per 3.5-ounce serving. Peaches contain 2 mg per serving, grapes 3 mg, and cantaloupe 12 mg.

77. **Correct answer: C**
Most fresh fish will be low in sodium. Pike has the lowest amount of sodium—only 51 mg sodium per 3.5-ounce serving. Chicken contains 60–80 mg of sodium per serving, canned beef hash 540 mg, and canned crab 1000 mg. Any canned or processed meat will contain some preservative. If it is not labeled as "low sodium," the sugar content should be scrutinized. For most people, eating fresh or fresh frozen meats, vegetables, and fruits will aid in limiting sodium, fat, and sugar intake.

78. **Correct answer: D**
Parmesan cheese has a sodium level of 1862 mg per serving, whereas Swiss cheese contains 260 mg per serving, cheddar cheese 620 mg, and mozzarella cheese 373 mg.

79. **Correct answer: B**
Overhydration is a common cause of hyponatremia. It is not a real hyponatremia, in that the sodium level falls below normal due to dilution, rather than a disease process or injury. Intake, orally or intravenously—causes an artificial drop in the sodium level. Correction of this imbalance is achieved through fluid restriction or decreasing IV rates. Other causes of hyponatremia include loss of sodium through sweating or vomiting, shock, bleeding, SIADH, renal failure (inability to save sodium), hypoxia, freshwater drowning, and excessive administration of hypotonic fluids.

80. **Correct answer: D**
The BUN may be elevated in patients who are taking steroids. The BUN may also be elevated in cases of GI or mucosal bleeding or excessive protein intake.

81. **Correct answer: D**
A renal transplant that results from humoral rejection or acute cellular rejection may be definitively diagnosed only via a renal biopsy. The renal biopsy is the gold standard for diagnosing rejection. Ultrasound results may be difficult to obtain or interpret due to ascites, obesity, or fluid in the retroperitoneal area. Doppler scans measure blood flow. This flow may be diminished due to either prerenal or intrinsic AKI. Nuclear scans are of limited value because the excretion rates may be slowed by disease.

82. **Correct answer: C**
Tetracycline decreases anabolism, thereby increasing BUN.

83. **Correct answer: D**
Medications that can decrease BUN levels include chloramphenicol and streptomycin. Neomycin, rifampin, chloral hydrate, furosemide, bacitracin, and gentamycin are all medications that increase BUN levels.

84. **Correct answer: A**
The normal creatinine range is 0.8 to 1.4 mg/dL. Females have less muscle mass than males, so they have lower levels of creatinine. The presence of abnormally high levels of creatinine may indicate pyelonephritis or eclampsia.

85. **Correct answer: B**
Allergic nephritis may result from the use of cimetidine. Cimetidine interferes with creatinine excretion in the renal tubules. Although renal function does not decrease, the creatinine level does rise. If diminished renal function exists, an allergic nephritis may develop.

86. **Correct answer: A**
This patient has hypercalcemia. A loop diuretic prevents reabsorption of calcium, and normal saline is administered to increase the patient's glomerular filtration rate. If a thiazide diuretic were used, it would actually decrease calcium excretion. Use of glucose, insulin, and Kayexalate is not indicated, because they are treatments for hyperkalemia.

87. **Correct answer: A**
The patient with an acute kidney injury cannot excrete ammonium or acid ions in the quantities necessary to aid in the excretion of hydrogen. The subsequent buildup of hydrogen causes the metabolic acidosis.

88. **Correct answer: B**
Renal infarction can occur with cocaine intoxication. Cocaine abuse can lead to any type of infarction, including MI. The proteinuria and RBCs in the urine are indicative of renal infarction, however.

89. **Correct answer: C**
Kenji is at a high risk for hyponatremia. Because of a defect in chromosome 7, patients with cystic fibrosis lose sodium through their skin and mucous membranes. This phenomenon results in a thickening of the mucus layers leading to infection and hyponatremia.

90. **Correct answer: A**
Sean is at risk for a deficit of sodium. Large amounts of extracellular fluids are found in the peritoneal cavity. If sodium is lost in this area, then it is no longer available to be absorbed into the vasculature.

91. **Correct answer: A**
Due to her medical condition, Leila became dehydrated, which in turn resulted in hemoconcentration. Her diabetes may have initiated additional renal injury. Because of the decreased blood flow through her kidneys owing to the CHF, Leila's kidneys were unable to filter the excess sodium from her body.

92. **Correct answer: B**
As aldosterone is secreted, potassium excretion increases. The reverse is also true: If aldosterone secretion is slowed, potassium excretion is slowed and more potassium is retained.

93. **Correct answer: C**
Hypokalemia may cause both respiratory and metabolic alkalosis. Potassium and hydrogen ions move in opposite directions to each other. When a patient is hypokalemic, hydrogen moves into the extracellular fluid, leading to both respiratory and metabolic alkalosis.

94. **Correct answer: A**
Oliguria is result of hyperkalemia. Renal disease, use of Lasix, and increased adrenal cortical hormones may all lead to hypokalemia.

95. **Correct answer: B**
Carrots contain the smallest amount of potassium (233 mg per serving) as compared to avocados (1484 mg), raisins (751 mg), and potatoes (610 mg).

96. **Correct answer: B**
Kaon is another name for potassium gluconate, a commonly used potassium replacement medication. Glucose and insulin, calcium gluconate, and bicarbonate all bind or push the potassium back into the cells from the intravascular space, thereby lowering extracellular potassium levels.

97. **Correct answer: C**
If the pH is high, potassium is driven into the cells, causing serum potassium levels to drop. Insulin will also force potassium back into the cells by stimulating the sodium–potassium pump.

98. **Correct answer: A**
Magnesium usually works synergistically with calcium to control neuromuscular function within all muscle groups.

99. **Correct answer: D**
Approximately 50% of the body's magnesium is within the bone marrow. The measured serum magnesium reflects only approximately 1% of the body's magnesium, and the remaining 49% is found in intracellular spaces.

100. Correct answer: C

Honey contains the smallest amount of magnesium. It is better to recommend consumption of foods such as leafy vegetables that have a deep, green color, whole grains, nuts, legumes, seafood, cocoa, and chocolate.

101. Correct answer: D

This patient is exhibiting signs and symptoms of hypermagnesemia. The dose should be held, the physician contacted, and the magnesium level evaluated.

102. Correct answer: C

Renal failure is one of the most common causes of hypermagnesemia. Patients with this condition are unable to excrete excess magnesium via the urine. Gastrointestinal bypass and fistulas will lead to hypomagnesemia.

103. Correct answer: B

Magnesium levels greater than 5 mEq/L produce vasodilation of the facial vessels.

104. Correct answer: B

The length of the removed PICC line should be compared to the length reported on insertion. Any discrepancy should be reported to the physician immediately and represents a surgical emergency. Any remaining catheter within the vessel could cause infarction and tissue necrosis by blocking blood flow. During removal, if the PICC line does not move easily or if any resistance is met, do not pull forcefully as this may tear either the catheter or the vessel. Instead, stop the removal immediately and notify the physician. It is possible for lines to spontaneously knot or kink in vessels. An X-ray will confirm placement and identify obstructions to removal. Once the PICC line is removed, the nurse should apply direct pressure to the site for 5 minutes to stop bleeding and prevent hematoma.

105. Correct answer: D

HCO_3^- is a buffer that binds with free hydrogen to form carbonic acid. Carbonic acid then breaks down into water and CO_2, which are removed via the lungs. Additional buffers include plasma proteins and hemoglobin. Acids are hydrogen donors, whereas bases are hydrogen receptors. When evaluating the primary causes of acid–base imbalances, respiratory imbalances are determined by evaluating PCO_2, and metabolic imbalances are determined by evaluating HCO_3^-.

106. Correct answer: D

Some individuals do not tolerate the sight of blood. Because CRRT occurs outside the body, blood is in full sight. To improve communication between the patient and his or her visitors, it is best for the patient to let visitors know when procedures are occurring so that they may visit at a time when the CRRT procedure is not occurring. There are some restrictions on how many people may fit in one room with the equipment. This will vary by facility. The more people in a room, the higher the risk that the equipment may be touched or disconnected. Visitors should be informed not to touch equipment while in the room. Simple hand washing can prevent many infections, and other infection control measures should be used based on the patient's specific disease process.

107. Correct answer: C

Continuous renal replacement therapy (CRRT) results in slower volume regulation to avoid rapid shifts in volume. This method results in continuous removal or regulation of solutes and volume.

108. Correct answer: C

Urea clearance in the blood is the best indicator for monitoring dialysis effectiveness. Electrolyte levels may be altered by fluid shifting and the distillate used. Blood pressure may fluctuate with fluid removal, so it is not the best measurement method. Urine creatinine clearance indicates residual renal function.

109. Correct answer: B

It is common for patients to have a feeling of abdominal fullness related to the 2–3 L of dialysate that is instilled into the abdomen and allowed to dwell there. The additional pressure may cause shortness of breath. Leaking at the insertion site must be reported to the physician, as the patient may develop peritonitis and the patients should be monitored closely for this complication. Dialysis cannot continue until the insertion site is repaired. If fluid is felt or seen in the groin, it indicates that the patient has a hernia. Any part of the bowel that enters the groin during the dwell phase and becomes trapped there when the dialysate is drained may be damaged by strangulation.

If a patient feels dizzy or has palpitations during the drain phase, it indicates a too-rapid fluid shift or triggering of the vagal nerve. The drain time may need to be lengthened.

110. Correct answer: C

Kinking, bends, and cracks in the tubing are the most likely causes of a decreased dialysate return. If fixing these problems does not correct fluid flow, then reposition the patient, assess for any subcutaneous fluid and fluid within the groin, double-check the amount of fluid instilled, and complete an assessment prior to reporting the situation to the physician.

111. Correct answer: C

The dialysate often contains a large amount of glucose. During diffusion, glucose may cross the membranes, causing the patient to develop hyperglycemia. It is important for the patient and family to monitor for this complication at home. Careful education will assist the family in managing any complications and teach them when to notify the physician.

112. Correct answer: B

Connie's tingling is caused by a decrease in the amount of calcium in her tissues. Citrate binds with calcium in the blood and metabolizes into sodium bicarbonate, thereby increasing sodium and phosphate alkaline concentrations. An ACT, measurement of ionized calcium levels, and ABGs will show the extent of binding.

113. Correct answer: B

Acidosis results in an increase in the amount of free ionized calcium in the blood. Acidosis inhibits calcium's binding ability with albumin, thereby increasing serum calcium.

114. Correct answer: D

It is quite easy for patients to become hypernatremic from water softeners. Many water softener systems filter out calcium and magnesium (these minerals make water "hard") and replace them with sodium. The longer the filter has been in place, the greater the sodium content of the water. Not all water softeners use sodium, so recommend to patients that they evaluate systems on this point before purchasing one. Instead of drinking tap water, Bobby might be better off drinking bottled water and eating foods that have been prepared with distilled or bottled water. The family might also consider replacing its water filter with a reverse osmosis system. Bobby is following his diet as prescribed and does not exhibit any signs of renal failure.

Hypertonic fluids would lead to higher sodium levels. Diabetes insipidus would lead to elevated sodium levels due to the lack of ADH.

115. Correct answer: C

With hyponatremia, sodium levels drop to less than 135 mEq/L. Twitching and seizures are common, as well as apnea (not tachypnea), irritability (lethargy is seen with hypernatremia), and generalized muscle weakness (a late sign). Flattened T waves are seen with hypokalemia.

116. Correct answer: C

The normal range for serum potassium in a neonate is 4.5–6.8 mEq/L.

117. Correct answer: D

The renal response to acidosis is to increase secretion of hydrogen ions in the distal tubules. Reabsorption of bicarbonate takes place in the proximal tubules. Production of ammonia serves to buffer the acid in the blood.

118. Correct answer: B

The presence of casts, tubular cells, and proteinuria in urine indicates intrinsic renal failure. Intrinsic renal failure may be caused by congenital anomalies, thromboembolic disease, infection, inflammatory disease, or acute tubular necrosis.

119. Correct answer: B

Urine output of less than 2 mL/kg/hr after furosemide administration indicates an intrinsic or postrenal cause of renal failure. Fluid boluses of 10–20 mL/kg are used to differentiate between intrinsic, prerenal, and postrenal causes of renal failure. If the cause of the renal failure is prerenal in nature, then the patient will respond to fluid challenges with a rapid and sustained diuresis that occurs within 1–2 hours after the fluid challenge.

120. Correct answer: A

Hydronephrosis is the dilation of the pelvis and calyces of one or both kidneys due to obstruction. Obstruction of the flow of urine from the kidney causes retrograde flow into the pelvis, resulting in dilation. This is the most common renal abnormality found during prenatal ultrasound, and its cause is not always known. Affected patients present with poor urinary output, a possible abdominal mass, and urinary tract infection.

121. Correct answer: C

The need for corrective surgery depends on the cause and severity of the hydronephrosis. This patient has unilateral hydronephrosis with moderately low urine output. Further testing and time will provide support for or against surgery. The decision to pursue surgery takes into account the level of kidney function, the presence of an obstruction, the presence (or absence) of hypertension, and any worsening in the hydronephrosis.

122. **Correct answer: D**
Adverse effects of bumetanide include hypochloremic alkalosis, hyponatremia, and hypokalemia. Bumetanide works by inhibiting chloride reabsorption and tubular sodium transport, resulting in hyponatremia and hypochloremia. In addition, there is urinary loss of potassium, calcium, and bicarbonate.

123. **Correct answer: A**
Diuril inhibits pancreatic insulin release, resulting in hyperglycemia. Bedside glucose monitoring should be performed at least daily to monitor for hyperglycemia. Additional monitoring should include sodium, potassium, magnesium, chloride, bicarbonate, and phosphorus due to the increased urinary loss.

124. **Correct answer: C**
Lasix solutions should be protected from light because light will cause degradation. Oral Lasix should be taken on an empty stomach to improve its absorption and IV Lasix should be given slowly to prevent muscle spasms.

125. **Correct answer: B**
If the return fluid is noted to be turbid (cloudy with sediment), then the nurse should inform the physician and request orders to obtain a CBC with differential and to send the fluid for Gram stain and culture. Peritonitis is a common and potentially deadly complication of peritoneal dialysis. If infection is suspected, prepare to administer antibiotics. Catheter sites should be sterile and covered with an occlusive dressing. To minimize respiratory distress from increased abdominal pressure on the diaphragm, position the patient in a supine or side-lying position, with the head of the bed elevated. The nurse must also ensure that the tubing is free of kinks. Accurate monitoring of dialysate flow provides early detection of fluid absorption, dehydration, and potential obstructions in the system.

126. **Correct answer: D**
Antidiuretic hormone (also known as ADH or vasopressin) is secreted by the pituitary gland when hyperosmolality and/or hypotension occurs. Renin and prostaglandin are secreted by the kidneys. ADH results in water reabsorption by making distal tubules permeable to water.

127. **Correct answer: B**
The normal specific gravity of urine should reflect a normal value of urine osmolality at 100–300 mOsm/L. This value is accurate if the patient does not have blood, glucose, or protein in the urine.

128. **Correct answer: D**
A capillary blood gas analysis will indicate metabolic acidosis when dehydration is present. Urine output should be less than 1 mL/kg/hr and the BUN and creatinine normal or elevated to support a diagnosis of dehydration.

129. **Correct answer: C**
Hyponatremia results in intravascular hypotonicity and fluid shifts into the cells, causing cellular edema and intravascular dehydration. Sodium is a major extracellular cation and movement across the cellular membrane occurs via the sodium–potassium pump. Hypernatremia causes intravascular hypertonicity and a fluid shift into the extracellular space, thereby producing cellular dehydration and intravascular overload.

130. Correct answer: C

Upon admission, it is important to obtain a CBC, chemistry panel, and blood glucose immediately to rule out fluid and electrolyte imbalances. A high-pitched cry, irritability, lethargy, and seizure activity may indicate hypernatremia in an infant. If the mother is exclusively breastfeeding, her milk production is probably insufficient. Both hypocalcemia and hypoglycemia may cause seizures if not managed rapidly. Lab draws may be completed while waiting for radiology staff to perform the chest X-ray.

131. Correct answer: B

Normal saline and lactated Ringer's solution are the most appropriate choices for fluid replacement in a dehydrated infant. Both solutions are isotonic crystalloids. As there is no indication of blood loss in this scenario, packed red blood cells should not be used, as the patient may become polycythemic. Although a patient may be hypoglycemic on admission related to poor intake or excessive diarrhea or vomiting, glucose solutions should not be used for fluid replacement, but rather for fluid maintenance.

RENAL REFERENCES

Aehlert, B. (Ed.). (2005). *Comprehensive pediatric emergency care.* St. Louis, MO: Mosby.

American Heart Association. (2010). Guidelines 2010 for cardiopulmonary resuscitation and emergency cardiovascular care. Retrieved from www.americanheart.org

Andreoli, S. P. (2009). Acute kidney injury in children. *Pediatric Nephrology, 24*(2), 253–263.

Baird, J. S. (2009). Extreme hyponatremia in a child with vegetative state and water intoxication. *Clinical Pediatrics, 48*(7), 767–769.

Burns, S. M. (Ed.). (2007). *American Association of Critical-Care Nurses (AACN): AACN protocols for practice: Healing environments* (2nd ed.). Sudbury, MA: Jones and Bartlett.

Canepa, A., Verrina, E., & Perfumo, F. (2008). Use of new peritoneal dialysis solutions in children. *Kidney International, 108*(suppl), S137–S144.

Chadha, V., Schaefer, F. S., & Warady, B. A. (2010). Dialysis-associated peritonitis in children. *Pediatric Nephrology, 25*(3), 425–440.

Chambers, M. A., & Jones, S. (Eds.). (2007). *Surgical nursing of children.* Philadelphia: Elsevier.

Chernecky, C., & Berger, B. (2004). *Laboratory tests and diagnostic procedures* (4th ed.). Philadelphia: Saunders.

Don, T., Friedlander, S., & Wong, W. (2010). Dietary intakes and biochemical status of B vitamins in a group of children receiving dialysis. *Journal of Renal Nutrition, 20*(1), 23–28.

Drake Melander, S. (Ed.). (2004). *Case studies in critical care nursing: A guide for application and review* (3rd ed.). Philadelphia: Saunders.

Edefonti, A., Mastrangelo, A., & Paglialonga, F. (2009). Assessment and monitoring of nutritional status in pediatric peritoneal dialysis patients. *Peritoneal Dialysis International, 29*(suppl 2), S176–S179.

Emergency Nurses Association & Newberry, L. (2005). *Sheehy's emergency nursing: Principles and practice* (6th ed.). St. Louis, MO: Mosby/Elsevier.

Fetal kidney volume and its association with growth and blood flow in fetal life: The Generation R Study. (2007). *Kidney International, 72*(8), 1034.

Fine, R. N. (2010). Etiology and treatment of growth retardation in children with chronic kidney disease and end-stage renal disease: A historical perspective. *Pediatric Nephrology, 25*(4), 725–732.

Gloor, J. M., Breckle, R. J., Gehrking, W. C., Rosenquist, R. G., Mulholland, T. A. Bergstralh, E. J., . . . Ogburn, P. L. (1997). Fetal renal growth evaluated by prenatal ultrasound examination. *Mayo Clinic Proceedings, 72*(2), 124–129.

Goldstein, S. L. (2009). Overview of pediatric renal replacement therapy in acute kidney injury. *Seminars in Dialysis, 22*(2), 180–184.

Gora-Harper, M. (1998). *The injectable drug reference.* Princeton, NJ: Bioscientific Resources.

Hardin, S. R., & Kaplow, R. (Eds.). (2004). *Synergy for clinical excellence: The AACN Synergy Model for Patient Care.* Sudbury, MA: Jones and Bartlett.

Hay, W. W. Jr., Levin, M. J., Sondheimer, J. M., & Deterding, R. R. (Eds.). (2007). *Current diagnosis and treatment in pediatrics* (18th ed.). New York: McGraw-Hill.

Hosseini, S., Gooran, S., Alizadeh, F., & Dadgari, S. (2009). Polycystic horseshoe kidney anomaly. *Applied Radiology, 38*(9), 38–39.

Indhumathi, E., Chandrasekaran, V., Jagadeswaran, D., Varadarajan, M., Abraham, G., & Soundararajan, P. (2009). The risk factors and outcome of fungal peritonitis in continuous ambulatory peritoneal dialysis patients. *Indian Journal of Medical Microbiology, 27*(1), 59–61.

Jain, S., Suarez, A. A., McGuire, J., & Liapis, H. (2007). Expression profiles of congenital renal dysplasia reveal new insights into renal development and disease. *Pediatric Nephrology, 22*(7), 962–974.

Jones & Bartlett Learning (2011). 2011 *nurse's drug handbook* (10th ed.). Sudbury, MA: Jones & Bartlett Learning.

Jones, K. L. (2006). Smith's recognizable patterns of human malformation (6th ed.). Philadelphia, PA: Elsevier.

Macksey, L. F. (2009). *Pediatric anesthetic and emergency drug guide.* Sudbury, MA: Jones and Bartlett.

Martin, B. (2010). Family presence during resuscitation and invasive procedures: AACN practice alert. Retrieved from http://www.aacn.org

Medina, J., & Puntillo, K. (2006). *AACN protocols for practice: Palliative care and end-of-life issues in critical care.* Sudbury, MA: Jones and Bartlett.

Mitra, S. C., Seshan, S. V. Salcedo, J. R., & Gil, J. (2000). Maternal cocaine abuse and fetal renal arteries: A morphometric study. *Pediatric Nephrology, 14*(4), 315–318.

Morris, S., Akima, S., Dahlstrom, J. E., Ellwood, D., Kent, A., & Falk, M. C. (2004). Renal tubular dysgenesis and neonatal hemochromatosis without pulmonary hypoplasia. *Pediatric Nephrology, 19*(3), 341–344.

Pace, R. C. (2007). Fluid management in patients on hemodialysis. *Nephrology Nursing Journal, 34*(5), 557–559.

Prenatal hydronephrosis: Researchers from McGill University report recent findings in prenatal hydronephrosis. (2009, August). *Gastroenterology Week,* 345.

Prescribing reference. (2009, Summer). *NPPR: Nurse Practitioner's Prescribing Reference, 16*(2).

Shroff, R., & Ledermann, S. (2009). Long-term outcome of chronic dialysis in children. *Pediatric Nephrology, 24*(3), 463–474.

Slota, M. C. (Ed.). (2006). *Core curriculum for pediatric critical care nursing* (2nd ed.). St. Louis, MO: Saunders.

Smeltzer, S., & Bare, B. G. (2003). *Brunner and Suddarth's textbook of medical–surgical nursing* (10th ed.). Philadelphia: Lippincott Williams & Wilkins.

Spratto, G. R., & Woods, A. L. (2001). PDR: *Nurse's drug handbook.* Montvale, NJ: Delmar & Medical Economics.

Trivits Verger, J., & Lebet, R. M. (Eds.). (2008). *AACN procedure manual for pediatric acute and critical care.* St. Louis, MO: Saunders.

Verrina, E., Cappelli, V., & Perfumo, F. (2009). Selection of modalities, prescription, and technical issues in children on peritoneal dialysis. *Pediatric Nephrology, 24*(8), 1453–1464.

Whyte, D. A., & Fine, R. N. (2008). Acute renal failure in children. *Pediatrics in Review, 29*(9), 299–307.

Young, T. E., & Magnum, B. (2009). *Neofax 2009.* Montvale, NJ: Thomson Reuters.

SECTION 10

Multisystem

1. **Seth is an 8 year old admitted to your unit after a burn injury. He was helping his father barbeque in the back yard when a sudden flame-up burned his chest, right shoulder, and chin. Which finding would be indicative of smoke inhalation in this patient?**
   A. PaO_2 81, met Hgb level of 2%
   B. PaO_2 76, pCO_2 26
   C. Increased CO_2
   D. CoHgb of 18%, burned chin

2. **Hypertonic solutions are frequently given to burn patients. An advantage of using this type of solution is**
   A. Its lower cost
   B. The decreased chance for sepsis
   C. Elimination of the need for vitamin replacements
   D. Minimization of wound edema

3. **Signs and symptoms of aspirin overdose include**
   A. Metabolic acidosis and tinnitus
   B. Bradycardia and respiratory acidosis
   C. Bradycardia and metabolic alkalosis
   D. Tachycardia and metabolic alkalosis

4. **The type of burn most likely to cause hemorrhage, thrombus formation, or generalized vascular disruption is a(n)**
   A. Chemical burn
   B. Electrical burn
   C. Direct flame burn
   D. Steam burn

5. **In patients with sepsis, endotoxins stimulate production of tumor necrosis factor (TNF). The TNF, in turn, stimulates**
   A. Neutrophil activation and platelet aggregation
   B. The parathyroid gland
   C. Increased CO_2 retention
   D. Increased CPP

6. **Acetaminophen overdose may cause hypoglycemia and should be treated with a**
   A. Continuous IV infusion of D_5W at 100 cc/hour
   B. Bolus of D_{10}, continuous infusion of 0.45% normal saline
   C. Bolus of D_{50}, continuous infusion of D_5W
   D. Continuous IV infusion of Lactated Ringers

7. **Your 15 year old patient is undergoing alcohol withdrawal and exhibits diplopia, peripheral neuropathy, confusion, recent memory loss, and hyperexcitability. You suspect that this patient is suffering from**
   A. Jorn's syndrome
   B. Leucine deficiency
   C. Increased caritine levels
   D. Wernicke-Kersakoff syndrome

8. **Sustained compartment pressures of _______ mmHg in a 15 year old patient are usually suggestive of compartment syndrome.**
   A. 15 mmHg
   B. 30 mmHg
   C. 40 mmHg
   D. 50 mmHg

9. **Phoebe was admitted to the PICU with recurrent *Pneumocystis carinii*. She is currently on protease inhibitors and nonnucleoside reverse transcriptase inhibitor. Which of the following herbal products may be contributing to her recurrent *Pneumocystis carinii*?**
   A. Ginkgo Biloba
   B. Ginseng
   C. St. John's Wort
   D. Thyme

10. **Gabriel was helping his mother clean out the garage yesterday. He developed a raised area that initially looked like a mosquito bite but is now red, pus filled, and inflamed. Gabriel is admitted to the unit with a necrotizing wound. You suspect a brown recluse spider bite. With this diagnosis, Gabriel may also exhibit all of the following signs and symptoms except**
    A. Dyspnea
    B. Nausea and vomiting
    C. DIC
    D. Hemolysis and thrombocytopenia

11. **Noah, a victim of a black widow spider bite, becomes obtunded, bradycardic, apneic, and hypotensive. You should**
    A. Administer morphine 2 mg IV
    B. Administer antivenin
    C. Tie a tourniquet around the affected leg
    D. Prepare to intubate

12. Nadeen is 16 and is preparing to go home after treatment with antivenin for a black widow spider bite. Which of the following discharge instructions is appropriate?

A. "You may experience muscle spasms for only a few days"
B. "You may experience tingling and weakness for several years"
C. "Call your doctor immediately if you have joint or abdominal pain or begin to have trouble breathing"
D. "It is normal to have a rash or fever in the next three days"

13. Many people are adding "exotic herbs" and supplements to their food and diets. Many of these substances may be very harmful. They may interact with medicines a child is taking or may result in serious or deadly complications of existing diseases. Serena is a 17 year old student who is experimenting with flavorings. She made a roast with Scotch Broom on it for her parents to try. After ingesting the roast, Serena began to feel light-headed, have palpitations, and feel weak. She is being treated in your unit post cardiac arrest in the emergency room. A priority of treatment would be to

A. Insert a nasogastric tube and provide gastric lavage with activated charcoal
B. Insert a Foley catheter
C. Continue quinidine medications taken at home
D. Continue the amiodarone infusion started in the ED

14. You are discussing herbal remedies at work when you are approached by the mother of your brain-injured patient with pneumonia. She asks if her daughter would benefit from drinking Ginkgo Biloba at home once discharged, because the mother had heard that it would decrease symptoms from the brain injury and improve memory. You tell her

A. "There is a lot of research, but nothing really supports its use"
B. "Sure, there are no interactions with other drugs, so she should be fine"
C. "Her doctor doesn't approve of any natural remedies, so don't tell him if you are using it"
D. "There could be very dangerous side effects if an herbal product is taken without consulting your daughter's physician. I will have him speak with you when he comes in"

15. You are treating 13 year old Enzo, a patient with long QT Syndrome. Which of the following herbs should he avoid ingesting after his discharge?

A. Marijuana
B. Ginkgo Biloba
C. Ginseng
D. Oregano

16. Molly was admitted to your unit after experiencing abdominal cramping, nausea, and severe diarrhea. Her EKG shows sinus tachycardia with frequent PVCs. She is currently on an amiodarone infusion. The only significant history was that Molly ate at a seafood restaurant three days ago. Molly is probably suffering from

A. Irritable bowel syndrome
B. Hypokalemia
C. Celiac disease
D. Shellfish poisoning

17. **Patients who are stung by bees numerous times are in danger of developing**
    A. Anemia
    B. Kidney failure
    C. Long QT interval
    D. Hydrocephalus

18. **A possible side effect of cocaine use is**
    A. Malignant hyperthermia
    B. Cherry red skin
    C. Paralytic ileus
    D. Constricted pupils

19. **Nicholas is receiving activated protein C. The actions of this drug include**
    A. Profibrinolytic action
    B. Antimicrobial agency
    C. Antiviral agency
    D. Blockade of Angiotensin II

20. **Which of the following drugs may promote anaphylaxis in a child receiving treatment for status asthmaticus?**
    A. Oxygen
    B. Acetylcysteine
    C. Codeine
    D. Guaifenesin

21. **A nursing consideration with administration of norepinephrine (Levophed) to a child would be**
    A. Do not administer this medication with alkaline solutions
    B. Do not administer this medication for low coronary artery perfusion states
    C. It is not indicated for vasogenic shock
    D. Do not use this medication for hypotensive states

22. **Levophed may cause tissue necrosis. You should treat extravasations with**
    A. An antihistamine
    B. Benadryl
    C. Phentolamine
    D. Hydralazine

23. **If your patient was in the early stage of septic shock, you would expect which of the following hemodynamic parameters?**
    A. SVR elevated, PAOP elevated, CO decreased
    B. CO decreased, RAP elevated, PAOP elevated
    C. RAP elevated, SVR decreased, PAOP increased
    D. CO increased, PAOP decreased, SVR decreased

24. Which of the following conditions would be contraindicated when scheduling a pediatric patient for a TEE (Transesophageal Echocardiogram)?

A. Cardiac tumors
B. Dysphagia
C. Vegetative endocarditis
D. Mitral valve regurgitation

25. Your patient was stabbed in the chest 6 days ago. The damage done to the heart required that the patient undergo a prosthetic mitral valve replacement. The patient is now experiencing transient chest pain and syncopal episodes. A TEE is ordered. You anticipate which of the following actions prior to this procedure?

A. Hold all meds 8 hours prior to procedure
B. Have the patient sit in a reclining chair two hours prior to the procedure
C. Administer prophylactic antibiotics
D. Position the patient on the right side

26. June has been scheduled for a pulmonary angiogram. Contraindications for a pulmonary angiogram would include

A. Perfusion deficits
B. Pregnancy
C. Pulmonary thromboembolism
D. Vascular filling defects

27. Acetaminophen overdose may take as long as two weeks to resolve. From 72 to 96 hours after ingestion of the overdose, symptoms will include

A. Pallor, lethargy, and metabolic acidosis
B. Jaundice, confusion, and coagulation disorders
C. Right upper quadrant pain and increased serum hepatic enzymes
D. Increased renal function

28. Which of the following statements about cocaine is false?

A. Cocaine use, even if only for one time, can cause rhabdomyolysis
B. Cocaine and tobacco use are associated with spontaneous abortion
C. Cocaine causes the placenta to shrink
D. Specimens should be kept on ice

29. An antidote for ethylene glycol toxicity is

A. Digoxin
B. Anisindione
C. Fomepizole
D. Narcan

30. GHB (Ecstasy) overdoses can lead to amnesia in what percentage of cases?

A. 13%
B. 21%
C. 24%
D. 32%

31. **Cadmium accumulates in the lungs, liver, and kidneys from exposure to**
    A. Cigarette smoke
    B. Asbestos
    C. Lead paint
    D. Fungicides

32. **Urine morphine levels may be affected in all of the following ways except**
    A. Poppy seed ingestion may produce false-positive results
    B. 10 mg MS IV may be detectable in urine for as long as 84 hours
    C. Use of a stealth adulterant will cause negative results in a positive sample
    D. High levels of lymphocytes will mask the presence of morphine in urine

33. **Phenytoin serum levels may be affected by**
    A. Holding tube feedings 30 minutes after oral phenytoin administration
    B. Waiting 2 hours before drawing a phenytoin peak level, after an oral dose
    C. After a change of dose, waiting 24 hours before drawing a phenytoin peak level
    D. None of the above

34. **Your patient's prothrombin time has an increased INR. You question the patient and determine that he has taken a medication that may have affected the INR level. Which of the following medications would have such an effect?**
    A. Antacids
    B. Herbs and natural remedies
    C. Antihistamines
    D. Diuretics

35. **Your patient underwent pulmonary function testing. The respiratory therapist tells you the preliminary result is a low peak expiratory flow rate (PEFR). This finding might indicate**
    A. Asthma
    B. Pneumothorax
    C. Pulmonary cysts
    D. Heart failure

36. **Your patient is undergoing a renal arteriogram. After the dye is injected, the patient complains of a "salty taste" in his mouth. You know**
    A. This effect is the first sign of an anaphylactic reaction
    B. This effect will result in termination of the arteriogram
    C. This effect is expected and should pass after about five minutes
    D. This effect is an emergency

37. **False-negative results for the sickle cell test will result from**
    A. Polycythemia
    B. High blood protein levels
    C. Anemia
    D. Multiple myelomas

38. Donna has had surgery to correct a ruptured appendix. The surgeon orders $ScvO_2$ monitoring. You know this type of monitoring is used for which of the following conditions?

A. Blood volume status
B. Late septic shock
C. Early septic shock
D. SVR status

39. Jose is an alcoholic admitted to your unit with cirrhosis. Why is thiamine added to his IV fluids?

A. Thiamine is a sedative and will ease agitation
B. Thiamine decreases the symptoms of DTs
C. Thiamine prevents the damage to the brain as a result of Wernicke's syndrome
D. Thiamine prevents complications of substance abuse

40. Leon is experiencing delirium tremens. Nursing interventions include keeping the room well lit and minimizing stimulation. Staff members continuously reorient Leon to time, place, and person. Haldol has been given as ordered and the patient is in 4 point restraints. Which of these nursing interventions should be discontinued?

A. Reorientation
B. Medication administration
C. Restraints
D. Controlling stimulation

41. Your patient is scheduled for implantation of a VAD. Approximately 20 minutes prior to the scheduled start of the procedure, the patient's mother informs you that she has concerns about side effects and the procedure itself. Your best nursing intervention would be to

A. See if the parent signed the consent form for the procedure
B. Notify the physician that the patient's mother does not have a full understanding of the procedure
C. Cancel the procedure
D. Answer the mother's questions yourself

42. What is the incubation period for inhalation anthrax?

A. 7–10 days
B. 5–7 days
C. 7–60 days
D. 20–30 days

43. Shawn works at a fast food restaurant. She finds an envelope that is torn and has white powder falling out of the tear. She and her fellow employees are sent to the hospital and admitted to the intensive care unit for possible inhalation anthrax. What is the treatment of choice for Shawn?

A. Penicillin G 2 million units intravenously every 6 hours
B. Ciprofloxacin 400 mg intravenously every 12 hours
C. Doxycycline 500 mg intravenously every 12 hours
D. Augmentin 875/125 mg intravenously every 12 hours

44. **What are the initial symptoms for inhaled anthrax?**
    A. Mild, flu-like symptoms
    B. Severe dyspnea and productive cough
    C. High fever, cough, and stridor
    D. Cutaneous lesions, cough, and high fever

45. **How long is antibiotic therapy continued for inhalation anthrax?**
    A. 10 days of intravenous antibiotics
    B. 14 days of intravenous, then oral antibiotics
    C. 30 days of intravenous, then oral antibiotics
    D. 60 days of combined intravenous and oral antibiotics

46. **Which form of isolation should be used for the patient with inhalation anthrax?**
    A. Full isolation with laminar air flow
    B. Droplet precautions
    C. Standard contact precautions
    D. Reverse isolation

47. **What is the causative organism in botulism poisoning?**
    A. *Clostridium deficile*
    B. *Clostridium botulinum*
    C. *Clostridium avium*
    D. *Botulinum botulinum*

48. **Your hospital is put on an external disaster notice after a ricin poisoning incident at a local train station. Your intensive care unit prepares to accept casualities. What makes ricin so toxic to humans?**
    A. Ricin causes respiratory failure
    B. Ricin causes renal failure
    C. Ricin inhibits protein synthesis, leading to cell death
    D. Ricin destroys the mitochondria in the cell, causing cell death

49. **Lisa is 17 years old and was admitted to the PICU with diffuse abdominal pain and confusion. In the ED, she had generalized seizures and bradycardia. Opioid overdose was suspected, and she was given naloxone with no discernible effect. Lisa is now lethargic, but does tell you that she is a "body packer" to help pay for beauty school. Lisa becomes hypotensive and bradycardic. Appropriate therapy would include**
    A. Bowel irrigations, intubation, mechanical ventilation, and anticonvulsants
    B. Sodium bicarbonate, activated charcoal, and hemodialysis
    C. Antiemetics, gastric lavage, and bronchodilators
    D. Activated charcoal, sodium bicarbonate, and vasopressors

50. **Polly is 13 years old and is admitted to your unit with tachycardia (146), RR 34, BP 90/60, and T 96.4 °F. Her white count is 15,000. Polly states that she was treated for a "kidney infection" two weeks ago while on vacation. She denies pain at this time. Polly probably has**
    A. MODS
    B. A kidney stone
    C. SIRS
    D. Appendicitis

51. Carl, age 11, was admitted to your unit because of increased respiratory effort and possible pneumonia. The blood culture revealed the presence of *E. Coli.* Which of the following antibiotics would have the best effect on the bacteria?

A. Ganciclovir

B. Gentamicin

C. Cytarabine

D. Cefoxitin

52. Your patient has pneumonia. You have just intubated him and placed him on mechanical ventilation. His urine output drops significantly. This effect is probably due to

A. Third spacing

B. Sepsis

C. Underresuscitation

D. MODS

53. A 16 year old male was pumping gas when a spark ignited the fumes. He suffered full thickness burns of the right arm. During your initial assessment, you note that eschar is present and the right radial pulse is not palpable. A Doppler pulse is also not discernible. Which of the following actions would be appropriate at this time?

A. Moving the patient's arm away from his torso and elevating it on a pillow

B. Escharotomy

C. Morphine 4 mg IV

D. Ice packs to reduce swelling

54. During the immediate post burn period, which of the following fluids would be most beneficial?

A. Normal saline

B. 0.45% normal saline

C. Lactated Ringers

D. Albumin

55. Your patient was in full arrest following a root canal. After a successful resuscitation, the patient has developed Ludwig's angina. This type of angina is defined as

A. A type of painful bradycardia in which the QT interval is lengthened

B. An infectious process

C. Dysrhythmia with severe pain secondary to inhalation of noxious gases

D. Cardiac ischemic post code syndrome

56. Children who have oral amphetamine overdoses should have which of the following substances used as part of their treatment regimen?

A. Ammonium chloride

B. Ipecac

C. Caffeine

D. Theophylline

57. **Gladys suffered severe respiratory depression following ingestion of a large amount of diazepam. She has now developed atrial fibrillation. Anticipated treatment would include**
    A. Amiodarone
    B. Lidocaine
    C. Adenosine
    D. Prostaglandin

58. **A 15 year old male was burned over the anterior chest, both arms, the anterior neck, and the lateral aspect of the right leg. The burns on his chest and right arm have a white, leather-like appearance, and the patient has no sensation in that area. What classification of burn is this?**
    A. First degree
    B. Second degree partial thickness
    C. Third degree full thickness
    D. Fourth degree full thickness

59. **If muscle is burned, what classification of burn is involved?**
    A. First degree
    B. Second degree partial thickness
    C. Third degree full thickness
    D. Fourth degree full thickness

60. **Your patient has burns on the right arm that are circumferential (all the way around the arm). What is a potential risk with this type of burn?**
    A. Infection in the bone
    B. Difficulty removing dead tissue
    C. Compartment syndrome
    D. Escharotomy

61. **You have been caring for Ziva in the PICU for terminal bone cancer. She has stopped eating due to nausea and vomiting. Her brother asks if he can bring in her favorite dessert to tempt her to eat. After clearing this action with the physician, he brings in the "special" brownies only for her. Within a few hours after her family members leave, Ziva is eating, but is noted to be shaking, anxious, and no longer oriented to time and place. You suspect**
    A. Ziva is exhibiting signs of brain metastasis
    B. Ziva is having a stroke
    C. Ziva has ingested marijuana and is exhibiting side effects
    D. Ziva is hypoglycemic and should continue eating

62. **Your patient has been receiving nitroprusside. When giving this medication, it is necessary to monitor for**
    A. Tachycardia
    B. Cyanide toxicity
    C. Retinal changes
    D. Ataxia

63. This morning, a fire broke out in your patient's home. Because it was a cold environment, the patient was surrounded by wool blankets and wool clothing from her closet. The patient did not suffer any burns, but did inhale large quantities of smoke. What would be the most potent toxin she might have inhaled?

A. Carbon monoxide
B. Smoke
C. Inhaled nitrates
D. Cyanide

64. Your patient lived in the country at a camp all summer and ate large quantities of deer and fish. He was admitted to the PICU for respiratory distress, weight loss, vomiting, and numbness around the mouth. He is also suffering from mouth sores and drools constantly. His probable diagnosis will be

A. Botulism
B. *Clamidia* infection
C. *Difficile* infection
D. Mercury poisoning

65. Your 17 year old patient was very anxious prior to undergoing a bronchoscopy. He received an IM injection of Versed. His blood pressure dropped from 142/80 to 88/56, and he became bradycardic. To counter this reaction, he should be given

A. Xanax
B. Ativan
C. Valium
D. Romazicon

66. Which of the following vasodilators should not be mixed with Ringer's lactate?

A. Nesiritide
B. Captopril
C. Cardene
D. Epinephrine

67. Jonathan is 16 years old. He got in a street fight with gang members and was stabbed in the right anterior chest. Jonathan lost approximately 1500 to 1600 mL of blood. Which of the following signs and symptoms would be expected with this volume of blood loss?

A. BP decreased, pulse pressure normal, RR 20–30/min
B. BP normal, RR increased, capillary refill normal
C. RR increased, BP normal, pulse pressure normal
D. BP decreased, RR increased, CO decreased

68. Peter lives on a ranch. Yesterday he complained of a stiff neck and was very lethargic. Last night he was found unconscious and had apparently vomited and possibly aspirated. Peter probably has

A. Pneumonia
B. West Nile virus
C. Western Equine Encephalitis
D. A brain tumor

69. Your patient is being treated for MRSA. She has been receiving vancomycin, and this morning her trough level result was > 20 ug/mL. This level

A. May cause ototoxicity
B. May cause nephrotoxicity
C. Is therapeutic
D. Indicates the current dosage is too low

70. Which of the following conditions would present with lab results showing a decreased sedimentation rate?

A. Anemia
B. Colon cancer
C. Infection
D. Congestive heart failure

71. Your patient has been on an amiodarone drip for atrial fibrillation. Today, the amiodarone serum level returned a result of 3.3 ug/mL. This result indicates

A. A therapeutic level
B. A subtherapeutic level
C. A panic level
D. Amiodarone levels are not measured this way

72. Pulmonary artery catheter infections may be best prevented by which of the following actions?

A. Use of an antibiotic coated catheter
B. Removal of the catheter within 48 to 72 hours of insertion
C. Administration of prophylactic antibiotics
D. Avoiding continuous heparin infusions

73. Joelle is 14 years old and just gave birth to a son. Because of complications with the delivery, she is now scheduled for a digital subtraction angiography procedure. Patient and family teaching for digital subtraction angiography includes

A. The length of the procedure is approximately 90 minutes
B. Women who are breastfeeding should substitute formula for breast milk for one or more days after the procedure
C. The patient will be able to change position frequently during the procedure
D. The patient will be free to move around during the procedure

74. Poisoning by arsenic may lead to which of the following symptoms?

A. Pneumonia, renal dysfunction
B. Tachycardia, hypertension
C. Paresthesia, cerebral edema
D. Convulsions

75. Your patient was admitted for severe flank pain and hematuria. He is scheduled for a kidney biopsy. Your patient and family teaching should include

A. Reporting any post procedure pain in the flank or abdomen
B. A small kidney stone may be passed after the procedure
C. The patient will be on bed rest for 24 hours
D. No teaching is necessary

76. Following a lung scan (V/Q), you should observe your patient for
A. 60 minutes following the study for possible reaction to the nucleotides
B. Signs and symptoms of pneumonia
C. 24 hours to measure urine output and maintain strict I&O
D. No observation is necessary

77. When preparing to obtain a wound culture for MRSA, which of the following tasks should not be performed?
A. Obtain a sterile, cotton-tipped culturette swab
B. Transport the sample on ice to the lab
C. Culture the site using a rotating motion for 10 seconds
D. Place the swab in a sodium chloride medium

78. Blood osmolality is decreased in
A. Uremia and dehydration
B. Alcoholism and burns
C. Diabetes insipidus
D. Hyponatremia and overhydration

79. Your 8 year old patient overdosed on metoprolol. As a PICU nurse, you know an appropriate nursing action would be to
A. Prepare for cardioversion
B. Administer activated charcoal
C. Have a pacer at the bedside
D. Prepare to administer beta blockers

80. Patients who are undergoing alcohol withdrawal are frequently hypoglycemic. Treatment should include
A. Bolus of $D_{10}W$, q 2 hour blood glucose monitoring
B. TPN with high concentrations of sugars, q 2 hour blood glucose monitoring
C. Maintenance fluids of $D_{25}W$ at 125 mL/h peripherally
D. Thiamine, then bolus with $D_{50}W$, then infusion of D_5W

81. The burn on your patient's right arm is pink and blistered. When touched, the patient screams with pain. This classification of burn is
A. First degree
B. Second degree partial thickness
C. Third degree full thickness
D. Fourth degree full thickness

82. Initially, a burned area can be estimated by the Rule of Nines, or using the palm as 1% of the body surface area. There are many ways to calculate the body surface area involved. If your patient was burned over 30% of his body and weighs 70 kg, calculate the total fluid requirements during the first 24 hours using the Parkland formula
A. 2100 mL
B. 6300 mL
C. 4500 mL
D. 8400 mL

83. **Calculate the fluid requirements (first 24 hours) for a patient who weighs 65 kg and is burned over 45% of his body using the Parkland formula**
    A. 29,250 mL
    B. 11,700 mL
    C. 26,000 mL
    D. 10,300 mL

84. **When utilizing the Parkland formula to calculate fluid needs, the preferred fluid for burn resuscitation is**
    A. Normal saline
    B. D_5W/ Isolyte M
    C. Lactated Ringers
    D. D_5W

85. **To minimize inflammation in burns, which of the following therapies may be used?**
    A. Vitamin C
    B. Hyperbaric therapy
    C. Prednisone
    D. Leaving burns open to the air

86. **Your male patient has been prescribed ergotamine. This drug was probably prescribed for**
    A. Erectile dysfunction
    B. Headache
    C. Pruritis
    D. Nausea

87. **Your patient was just transferred to the PICU because he became septic following an appendectomy one week ago. During his course of treatment, he is prescribed naloxone. The purpose of the naloxone is**
    A. To block prostaglandins
    B. To stabilize the cell membrane
    C. To block endorphins
    D. To block histamine

88. **Your patient has a history of cluster migraine headaches and has been treated with lithium. Her lithium level on admission was 1.8 mmol/L. This level would correspond with her symptoms of**
    A. Somnolence and coma
    B. Ataxia and diarrhea
    C. Seizures and flattened T waves
    D. Manic-depressive behavior

89. **The antidote for digoxin overdose is**
    A. Calcium gluconate
    B. Digoxin immune Fab
    C. Glucagon
    D. Potassium chloride

90. Your patient has been scheduled for a PET scan. Your patient and family teaching should include

A. The patient is to remain NPO
B. The test will require the patient to change position several times during the test
C. The patient should avoid consuming large quantities of fluids within 2 hours prior to the PET scan
D. Lactating women should not breastfeed for at least 48 hours after a PET scan

91. Rocky Mountain spotted fever is caused by

A. A parasite
B. Fleas
C. Rotavirus
D. Fungi

92. Your hospital has just received word of a mass-casualty incident. You are called on to report to the ED and assist with triage of the pediatric patients. The preliminary report states that you will be receiving as many as 40 patients. The first patient you see is a male, approximately 10 years old, with multiple lacerations. He is awake and alert and complaining of pain in the right chest and right upper quadrant. There is no rebound tenderness. You confirm that ribs 7–9 are fractured. You would suspect which of the following underlying conditions/injuries?

A. Flail chest
B. Liver laceration
C. Pneumothorax
D. Mesenteric infarction

93. The second patient you see during a mass-casualty incident is a 17 year old female who was trapped in her car for almost two hours by the steering column. She complains of left shoulder pain and left upper quadrant rebound tenderness, and presents with an obviously fractured lower leg that was splinted by paramedics. The paramedics had listed her as stable and stated that she had no rebound tenderness or guarding at the accident scene. The patient is tachycardic at 128 and has fractures of ribs 9–10. You suspect a

A. Ruptured pancreas
B. Diaphragm rupture
C. Spleen injury
D. Lacerated liver

94. The third patient you triage from a mass-casualty event is a 4 year old girl. She is confused, but complains of back pain at the level of L3. She is hypotensive and has swelling at the level of L1–L3. You would suspect which type of injury?

A. Splenic rupture
B. Kidney laceration
C. Large bowel rupture
D. Retroperitoneal liver injury

95. Raj was a spectator at a golf tournament when he was struck by lightning. He was thrown approximately 10 feet into a tree. Raj suffered a fractured left radius and ulna, a concussion, and burns on his left arm, chest, and right leg. He has been somewhat confused since the accident. Which of the following statements about lightning injuries is true?

A. Internal burns are common
B. Barotrauma is rare
C. Myoglobinuria is rarely seen
D. DC current will most likely cause ventricular fibrillation

96. Cathy is an 8 year old girl who lives on a farm. She frequently helps her mother home-can meat and vegetables every year. Cathy is admitted to the intensive care unit with profound weakness, double vision, slurred speech, and dysphagia. Her initial diagnosis is Guillain-Barré syndrome. While you are interviewing her family, you learn that a few days ago Cathy ingested some home-canned green beans that were several years old. No other family members ate the beans because the color was odd. What do you do with this information?

A. Do nothing; it is of no consequence
B. Notify the physician immediately; Cathy may have botulism
C. Tell the physician tomorrow during rounds
D. Continue the interview

97. Opioids are frequently used for regional anesthesia via the epidural route. These agents provide anesthesia by binding to receptors in the dorsal horn of the spinal cord and

A. Affect sensory neurons without affecting motor or sympathetic activities
B. Alter neurologic sensory pathway via parasympathetic tract
C. Eliminate the need for continuous dosing
D. Are lipophilic and will stay in the lower spinal tract to provide anesthesia

98. A possible adverse effect of morphine is

A. Ileus
B. Hyperactive bowel tones
C. Ototoxicity
D. Increased venous capacitance

99. A possible adverse effect with the use of fentanyl is

A. Neutropenia
B. Chest wall rigidity
C. Hyperthyroidism
D. Tachypnea

100. Fentanyl administered intravenously is incompatible with

A. Piperacillin
B. Phenytoin
C. Esmolol
D. Morphine

101. A contraindication for the use of fentanyl is

A. Asthma

B. Urinary tract infection

C. Concomitant use of penicillin

D. Open heart surgery

102. You are preparing to administer ampicillin IV to your patient. Which of the following statements is true?

A. Ampicillin can be given with aminoglycosides

B. Reconstituted ampicillin is stable for 4 hours if stored in the refrigerator

C. Ampicillin may be infused with intralipids at the terminal injection site of venous access

D. You should administer ampicillin rapidly with a 1 mL saline flush afterward

103. Gentamicin was started on an infant 20 days ago. You note that the patient's urine output has dropped to 1 mL/kg/hr, and the urine is an amber color in the diaper. The grasp reflex is weak and the infant appears lethargic. You would

A. Administer Lasix 1 mg/kg IV

B. Give a 10 mL/kg bolus of normal saline

C. Administer the next dose of gentamicin immediately

D. Check the last gentamicin peak and trough results

104. Your 14 year old patient tells you she smokes pot. How is today's marijuana different from the marijuana of 20 years ago?

A. Pot today is purer than pot was 20 years ago

B. There is no difference

C. Pot 20 years ago was safer

D. Today's pot has delayed effects of 3 hours

105. You are assessing a 17 year old who is 14 weeks pregnant and who is addicted to energy drinks. When speaking to her about complications for her baby, what effects would you discuss as potential complications in the neonate?

A. Complications similar to fetal alcohol syndrome

B. Complications similar to heroin addiction

C. Complications similar to trisomy 13

D. There are no effects

106. Addiction and abuse are terms often used interchangeably in conversation with parents and family members. Which statement best defines these terms?

A. They are the same terms

B. Addiction is when the user cannot stop using the drug or substance without experiencing mild symptoms of withdrawal, and abuse is when the user cannot live without the substance or drug

C. Addiction is when a user cannot live or function without the drug or substance and without experiencing severe or life-threatening withdrawal; abuse is when the user uses the drug or substance in amounts or functions not intended

D. Addiction is when the user uses the drug or substance in a way not intended, and abuse is when the user uses the drug or substance without the knowledge of other people

107. Which illegal drug of addiction is the most commonly abused?

A. Marijuana
B. Toluene
C. Cocaine
D. Heroin

108. Helen tells you that she uses witch hazel. Your first question after hearing this statement should be

A. "Why did you take witch hazel?"
B. "How did you obtain the witch hazel?"
C. "How much and how often did you use witch hazel?"
D. "Do your parents know?"

109. Mara is a 16 year old who was brought into the emergency room after collapsing at a party. Mara's cardiac and neurologic work-up is negative. Her urine drug screen is negative. What do you suspect caused her collapse?

A. Respiratory depression
B. Dehydration
C. Hyperthermia
D. Toxic ingestion

110. You are assessing a 17 year old patient named Brenna. Brenna appears euphoric and confused. While looking around the room, you note a chewed-up pacifier in the bed with her. Why would the pacifier be significant?

A. It was from a previous patient
B. Brenna may have been using the pacifier prior to you entering the room
C. The pacifier was caught in the railing and torn
D. Brenna's other children were in the room just before you arrived

111. You are caring for a 40 week gestation infant who was born to a mother addicted to methamphetamines. Which complications are you most likely to see?

A. Cleft palate and hypoglycemia
B. Hyperglycemia and bradycardia
C. Feeding intolerance and hypothermia
D. Feeding intolerance only

112. Rosa is a 14 year old admitted for delirium. During her physical assessment, you note that Rosa is combative, red faced, and talking to the walls. You approach the family to obtain a history, and her father reports that Rosa has been sick with a severe cough and allergies for 4 days. The mother went to the store this morning for Benadryl® and Robitussin®, as Rosa had not slept soundly for 2 days. Rosa took both medications every 2 hours for the past 8 hours. You suspect her lab results and vital signs will also reflect

A. Dehydration
B. Overhydration
C. Hypotension
D. Metabolic alkalosis

113. Which of the following drugs are classified as stimulants?
A. Doriden, methadone, and ketamine
B. Cocaine, marijuana, and yellow jackets
C Caffeine, methadone, and ketamine
D. Modafinil, caffeine, and amphetamines

114. Your patient is being weaned off IV morphine. The doctor tells you that today the patient will switch from IV morphine to oral morphine. You expect the oral dosage to be
A. Three to five times the IV dose
B. Twice the IV dose
C. There is no change in dosing or frequency
D. The same as the IV dose, but more frequent

115. Which of the following statements is false regarding the use of activated charcoal for suspected or confirmed poisoning?
A. Activated charcoal adsorbs most poisons
B. Activated charcoal adsorbs metals
C. Activated charcoal cannot be mixed with ice cream
D. Single doses of activated charcoal are indicated for serious poison exposures

116. Multiple doses of activated charcoal should be used for ingestions of
A. Theophylline
B. Gentamicin
C. Aspirin
D. Acetaminophen

117. Exchange transfusions may be used to treat "gray baby syndrome." This syndrome is induced by
A. Lithium
B. Salicylates
C. Methanol
D. Chloramphenicol

118. Hemoperfusion may be used in the treatment of
A. Ethylene glycol
B. Sorbitol
C. Magnesium citrate
D. Theophylline

119. Acetaminophen is metabolized by the
A. Spleen
B. Kidneys
C. Liver
D. Lungs

120. A side effect of ethanol in young children is to

A. Cause supraventricular tachycardia
B. Suppress the liver's ability to produce glucose
C. Cause corneal burns
D. Cause hyperglycemia

121. Quinn is 7 years old. He was admitted to the PICU for intractable cyanosis. The cyanosis does not improve with oxygen, and his blood appears brown when placed on white paper. You suspect Quinn is suffering from

A. Tricyclic overdose
B. Gentamicin overdose
C. Methemoglobinemia
D. GI bleeding

122. Methemoglobinemia may be treated with

A. Sodium bicarbonate
B. Packed RBCs
C. Methylene blue
D. Whole blood

123. The drug of choice for treatment of tricyclic antidepressant overdose is

A. Atropine
B. Imipramine
C. Doxepin
D. Sodium bicarbonate

124. A cyclic antidepressant that may cause cardiovascular effects and will probably cause status epilepticus is

A. Amoxapine
B. Amitriptyline
C. Desipramine
D. Doxepin

125. The specific antidote for a benzodiazepine overdose is

A. Calcium chloride
B. Flumazenil
C. Atropine
D. Calcium gluconate

126. The acid–base imbalance likely to be seen with an iron overdose is

A. Respiratory acidosis
B. Metabolic alkalosis
C. Metabolic acidosis
D. Respiratory alkalosis

127. The antidote for iron poisoning is

A. No antidote is available, treat symptoms only
B. Chelation
C. Deferoxamine
D. Activated charcoal

128. The triad of symptoms usually associated with opioid overdose is

A. Respiratory depression, miosis, and coma
B. Obtundation, hypotension, and ventricular arrhythmias
C. Confusion, slurred speech, and seizures
D. Stupor, respiratory alkalosis, and hypotension

129. Which of the following drugs has a half-life of approximately 24 hours and requires continuous doses of naloxone in the event of overdose?

A. Demerol
B. Heroin
C. Cocaine
D. Methadone

130. Symptoms of salicylate poisoning include

A. Respiratory acidosis and bradycardia
B. Lethargy and hypotension
C. Abdominal cramping and hyperglycemia
D. Tachycardia and hyperthermia

131. Which of the following substances contain large amounts of alkali?

A. Toilet bowl cleaners
B. Swimming pool chemicals
C. Oven cleaners
D. Metal cleaners

132. Which statement is true regarding alkaline substances?

A. Their pH is lower than 2
B. Vascular thrombosis may result
C. Eschar forms over the burn
D. Alkalines dehydrate tissues

133. An acid that is absorbed even through intact skin, causing local and systemic effects, is

A. Hydrochloric acid
B. Hydrofluoric acid
C. Carbonic acid
D. Acetic acid

134. The toxic ingredient in automobile antifreeze is

A. Freon
B. Ethanol
C. Methanol
D. Ethylene glycol

135. After a child ingests toxic levels of iron, there is a latent asymptomatic phase. This phase may cause caregivers to underestimate the continuing risk to the patient. This latent phase usually occurs ______ hours after ingestion

A. 1–4
B. 2–12
C. 8–16
D. 12–24

136. The body's systemic inflammatory immune hormonal response to severe injury or illness arising from a variety of causes is known as

A. MODS
B. SSCM
C. SIRS
D. PACC

137. Which of the following substances is not considered a highly influential mediator of gram-negative septic shock?

A. Myocardial depressant factor
B. TNF
C. Interleukin-1
D. Endotoxin

138. The area of a burn that has the closest contact with the heat source and sustains the most damage is the

A. Zone of stasis
B. Zone of hyperemia
C. Zone of erythemia
D. Zone of coagulation

139. A burn that involves muscle, fat, or bone is classified as a

A. First degree partial thickness burn
B. Second degree partial thickness burn
C. Third degree full thickness burn
D. Fourth degree full thickness burn

140. Use of 0.5% silver nitrate solution is a good treatment for burns because of its broad-spectrum antibacterial action. As a PICU nurse, you know that use of this medication has which of the following disadvantages?

A. Metabolic acidosis
B. Hypochloremia and hyponatremia
C. Transient leucopenia
D. Limited penetration of eschar

141. An example of a primary blast injury would be

A. A hemorrhagic contusion
B. A fractured femur
C. An arm impaled by a stick
D. A gunshot wound

142. A blast injury that occurs when a body is hurled though the air and struck by another object is known as

A. A primary blast injury
B. A compound blast injury
C. A secondary blast injury
D. A tertiary blast injury

143. Your patient is irritable, confused, and has paresthesias around the mouth. He is having watery rice-like diarrhea, nausea, and vomiting. These symptoms are indicative of

A. Arsenic poisoning
B. Digoxin toxicity
C. Methanol poisoning
D. Insecticide poisoning

144. When treating salicylate overdose, which of the following goals is appropriate?

A. A hypocalcemic state
B. Urine pH of 7 to 8
C. Resolution of jaundice
D. Entry of salicylate into the CNS

145. Children require special considerations during a disaster or terrorism event. Which of the following statements is false?

A. Children are more susceptible to the effects of radiation exposure
B. A child's cognitive and developmental levels may limit his or her ability to escape
C. A child cannot be decontaminated in an adult decontamination unit
D. Children are less vulnerable to chemicals absorbed through the skin

146. The type of device made by combining radioactive materials and an explosive is known as a(n)

A. Improved nuclear device
B. Radiologic dispersal device
C. Simple radiological device
D. Improved explosive device

147. The type of chemical agent that can cause blistering is called a(n)

A. Vesicant
B. Contaminant
C. Intoxicant
D. Nerve agent

148. Which of the following is not a form of anthrax?

A. Nonspecific
B. Cutaneous
C. Pulmonary
D. Gastrointestinal

149. Which of the following statements about plague is incorrect?

A. Plague is caused by *Yersenia pestis*
B. Aerosol droplets may spread plague from person to person
C. Plague is usually transmitted by rats
D. Plague is seen on a gram stain as a gram positive rod

150. If your 10 year old patient is in cardiogenic shock, which of the following sets of parameters would be expected?

	HR	CI	SVR	PVR
A.	↑	↓	↑	Normal or ↑
B.	↓	↑	↑	↓
C.	↑	↓	↑	↓
D.	↑	↑	↑	↓

151. The classic presentation of septic shock is

A. Tachypnea, vasoconstriction, and tachycardia
B. Fever, tachycardia, and vasodilation
C. Pale, cool skin, positive blood culture, and tachycardia
D. Vasoconstriction, hypothermia, and cool skin

152. SIRS is the acute development of two or more of the following criteria, which are

A. Hypothermia ($< 36°$ C) and bradycardia (age related)
B. Fever ($> 38°$ C) and leukocytosis (WBC $>12{,}000/mm^3$)
C. Leukopenia (WBC $>10{,}000/mm^3$) and tachypnea
D. Weak central pulses and neutropenia

153. Brad was admitted to the pediatric ICU with periorbital cellulitis. He has injection of the conjunctiva with lid swelling and exophthalmos. Which condition do you suspect?

A. Thyrotoxicosis
B. Cavernous sinus syndrome
C. Severe sinusitis
D. Pituitary tumor

154. What are the common symptoms of early cavernous sinus syndrome?

A. Conjunctival injection, fever, eye pain
B. Fever, loss of vision, vomiting
C. Fever, meningeal irritation signs, nuchal rigidity
D. Fever, ptosis, decreased level of consciousness

155. What are the expected treatments for cavernous sinus syndrome?

A. Antibiotic therapy, VP shunt
B. Antibiotic therapy, intraventricular drain
C. Antibiotic therapy, surgical drainage of the initial infection
D. Antibiotic therapy is the only treatment necessary

156. What are the four components of $ScvO_2$ monitoring?

A. Cardiac output, serum hemoglobin, SaO_2, vO_2

B. Serum hemoglobin, heart rate, SaO_2, PCO_2

C. Cardiac output, PCO_2, VO_2, hemoglobin

D. Serum hematocrit, SaO_2, respiratory rate, heart rate

SECTION 10

Multisystem Answers

1. **Correct answer: D**
   When a sudden flame-up comes near the face, the first instinct is to gasp. This inhalation of superheated air will cause swelling of the tissues in the air passages. Seth was probably very near the flame, given that his chin was burned. He is at great risk of a compromised airway and may need intubation.

2. **Correct answer: D**
   Hypertonic solutions minimize wound edema in burn patients.

3. **Correct answer: A**
   Aspirin is an acid and causes a profound metabolic acidosis and a respiratory alkalosis. Tinnitus may also be present.

4. **Correct answer: B**
   Electrical burns are insidious and follow the path of least resistance. Muscle tissue breaks down and causes rhabdomyolysis from the myoglobin that was released into the circulation.

5. **Correct answer: A**
   In patients with sepsis, endotoxins stimulate production of tumor necrosis factor (TNF). The TNF, in turn, stimulates neutrophil activation and platelet aggregation. In addition, TNF increases capillary permeability and promotes release of IL-1, IL-6, and IL-8.

6. **Correct answer: C**
   Acetaminophen overdose may cause hypoglycemia and should be treated with a bolus of $D_{50}W$, followed by continuous infusion of D_5W. Hypoglycemia occurs because of the hepatotoxic effects of acetaminophen. Infusions must also be based on the patient's blood glucose results.

7. **Correct answer: D**
   The patient who is undergoing alcohol withdrawal and who exhibits diplopia, peripheral neuropathy, confusion, recent memory loss, and hyperexcitability has Wernicke-Kersakoff syndrome. Wernicke-Kersakoff syndrome is a thiamine deficiency and a metabolic encephalopathy.

8. **Correct answer: B**
   Sustained compartment pressures of 30 mmHg in a 15 year old patient are usually suggestive of compartment syndrome. This level of sustained pressure requires a release to be performed by a physician. If the compartment pressure reaches 40 mmHg, it requires an immediate escharotomy or fasciotomy. In most burn units, some sort of electrocautery device is available at the bedside or close by. The patient should

be sedated and medicated for pain if hemodynamically stable. When assessing a burned patient, if a weak pulse is noted, it is probably due to underresuscitation.

9. **Correct answer:** C
St. John's Wort is contraindicated in patients with HIV/AIDS, as this herb interferes with the metabolism of protease inhibitors and nonnucleoside reverse transcriptase inhibitors.

10. **Correct answer:** A
Patients presenting post recluse spider bites may not initially know that they were bitten and may not seek medical help until 12 to 36 hours after the initial bite. Because treatment is delayed, symptoms may be difficult to treat. The majority of patients may present with flu-like symptoms, such as nausea and vomiting. DIC, hemolysis, and thrombocytopenia are severe symptoms. Treatment includes using ice to control inflammation, keeping the area clean and protected, and treating symptoms. No specific treatment has been proven to be 100% effective. Dapsone has limited support for preventing necrosis. Nitroglycerin patches counter the vasoconstrictive properties of the venom; they lead to hemodilution in the bloodstream and promote increased bleeding at the site to wash the venom out.

11. **Correct answer:** D
Noah is apneic and bradycardic. Priorities are to maintain the airway to provide ventilation and oxygen therapy. The next step is to administer antivenin as soon as available. Morphine may help with pain, but will worsen the patient's bradycardia and hypotension. It is a myth that tying a tourniquet around the affected limb will stop the venom from reaching the bloodstream or lymphatic system. At this point, the venom is already systemic. In minor cases involving healthy patients, symptoms may be managed with pain control, muscle relaxants, and comfort measures. Symptoms should dissipate during the first 3 days after exposure.

12. **Correct answer:** C
Nadeen suffered a black widow spider bite. Her discharge instructions should include the need to contact her physician immediately if she has joint or abdominal pain or difficulty breathing. Joint and abdominal pain (pain related to splenomegaly) as well as dyspnea may be signs of anaphylaxis or serum sickness up to 2 to 4 weeks after antivenin administration. Patients should be taught to contact their physicians immediately so early treatment can be initiated to prevent complications. Administration of corticosteroids and antihistamines will aid in combating the inflammatory response to the animal proteins in the antivenin. The neurotoxin may cause residual muscle spasms, tingling, weakness, and nervousness for weeks to months after the exposure to the venom. Patients may need to slowly increase their level of activity during their recovery.

13. **Correct answer:** A
The priority of care would be to insert a nasogastric tube and provide gastric lavage with activated charcoal. Scotch Broom contains sparteine, which has very powerful cardiovascular effects. Arrhythmias, blood pressure changes (increased or decreased), coagulation changes, and vision changes are possible side effects of this herb. The best action listed would be to lavage the stomach to remove any undigested or partially digested Scotch Broom. You will need to insert a Foley catheter, as this herb does have

diuretic properties, but this step is not a priority. Quinidine and amiodarone should be stopped immediately, as they will interact with the Scotch Broom to cause further cardiovascular collapse by increasing the toxicity of the Scotch Broom.

14. **Correct answer: D**
Although they are natural products, many herbal supplements may have deleterious side effects. These products are not regulated, so different preparations may have different strengths. Regardless of the nurse's personal beliefs, it is vital that the treating staff be made aware of any herbal supplements taken either separately or in drinks or foods. Although some research has favored Ginkgo's use in increasing cerebral blood flow, cases of severe bleeding, seizures, glucose instability, and allergic reactions to this herb have been documented. Extreme caution should be used with patients on anticoagulation therapy, antiplatelet therapy, anti-inflammatory drugs, diabetic regimen, MAO inhibitors, antipsychotic drugs, and antiseizure medications.

15. **Correct answer: C**
Ginseng has been known to increase the QT interval, placing this patient at greater risk for cardiac rhythm complications. Advise patients and their families to carefully read the labels of any sports or high-energy drinks, as many now contain various herbs and high levels of caffeine. Ginseng may also cause breast tissue enlargement in men as well as erectile dysfunction. In females, it may lead to increased menstrual bleeding or hormone imbalances in women with breast cancer, uterine cancer, and endometriosis. This may be due to similar effects to estrogen. Ginseng may also cause complications or interactions with anticoagulation therapy, calcium channel blockers, and diabetes management, and it increases the potency of some sedatives.

16. **Correct answer: D**
Shellfish poisoning can exhibit symptoms days after ingestion. The toxin contained in shellfish, clams, and oysters is called saxotoxin and is not affected by steaming or cooking. It inhibits sodium channels of membranes, blocking propagation of nerve and muscle action potentials. If the nerves are involved, there may be parasthesias of the lips, tongue, gums, and face. The parasthesias may spread to the trunk and lead to paralysis and respiratory arrest. There is no definite treatment. Care is driven by treating symptoms and psychological support.

17. **Correct answer: B**
Patients who are stung by bees numerous times are in danger of developing kidney failure. Bee stings have proteins in the venom that act as enzymes. The enzymes lyse the cells, with the cellular debris accumulates very quickly and actually clogs the kidneys. The patient ultimately dies from kidney failure. Any patient who has been stung multiple times needs to be monitored for alterations in kidney function at least two weeks following the incident.

18. **Correct answer: A**
A possible side effect of cocaine use is malignant hyperthermia, for which the antidote is dantrolene. Malignant hyperthermia is usually seen in patients who are receiving anesthetics. This patient may also require ice packs and a hypothermia blanket. On occasion, bowel irrigations with cold water and cold NG tube irrigations have been necessary. Cherry red skin is a possible effect with carbon monoxide poisoning.

19. **Correct answer: A**
Activated protein C (Xigris) inhibits factors Va and VIIIa. In addition, it inhibits human tumor necrosis factor production by monocytes. It also limits thrombin-induced inflammatory responses.

20. **Correct answer: B**
Anaphylaxis may be caused or exacerbated by the use of *N*-acetyl-cysteine (Mucomyst). Mucomyst may actually cause bronchospasm, so it must be used with a bronchodilator. Usually, Mucomyst is contraindicated. Codeine is generally not used in status asthmaticus. Guaifenesin is Robitussin, a mild cough syrup.

21. **Correct answer: A**
Alkaline solutions may cause the norepinephrine to precipitate. Also, do not use it if the solution is discolored. Norepinephrine is used for low coronary perfusion states, vasogenic shock, and hypotension.

22. **Correct answer: C**
Regitine (phentolamine) is used to counteract tissue necrosis caused by Levophed. It should be administered subcutaneously around the area of extravasation.

23. **Correct answer: D**
A patient in the early stages of septic shock may have a mild fever and will be in a hyperdynamic state. The endotoxins that are circulating will have vasodilatory effects, so RAP, PAOP, and SVR are decreased. The increase in CO is compensatory.

24. **Correct answer: B**
When undergoing a TEE, the patient is sedated and the gag reflex is reduced by an oral numbing spray. A gastroscope is advanced, and the patient would swallow it. The tube is positioned directly behind the heart and allows for sound waves to be reflected off the heart chambers and valves. The left mainstem bronchus can interfere with the view. Some of these types of scopes can generate a three-dimensional picture.

There is a risk with this procedure for the patient to have a reflex bradycardia, an esophageal perforation, transient hypoxia, drug-initiated tachycardia, or be over sedated. Additional contraindications would include stenosis and obstruction of the esophagus, penetrating chest injuries, and central nervous system depression (no sedatives). Patients who cannot lie flat are another contraindication.

25. **Correct answer: C**
The patient should receive prophylactic antibiotics to mitigate possible endocarditis, which may be the cause of his transient chest pain and syncopal episodes.

26. **Correct answer: B**
This test requires iodine-based radiographic contrast dye to be injected into the antecubital or femoral vein via a catheter placed in the pulmonary artery. The pulmonary vasculature can be visualized. The radioactive iodine crosses the blood–placental barrier, which explains why it is contraindicated in pregnancy. Other contraindications include allergy to shellfish, iodine, radiographic dye, and renal insufficiency.

27. **Correct answer: B**
From 72 to 96 hours after acetaminophen ingestion, symptoms of an overdose will include jaundice, confusion, and coagulation disorders. Renal function may be decreased, and the patient may have increased ALT and AST levels. Approximately 4 days to 2 weeks after the ingestion, the symptoms abate.

28. **Correct answer: C**
Cocaine may cause the placenta to shrink. Cocaine is a Schedule II central nervous system stimulant. It acts as a local anesthetic, a bronchodilator, and a vasoconstrictor. Cocaine compromises the heart's antioxidant defense system, so an overdose can cause an MI. Cocaine can also cause aortic dissection, stroke, intestinal ischemia, hallucinations, and adverse effects in fetuses.

29. **Correct answer: C**
Fomepizole is an antidote for ethylene glycol toxicity. Ethylene glycol is the key compound found in antifreeze. After ingestion, it is converted to oxalic acid, which is then excreted by the kidneys. This process causes crystals to form in the urine, and it leads to acidosis, tetany, and renal failure. Hemodialysis and peritoneal dialysis will remove ethylene glycol.

30. **Correct answer: A**
Ecstasy overdose can lead to amnesia in approximately 13% of patients. Ecstasy can also cause ataxia, central nervous system depression, coma, bradycardias, hypothermia, hypotension, hypothermia, respiratory depression, and respiratory acidosis.

31. **Correct answer: A**
Cadmium is found in cigarettes. Cadmium is a heavy metal with a half-life of 15 to 20 years. As a respiratory irritant, it can produce pulmonary edema, interstitial pneumonia, and cardiovascular collapse if inhaled. Cadmium is used in the manufacture of storage batteries, in alloys, and in electroplating. If it is ingested, the individual will develop severe gastrointestinal symptoms within 30 minutes. Most cadmium collects in erythrocytes and kidney tissues; it is not metabolized in the body.

32. **Correct answer: D**
It is untrue that high levels of lymphocytes will mask the presence of morphine in urine. The stealth adulterant will mask morphine in the urine, causing a false-negative response. When heroin is taken, it breaks down into morphine. 10 mg of morphine is detectable in urine for 84 hours and can be measured in corpses for approximately a week.

33. **Correct answer: D**
Phenytoin is metabolized in the liver and excreted in bile and urine. It is used as an anticonvulsant and antidysrhythmic. Tube feedings should be held before the test for 2 hours. Peak levels should be drawn 3 to 9 hours after oral use. As much as 5 days must be allowed before a change in dose will change results.

34. **Correct answer: B**
Many herbs and natural remedies affect the INR because they are oral anticoagulants. These ingredients include dan shen, dang gui, dong quai, Gingko biloba, garlic, ginseng, and ginger.

35. **Correct answer: A**
Because of air trapping, a patient with asthma has a low peak flow rate during expiration.

36. **Correct answer: C**
The salty taste after a renal arteriogram is normal. The patient may be slightly nauseous, feel an urge to cough, or feel flushed. This sensation will pass in approximately five minutes.

37. **Correct answer: C**
False-negative results on the sickle cell test may be due to anemia or the fact that less than 7 mL of blood was drawn for the test. False-positive results may be caused by polycythemia.

38. **Correct answer: C**
$ScvO_2$ monitoring assesses for the onset of early septic shock before the patient exhibits a demonstrable change in vital signs. Sepsis is an interruption of the oxygen demand and delivery due to infection. This allows for rapid hemodynamic treatment of shock and reduces mortality by 25% -30%. Early goal-directed therapy (EGDT) aims to keep $ScvO_2$ at 70% or greater to reduce mortality from sepsis.

39. **Correct answer: C**
Wernicke's syndrome is a result of thiamine deficiency. It will result in brain damage if not treated immediately.

40. **Correct answer: C**
Restraints should be used only if alternative methods for behavioral correction are ineffective. There is no indication that the patient is violent or has caused any threat to staff or self. Restraints should only be used as a last resort to prevent injury to self and staff. Reorientation, medication, and controlling external stimulation are all effective methods for controlling behavior.

41. **Correct answer: B**
Even if the patient's mother signed the consent form, she is not certain about the procedure or is not fully informed. The nurse must act as her advocate and notify the physician.

42. **Correct answer: C**
Inhalation anthrax has an incubation period ranging from 7 days to as long as 60 days after exposure. Symptoms are initially vague and flu-like, such as malaise, low-grade fever, and nausea. These symptoms quickly progress to profound diaphoresis, chest discomfort, and rhonchi. The mild symptoms occur in the first 5 days of the illness and are followed by a brief period of improvement. An abrupt onset of high fever and severe respiratory distress is then noted. Death may occur as early as 24 to 36 hours after symptoms begin.

43. **Correct answer: B**
Ciprofloxacin, a fluoroquinolone antibiotic, is the drug of choice for inhalation anthrax. Doxycycline, a tetracycline derivative, may also be used, but the dosage in this question is incorrect. Penicillin G is not an option as the bacterium in this case, *Bacillus anthracis,* becomes beta lactamase positive, making the penicillin ineffective against it. Augmentin would not be used for this situation; it is always given orally.

44. **Correct answer: A**
Inhalation anthrax starts with mild, nonspecific symptoms such as malaise, low-grade fever, fatigue, and cough. If it is left untreated, death occurs within 24 to 36 hours from respiratory failure.

45. **Correct answer: D**
Antibiotics for inhalation anthrax are continued for 60 days after exposure, even if the exposure is simply suspected. Treatment is initially intravenous, but is then changed to

oral dosing for the remaining time. The two antibiotics most commonly given are ciprofloxacin and doxycycline.

46. **Correct answer: C**
According to the CDC, contact precautions are all that is required for inhalation anthrax. Standard precautions may include the use of a face mask if the patient has a productive cough.

47. **Correct answer: B**
Clostridium botulinum is a rod-shaped bacterium and is the causative organism of botulism. Only 25% of the United States cases of botulism are from food products, and most of these are from home-canned foods. The majority of cases are infant botulism, comprising over 70% of the yearly cases of botulism in the United States. The third type of botulism is seen in wounds contaminated by soil containing the botulism spores. Babies less than one year old should not consume honey, especially raw or home-grown honey, because it may contain botulism spores.

48. **Correct answer: C**
Ricin is made from castor beans and is one of the most toxic substances known. It interferes with protein synthesis and causes cell death. Chewing castor beans may cause some symptoms, but the most lethal form of ricin is inhaled. The toxin is not spread by casual contact. The most likely victims would be seen in enclosed areas such as subway trains, buses, or small rooms. When used as a bioterrorism agent, ricin is typically aerosolized with some liquid such as water or a weak acid.

49. **Correct answer: A**
"Body packer" is a term used to describe people who transport narcotics in their body cavities. In this case, it is probable that a packet may have ruptured in the patient's body. Treatment may require bowel irrigations, intubation, mechanical ventilation, and anticonvulsants. More doses of naloxone may be necessary, along with supportive treatment for opioid overdose. Be alert for bradycardia, hypotension, respiratory depression, and hypothermia.

50. **Correct answer: C**
SIRS is a systemic infection that can present with hypothermia and even a WBC of < 4000 or $> 12{,}000$. MODS is usually the result of a direct injury to an organ. A kidney stone or appendicitis should present with pain and tenderness

51. **Correct answer: B**
Gentamicin is an aminoglycoside, as are tobramycin and amikacin. These drugs are used to combat gram-negative bacterial infections such as E. Coli, but they must be used with caution because they can cause nephrotoxicity.

52. **Correct answer: C**
The underresuscitation in this patient is probably due to miscalculation of possible insensible losses and third spacing.

53. **Correct answer: B**
This question describes an emergency situation. There is no discernable radial pulse either by palpation or by Doppler. The pressure must be relieved via an escharotomy—that is, an incision through multiple layers of tissue. Any circumferential burn of the body may lead to impaired function and escharotomy.

54. Correct answer: C
Lactated Ringers solution is used for burn patients because it is used with many of the formulas for burn resuscitation. It is preferred for large volume resuscitation because LR contains 130 mEq/L of sodium, compared to normal saline that has 154 mEq/L. LR has a higher pH (6.5) compared to normal saline (5.0). The pH of the LR is close to a normal pH. The patient will be in metabolic acidosis, so the metabolized lactate will buffer the acidosis. LR is also an isotonic crystalloid.

55. Correct answer: B
Ludwig's angina is a submaxillary infection. It is a cellulitis of the neck and floor of the mouth that usually occurs with, or after, dental disease.

56. Correct answer: A
Ammonium chloride is converted to ammonia and HCl in the liver, a process that will indirectly correct metabolic alkalosis. However, the ammonia generated may produce encephalopathy.

57. Correct answer: A
Amiodarone is useful in the treatment of atrial fibrillation because the drug decreases sinus rate, increases PR and QT intervals, and results in the development of U waves.

58. Correct answer: C
Third degree full-thickness burns destroy nerve endings because they extend into subcutaneous tissue. The affected tissue may have a whitish color and will be somewhat firm with a leather-like appearance. Sometimes you can see clotted vessels through the eschar.

59. Correct answer: D
This is a fourth degree burn. Not many people are familiar with this classification, which describes a burn that not only involves muscle but also extends through muscle and bone.

60. Correct answer: C
The highest risk at this time is compartment syndrome. As a nurse, you must constantly assess for quality of pulses. Edema may be so great as to completely cut off circulation in a limb and cause a myoglobin-related renal failure. Escharotomy is a procedure, not a direct risk. Elevating the limb may help drain fluid and mitigate further edema. If the pulse is lost, it still may not mean compartment syndrome is the cause. It could be due to not replacing lost volume secondary to the burn.

61. Correct answer: C
Based on the history presented, it is suspicious that Ziva's behavior toward food and her psychomotor skills would be altered so soon after she ingested a home-made meal. The brownies should be tested for marijuana or other toxic substances. Additional side effects of marijuana consumption may include paranoia, sleeplessness, short-term memory impairment, nausea, respiratory depression, and headaches.

Each state has specific regulations regarding marijuana use for medicinal purposes. Regardless, the staff should have a family conference with the patient to determine the best course of treatment regarding Ziva's symptoms. Self- or family-prescribing should not be permitted during hospitalization. If marijuana use for medicinal purposes is illegal within your state, local law officials may need to be contacted.

62. **Correct answer: B**
Sodium nitroprusside, when used in high doses (10 ug/Kg/min) or over a period of days, can raise blood concentrations of cyanide to toxic levels. Patients who are malnourished or are stressed from surgery may have low thiosulfate reserves. These patients are at increased risk for developing symptoms, even with therapeutic dosing. These patients may become agitated and combative, and these symptoms may be mistaken for PICU psychosis. If patients are given hydroxocobalamin or sodium thiosulfate along with the nitroprusside, the symptoms may be prevented or at least mitigated.

63. **Correct answer: D**
Wool and silk give off cyanide gas when burned. Nitriles, found in the gloves nurses wear, will also give off cyanide gas when burned. Household plastics such as melamine dishes, plastic cups, polyurethane foam in furniture cushions, and many other synthetic compounds may produce lethal concentrations of cyanide when burned under appropriate circumstances.
Cyanide inhibits cellular respiration, even with enough oxygen stores. Cellular metabolism changes from aerobic to anaerobic and produces lactic acid. The organs with the highest oxygen requirements are those most affected by cyanide inhalation.

64. **Correct answer: D**
Fish can contain large amounts of mercury. In fact, the concentration in fish can be more than 1000 times greater in the fish than in the surrounding water. For this reason, people who eat fish as a main component of their diet may be at risk.
Organic mercury compounds are very toxic. They are taken into the body by ingestion, inhalation, skin, and eye contact. These mercury compounds can attack all body systems. They can cause nausea, lack of appetite, abdominal pain, kidney failure, swollen gums and mouth sores, numbness and tingling in the lips, mouth, tongue, hands, and feet, tremors, and seizures. The patient can become very uncoordinated and feel disconnected from their surroundings. They may lose part or all of their vision and hearing. Additional neurological issues with mercury poisoning may include memory loss, personality changes, and headache. Organic mercury can pass to a baby via breast milk. Methyl mercury may cause serious birth defects.

65. **Correct answer: D**
The patient had a reaction to Versed. To counter this reaction, he should be given Flumazenil (Romazicon), a benzodiazepine antagonist. Xanax, Valium, and Ativan are also benzodiazepines, as is Versed.

66. **Correct answer: C**
Cardene cannot be mixed with Ringer's lactate or sodium bicarbonate infusions. According to studies, although the combination does not cause a precipitate, the Ringer's lactate inactivates 15% to 42% of the drug.

67. **Correct answer: D**
This patient is in hypovolemic shock. The normal blood volume in an adolescent is about 5000 mL. 1500 mL of blood loss would be equal to about one-third of the total blood volume. You would expect the HR to increase to 120-150, cardiac output and BP to decrease, a narrowed pulse pressure will occur, the RR to increase to 25-40, and delayed capillary refill will be observed. The skin would be cool and clammy, and some neurological issues might be observed, such as restlessness, anxiety, and confusion.

68. **Correct answer: C**
Western Equine Encephalitis is a type of encephalitis that is caused by an arbovirus (togovirus). An arbovirus is carried by arthropods. In this case, a horse or small mammal was probably infected and the virus was vectored by a mosquito. This type of encephalopathy is not directly transmitted by human-to-human contact. This patient is at high risk for aspiration pneumonia and ARDS.

69. **Correct answer: B**
This is actually a panic level at > 20 ug/ml and if not addressed will cause nephrotoxicity. Ototoxicity usually occurs if levels are prolonged at > than 30 ug/mL. Vancomycin may cause hypertension, thrombocytopenia, tubular necrosis, colitis, and deafness. The patient may require hemodialysis, hemofiltration, or peritoneal dialysis. Note: charcoal hemofiltration does not remove vancomycin.

70. **Correct answer: D**
Congestive heart failure would present with lab results showing a decreased sedimentation rate. The sed rate may also be decreased in patients with poikilocytosis. Other potential causes of a low sed rate include cortisone, lecithin, and corticotrophin.

71. **Correct answer: C**
An amiodarone serum level that returned a result of 3.3 ug/ml is a panic level.

72. **Correct answer: B**
One of the major complications with placement of pulmonary artery catheters is infection. If the catheter remains in place for more than 72 hours, there is significant risk of infection. Studies have shown that the initial source of the infection typically involves a colonization of the skin, with bacteria migrating down the catheter. Additional studies have shown that coating the catheter with antibiotics is not a particularly effective means of preventing infection. The point of insertion (subclavian or jugular) also has been found to have no bearing on the risk of infection. Heparin may keep the catheter from clotting, but does not have any bearing on potential infections. Prophylactic antibiotics will not prevent catheter-related infections and, in fact, may lead to more antibiotic-resistant strains colonizing the catheter.

73. **Correct answer: B**
Patient and family teaching for digital subtraction angiography includes the fact that women who are breastfeeding should substitute formula for breast milk for one or more days after the procedure. This test can be done to diagnose aneurysms, aortic valve stenosis, carotid stenosis, pulmonary emboli, ulcerative plaques, hepatocellular carcinomas, and many other conditions. There are risks to the procedure—allergic reactions to the contrast dye, anaphylaxis, aphasia, hemiplegia, paresthesias, hemorrhage, infection, renal toxicity, and thromboemboli.

74. **Correct answer: D**
Patients poisoned by arsenic may exhibit convulsions. Arsenic is found in all human tissues as a trace element. These levels may become elevated with exposure. Approximately 60% of ingested arsenic is excreted in the urine. Arsenic may be found in well water, pesticides, paints, cosmetics, treated wood, and coal. Chronic exposure can lead to cancers.

75. **Correct answer: A**
The biopsy may cause bleeding from highly vascular tissue. Flank or abdominal pain may be the first sign, so your teaching should be directed toward reporting pain in these areas.

76. **Correct answer: A**
Following a lung scan (V/Q), you should observe your patient for 60 minutes following the study for possible reaction to the nucleotides. An additional consideration is that when you are discarding the patient's urine, you should wear gloves for 24 hours after the test. You must also wash the gloves with soap and water before removing the gloves. Then, wash your hands again. Many nurses have needlessly exposed themselves because in their haste to empty fluids for I&Os at shift change, they forgot to wear gloves.

77. **Correct answer: B**
Wound cultures for MRSA do not have to be placed on ice for transport. They may be kept as long as 8 hours at room temperature.

78. **Correct answer: D**
Hyponatremia and overhydration will decrease blood osmolality. Uremia, dehydration, alcoholism, burns, and diabetes insipidus are all causes of increased blood osmolality.

79. **Correct answer: C**
A pacer should be kept at the bedside for any patient with metoprolol overdose, because bradycardia, AV block, and hypotension will probably occur.

80. **Correct answer: D**
Administer thiamine, then give a bolus of $D_{50}W$, and finally start an infusion of D_5W.

81. **Correct answer: B**
The burn on your patient's right arm is pink and blistered. This type of burn (second degree) may be either superficial or a deep partial-thickness burn. The nerve endings are still intact and this burn is very painful. Sometimes burns can be deceptive. For example, a reddened area diagnosed as a first-degree burn may be overlooked when the staff is calculating requirements for fluid and nutrient resuscitation. After a few hours, these areas can develop blisters, only then being recognized as dermal burns. A new way of assessing burn levels involves the use of a laser Doppler scan during the first week of treatment.

82. **Correct answer: D**
The Parkland formula was developed by Dr. Charles Baxter at Parkland Hospital in Dallas, Texas, in the 1960s and is still used today as a standard for fluid resuscitation. Although many other formulas are employed for this purpose, this one is widely known and will probably be on the CCRN examination. The formula is

$$4 \text{ mL fluid} \times \text{pt's weight in Kg} \times \% \text{ of burn, so}$$
$$4 \times 70 = 280 \times 30 = 8400 \text{ mL fluid requirement for the first 24 hours.}$$

Half of the calculated volume is given in the first 8 hours, then the remaining volume is given over the next 16 hours. Remember to calculate from the time the burn occurred.

83. **Correct answer: B**
The formula is $4 \times 65 = 260 \times 45 = 11{,}700$

84. **Correct answer: C**
Lactated Ringers is used with the Parkland formula for burn resuscitation. It is preferred for large-volume resuscitation because LR contains 130 mEq/L of sodium, compared to normal saline that has 154 mEq/L. LR has a higher pH (6.5) compared to normal saline (5.0). The pH of the LR is close to a normal pH. The patient will be in metabolic acidosis, so the metabolized lactate will buffer the acidosis. LR is also an isotonic crystalloid.

85. **Correct answer: A**
This topic will probably not be on the exam, but it may show up as a question within the next year or so. The Vitamin C is an antioxidant and it is used to counter oxidant-mediated effects on the inflammatory cascade. There have been studies with animals that if the Vitamin C is given within 6 hours of the burn, up to 50% of the fluid needed for resuscitation can be eliminated.

Always remember that if you have a burn patient, you should start at least two large bore IVs.

Another new treatment involves the use of subatmospheric pressure dressings. These dressings may aid in removing excess fluid and help save areas that would otherwise have to be grafted or removed.

86. **Correct answer: B**
Ergotamine (Ergot) is used quite often for migraine headaches. In females, it may be administered to promote uterine contraction in childbirth. Because ergotamine promotes the contraction of smooth muscles, it can be used to control bleeding.

In large doses, ergotamine paralyzes the motor nerve endings of the sympathetic nervous system. It can cause disorientation, confusion, convulsions, seizures, severe muscle cramping, and dry gangrene of the extremities. LSD (lysergic acid diethylamide) is chemically related to ergotamine.

87. **Correct answer: C**
The purpose of the naloxone is to block endorphins. Excess endorphins need to be mediated. Prostaglandin is blocked by ibuprofen. Corticosteroids are used to stabilize the cell membrane by modifying mediators.

88. **Correct answer: B**
The patient's lithium level on admission was 1.8 mmol/L. This level would correspond with her symptoms of ataxia and diarrhea. Toxic levels occur at 1.5 mmol/L. Lithium is an alkaline, metal salt used mostly in the treatment of bipolar disorder and is sometimes used in the treatment of cluster migraine headaches. In bipolar disorder and alcohol withdrawal, lithium works by altering the sodium transport mechanisms in nerves and muscles, which helps stabilize mood.

89. **Correct answer: B**
The antidote for digoxin overdose is digoxin immune Fab, which reverses hyperkalemia and most dysrhythmias. Patients in renal failure may require dialysis to remove the digoxin immune Fab.

90. Correct answer: C

Patients may eat prior to undergoing the PET scan, but they should not drink large quantities of fluid within 2 hours of the scan unless the patient has, or will have, an indwelling catheter. Caffeinated drinks should also be avoided within 2 hours of the test. It is important to inform lactating teenagers not to breastfeed for at least 20 hours after the scan.

91. Correct answer: C

Rocky Mountain spotted fever is spread by ticks that carry a rotavirus. Symptoms include a sudden-onset fever that lasts for 2 to 3 weeks and a rash that may cover the entire body. Treatment must include both chloramphenicol and tetracycline.

92. Correct answer: A

The liver may be lacerated by either blunt or penetrating trauma. In blunt trauma, there will often be fractures of the 7th–9th ribs overlying the liver. We do not have a good history for this patient's mechanism of injury. Right upper quadrant tenderness will be present with a liver laceration. Rebound sensitivity and guarding will not be present because blood has not been in the abdomen at least 2 hours (long enough to cause peritoneal irritation).

Suspect a liver laceration when penetrating trauma involves the right lower chest or right upper abdomen, or when right upper quadrant tenderness accompanies blunt trauma. This patient needs a CT scan to confirm the diagnosis.

93. Correct answer: C

Splenic injury should be suspected when the 9th–10th ribs on the left side are fractured, or when left upper quadrant tenderness and tachycardia are present. This patient has complained of pain in the left shoulder, which is a common complaint. Peritoneal signs such as rebound sensitivity and guarding are delayed until the blood has had enough time to cause local irritation of the peritoneum (this patient was trapped in her car for almost 2 hours). Hypotension is a sign of an active bleed.

94. Correct answer: B

The kidneys are in the retroperitoneal space at the level of T-12 to L-3. Kidneys can be damaged by shearing or compression forces and cause laceration or contusion. Renal injuries must be suspected with fractures to the posterior ribs or lumbar vertebrae. Rupture of the renal artery with a deceleration injury like a crash may cause hypovolemia. There is little collateral circulation to the kidney, and damage to the renal artery may lead to acute tubular necrosis and intrarenal failure. Sometimes, the signs of a kidney injury can be confused with a pancreatic injury. However, you do not generally have hematuria with a pancreatic injury. You will have common signs such as Grey-Turner's Sign (flank ecchymosis), Cullen's sign (periumbilical bruising), and flank pain. This patient also is exhibiting confusion, which could be a simple concussion to an acute brain injury. The patient needs immediate evaluation.

95. Correct answer: C

Myoglobinuria is rarely seen with lightning burns. AC current usually causes ventricular fibrillation, and DC current usually causes asystole. In some cases, arrhythmias are delayed for up to 12 hours. The mechanism of lightning strikes is quite complex. There are several ways that lightning can injure a person.

A side splash from another object is probably the cause of this patient's injuries. The lightning hits something like a tree, then bounces off. A direct strike may also have occurred. Another type of strike can occur when the person is touching an object that is struck. Ground current effect occurs when energy spreads out across the surface of the earth. Lightning has two strokes, upward and downward. If they do not meet, energy can be directed outward.

Internal burns from lightning are rare and myoglobinuria rarely occurs. Generally, lightning will cause cardiac and respiratory arrest, burns from metals touching the victim (watches, necklaces, etc.), and neurological damage.

96. **Correct answer: B**
Sometimes families do not have enough education to make proper decisions or understand the nature of a disease. It is likely that this patient has botulism.

97. **Correct answer: A**
Opioids are frequently used for regional anesthesia via the epidural route. These agents provide anesthesia by binding to receptors in the dorsal horn of the spinal cord and affect sensory neurons without affecting motor or sympathetic activities. Morphine is actually hydrophilic and will stay in the cerebrospinal fluid longer and tends to travel toward the brain.

98. **Correct answer: A**
Possible adverse effects of morphine include respiratory depression, ileus, abdominal distension, delayed gastric emptying, hypotension, bradycardia, and urine retention.

99. **Correct answer: B**
Possible adverse effects of fentanyl include respiratory depression, chest wall rigidity, apnea, laryngospasm, abdominal distension, loss of bowel sounds, and generalized muscle rigidity.

100. **Correct answer: B**
Fentanyl administered intravenously is incompatible with phenytoin, azithromycin, and pentobarbital.

101. **Correct answer: A**
Contraindications for the use of fentanyl include increased intracranial pressure, severe respiratory disease or depression including acute asthma (unless the patient is mechanically ventilated), and seizures. Additional contraindications include CNS depression, paralytic ileus, severe liver or renal insufficiency, and hyperglycemia (fentanyl may elevate blood glucose). Fentanyl is used in open heart surgery.

102. **Correct answer: C**
Ampicillin is a broad-spectrum antibiotic that is commonly used in prophylactic and ongoing treatment for bacterial infections. It is compatible at the terminal injection site with intralipids, but not with dextrose/amino acid solution. Once reconstituted, ampicillin should be administered within 1 hour by IV push slowly over 3–5 minutes. Ampicillin should not be given with aminoglycosides. If the two medications must be given together, use separate IV sites or administer at least 1 hour apart, with flush prior to administering the second medication.

103. **Correct answer: D**
The nurse should check the last peak and trough values for the gentamicin prior to contacting the physician. This infant is exhibiting signs and symptoms of nephrotoxic-

ity and neurotoxicity, as indicated by the decreased urine output and muscular weakness. Although a patient may recover from gentamicin nephrotoxicity, the ototoxic and neurotoxic effects are irreversible.

104. Correct answer: C
Pot (marijuana) produced 20 years ago was more natural and purer with fewer additives. Pot grown and sold in today's market contains 20 times more ammonia and 5 times more hydrogen cyanide, formaldehyde, and PCP. The goal with today's brand of pot is to obtain a more profound, faster, and sustained high. Within a few minutes of ingestion or inhalation, the user's heart rate may increase from 20 to 80 beats per minute above baseline, and memory loss will occur. The individual may also experience an inability to concentrate, confusion, dry mouth, and an increased appetite. The effects may be compounded and varied if other drugs are cut or mixed with the marijuana.

105. Correct answer: A
Energy drinks contain massive amounts of caffeine and a variety of ingredients that will break down into methamphetamines and amphetamines with effects on the fetus similar to fetal alcohol syndrome. Immediate presentation includes small for gestation, dehydration, poor coordination for suck and swallow, hyperactive behavior, and sleep disturbances. Long-term effects include learning disabilities, speech and language delays, poor judgment, and low intelligence quotient.

106. Correct answer: C
The correct definition of addiction is when the user cannot live or function without the use of a substance or drug. Addiction withdrawals can be severe or life threatening. Abuse occurs when the user uses a substance or drug in an amount or function that was not originally intended. An individual who abuses a drug might not be an addict. For example, an individual who uses Benadryl to fall asleep when no allergy symptoms are present is abusing the drug. An addict is usually an abuser by both function and amount of the substance or drug used. Substances or drugs abused range from the obvious (alcohol, marijuana, oxycodone, heroin, and cocaine) to the unexpected (glue, spray paint, nail polish remover, energy drinks, ibuprofen, and cough syrups).

107. Correct answer: A
Marijuana is the most commonly used illegal drug in the world. In many countries and some states, medicinal marijuana has been legalized but closely regulated. To obtain more information regarding statistics for a specific area and its current ranking in terms of substance abuse, visit the U.S. government's websites at www.dea.gov and www.nida.nih.gov, both of which are updated frequently.

Toluene is the addictive chemical in glue.

108. Correct answer: A
Although you may ask all of these questions, the first question should be to determine if Helen was using actual witch hazel for acne or facial cleaning, or if she is using the slang term witch hazel for heroin. Many street drugs may present with innocuous names. Heroin may also be referred to as smack, nose drops (liquid heroin), dragon rock (mixed with cocaine), A-bomb (mixed with marijuana), big H, brown sugar, brown tape, diesel, and old navy. If the patient was referring to heroin, monitor the patient for additional signs and symptoms of heroin abuse such as venous tracks, bruising, and burnt fingertips from holding a roll lighter to smoke the heroin.

109. **Correct answer: D**
The sudden collapse of a young woman at a party without explanation is suspicious for gamma hydroxybutyrate (GHB) or ketamine ingestion. Both of these drugs are known date or party rape drugs. Due to the anesthetic and amnesic effects of the drug, an affected female may be unable to describe the events leading up to the collapse. To determine her exposure, the drug screen should be repeated, looking specifically for gamma hydroxybutyrate and/or ketamine.

110. **Correct answer: B**
A chewed-up pacifier and presentation of euphoria and confusion should lead the staff to consider Ecstasy addiction and abuse. Ecstasy, or methylenedioxymethamphetamine (MDMA), causes trismus, or teeth grinding. Users may chew on pacifiers to preserve their teeth and hide the grinding from others. Most children using pacifiers will not chew the pacifiers, but rather suck on them.

111. **Correct answer: A**
Methamphetamines create an increased risk for cleft palate/lip, hypoglycemia, seizures, poor sucking, and feeding intolerance in infants. Cardiac rhythm disturbances such as supraventricular tachycardia may occur. In addition, the baby may have hyperthermia, agitation, tremors, intraventricular hemorrhages, and a high-pitched cry.

112. **Correct answer: A**
Diphenhydramine (Benadryl) and guaifenesin (Robitussin) both contain antihistamines and have anticholinergic effects. Rosa appears to have overdosed on cough and cold remedies, causing her to become severely dehydrated, hyperthermic, and have hallucinations. The classic presentation of anticholinergic overdose is described as follows: "dry as a bone, red as a beet, hot as a pistol, mad as a hatter, and loony as a toon." Due to hallucinations, patients who present with anticholinergic overdose must be protected from others and from themselves. They may be very agitated and difficult to treat. Emergency management consists of fluids and benzodiazepines.

113. **Correct answer: D**
Modafinil, caffeine, and amphetamines are all classified as stimulants. Other stimulants include cocaine cathinone, ephedrine, phentermine, and theophylline. Effects of marijuana range from stimulation to depression, depending on the amount and frequency of use as well as the chemicals cut or mixed in for smoking. Yellow jackets, methadone, and ketamine are depressants.

114. **Correct answer: A**
Oral morphine doses may be administered at three to five times that of intravenous doses, as absorption rates and times of onset of effect differ. Ongoing visual (including via monitor) respiratory assessment should be continuous to evaluate for response to treatment and respiratory depression.

115. **Correct answer: B**
Activated charcoal does not adsorb metals. Activated charcoal adsorbs most poisons. Activated charcoal cannot be mixed with ice cream or syrups because the charcoal adsorbs many of these agents and would be less effective. Single doses of activated charcoal are indicated for serious poison exposures.

116. **Correct answer: A**
Multiple doses of activated charcoal should be used for ingestions of theophylline. Additional drugs for which multiple doses are indicated include digoxin, phenobarbital, and amitriptyline.

117. **Correct answer: D**
"Gray baby syndrome" is induced by chloramphenicol.

118. **Correct answer: D**
Hemoperfusion may be used in the treatment of theophylline.

119. **Correct answer: C**
Acetaminophen is metabolized by the liver. In children younger than 10 years, a different metabolic pathway may be followed. Some renal metabolism of acetaminophen occurs, so renal injury is a possibility.

120. **Correct answer: B**
In young children, the effect of ethanol is to suppress the liver's ability to produce glucose. Other symptoms of ethanol ingestion include hypoglycemia, altered mental status, hypothermia, respiratory depression, slurred speech, gastric irritation with vomiting, bradycardia, and vasodilation.

121. **Correct answer: C**
Patients with methemoglobinemia present with intractable cyanosis unresponsive to oxygen administration. Their blood will appear brown when placed on white paper. Methemoglobin is the portion of normal hemoglobin that has been converted and cannot carry oxygen.

122. **Correct answer: C**
Methylene blue is used to treat methemoglobinemia. Toxicity and other symptoms are treated as they occur.

123. **Correct answer: D**
Sodium bicarbonate is used to treat tricyclic antidepressant overdose. Imipramine and Doxepin are both tricyclics.

124. **Correct answer: A**
Amoxapine is a cyclic antidepressant that may cause cardiovascular effects and will probably cause status epilepticus. The patient often requires intubation and muscular paralysis because of seizures.

125. **Correct answer: B**
Flumazenil is a specific antidote for benzodiazepine overdose. This drug should not be given to patients who overdose on tricyclic antidepressants because it increases their risk of seizures.

126. **Correct answer: C**
Metabolic acidosis is likely to be seen with an iron overdose. After iron is metabolized, free hydrogen is released and leads to metabolic acidosis.

127. **Correct answer: C**
Deferoxamine is used to treat iron poisoning by chelation. It is also possible that the child may have to be treated with GI tract decontamination, which may involve either gastric lavage or whole bowel irrigation.

128. **Correct answer: A**
Respiratory depression, miosis, and coma are the triad of symptoms associated with opioid overdose.

129. **Correct answer: D**
Methadone has a half-life of approximately 24 hours. Continuous doses of naloxone are needed to prevent respiratory depression until the methadone is fully eliminated from the child's system.

130. **Correct answer: D**
Symptoms of salicylate poisoning include tachycardia and hyperthermia. Additional symptoms include tinnitus, tachypnea, LOC changes, respiratory alkalosis, metabolic acidosis, or mixed acid–base abnormalities. Occult GI tract bleeding may occur as well.

131. **Correct answer: C**
Oven cleaners contain large amounts of alkali. Other highly alkaline substances include dishwasher detergents, laundry detergents, drain openers, and ammonia capsules.

132. **Correct answer: B**
Vascular thrombosis may result from alkaline substances and liquefaction necrosis. Serious injury results from products with a pH higher than 12.

133. **Correct answer: B**
Hydrofluoric acid is absorbed even through intact skin, causing local and systemic effects. Hydrofluoric acid is used as rust removers, metal cleaners, and to etch glass.

134. **Correct answer: D**
Ethylene glycol is the toxic ingredient in automobile antifreeze.

135. **Correct answer: B**
After a child ingests toxic levels of iron, there is a latent asymptomatic phase that occurs 2–12 hours after ingestion. After about 12 hours, the child may enter the next phase, which is an abrupt cardiovascular collapse.

136. **Correct answer: C**
SIRS is the body's systemic inflammatory immune hormonal response to severe injury or illness arising from a variety of causes. Although SIRS is not dependent on the presence of an infection for its emergence, it is accompanied by an infectious process (sepsis).

137. **Correct answer: A**
Myocardial depressant factor is not considered a highly influential mediator of gram-negative septic shock.

138. **Correct answer: D**
The area of a burn that has the closest contact with the heat source and sustains the most damage is known as the zone of coagulation. Coagulation necrosis is usually the result of most burn injuries.

139. **Correct answer: D**
A fourth degree full thickness burn involves muscle, fat, fascia, or bone. This type of burn usually occurs as a result of deep thermal or electrical burns.

140. Correct answer: B
Hypochloremia and hyponatremia are disadvantages of using 0.5% silver nitrate solution for burn patients.

141. Correct answer: A
Hemorrhagic contusion is an example of a primary blast injury. A blast injury occurs after an explosion that causes sudden changes in atmospheric pressure.

142. Correct answer: D
A tertiary blast injury occurs when a body is hurled though the air and struck by another object.

143. Correct answer: A
Watery rice-like diarrhea, nausea, vomiting, irritability, confusion, and paresthesias around the mouth are symptoms of arsenic poisoning. Additional symptoms include headache, a metallic taste, palpitations, and EKG changes.

144. Correct answer: B
A urine pH of 7 to 8 is an appropriate goal for a patient treated for salicylate overdose.

145. Correct answer: D
Children require special considerations during a disaster or terrorism event. They are more—not less—vulnerable to chemicals absorbed through the skin. Other issues to consider include the facts that children are more susceptible to the effects of radiation exposure, and their cognitive and developmental levels may diminish their ability to escape. Children cannot be decontaminated in an adult decontamination unit.

146. Correct answer: B
The type of device made by combining radioactive materials and an explosive is known as a radiologic dispersal device.

147. Correct answer: A
The type of chemical agent that can cause blistering is called a vesicant.

148. Correct answer: A
Nonspecific is not a form of anthrax. Cutaneous, pulmonary, and gastrointestinal are all forms of anthrax.

149. Correct answer: C
Plague is not transmitted by rats. Plague is transmitted by fleas, and aerosol droplets may spread the disease from person to person.

150. Correct answer: A
A child in cardiogenic shock would present with these parameters:

	HR	CI	SVR	PVR
A.	↑	↓	↑	**Normal or** ↑

151. **Correct answer: B**
The classic presentation of septic shock is fever, tachycardia, and vasodilation.

152. **Correct answer: B**
SIRS is the acute development of two or more of the following criteria, which are fever (> 38°C) and leukocytosis (WBC > 12,000/mm^3).

153. **Correct answer: B**
Cavernous sinus syndrome is a rare, but life-threatening condition. Symptoms include periorbital cellulitis, conjunctiva with lid swelling, and exophthalmos. It is usually the result of some form of infection from sinusitis, furuncles, dental infections, trauma, or neoplasm. Staphylococcus or streptococcal infections are two of the main causative organisms. Severe sinusitis and pituitary tumors can also lead to this syndrome.

154. **Correct answer: A**
The early signs of cavernous sinus syndrome are quite varied, but typically include the conjunctival injection, eye pain, and fever. Other symptoms include ptosis, changes in the extraocular exam, meningitis signs, or sepsis.

155. **Correct answer: C**
If the cause of the cavernous sinus syndrome is a bacterial infection, recovery may be rapid following the administration of appropriate antibiotics. Surgical correction involves drainage of the infection without touching the cavernous sinus. Neurosurgery or oncology specialists should be consulted about neoplasms. Mortality is approximately 30% with this condition, and relapses may occur.

156. **Correct answer: A**
$ScvO_2$, or central venous oxygen saturation, is comprised of the following components: cardiac output, serum hemoglobin, oxygen saturation (SaO_2), and cellular oxygen use/demands (vO_2). $ScvO_2$ monitoring allows for early detection and treatment of septic shock.

MULTISYSTEM REFERENCES

Aehlert, B. (Ed.). (2005). *Comprehensive pediatric emergency care.* St. Louis, MO: Mosby.

Ahmed, I., & Beckingham, IG. (2007). Liver trauma. *Trauma, 9*(3), 171–180.

Allen, E., Freeman, S., & Druschel, C. (2009). Maternal age and risk for trisomy 21 assessed by the origin of chromosome nondysjunction: A report from the Atlanta and National Down Syndrome Projects. *Human Genetics, 125*(1), 41–52.

Allen, S. F., Pfefferbaum, B., Cuccio, A., & Salinas, J. (2008). Early identification of children at risk for developing posttraumatic stress symptoms following traumatic injuries. *Journal of Psychological Trauma, 7*(4), 235–252.

American Heart Association. (2010). Guidelines 2010 for cardiopulmonary resuscitation and emergency cardiovascular care. Retrieved from www.americanheart.org

Antunez, C., Martin, E., Cornejo-Garcia, J. A., Blanca-Lopez, N., Pena, R. R., & Mayorga, C. (2006). Immediate hypersensitivity reactions to penicillins and other betalactams. *Current Pharmaceutical Design, 12*(26), 3327–3333.

Balmadrid, C., & Bono, M. J. (2009). Recognizing and managing lead and mercury poisonings. *Emergency Medicine, 41*(9), 35–43.

Benachi, A., & Costa, J. M. (2007). Non-invasive prenatal diagnosis of fetal aneuploidies. *Lancet, 369*(9560), 440–442.

Bhana, D. (2008). Beyond stigma? Young children's responses to HIV and AIDS. *Culture, Health & Sexuality, 10*(7), 725–738.

Bondy, C. A. (2007). Care of girls and women with Turner syndrome: A guideline of the Turner Syndrome Study Group. *Journal of Clinical Endocrinology and Metabolism, 92,* 10–25.

Bulloch, B., Garcia-Filion, P., Notricia, D., Bryson, M., & McConahay, T. (2009). Reliability of the color analog scale: Repeatability of scores in traumatic and nontraumatic injuries. *Academic Emergency Medicine, 16*(5), 465–469.

Burns, S. M. (Ed.). (2007). *American Association of Critical-Care Nurses (AACN): AACN protocols for practice: Healing environments* (2nd ed.). Sudbury, MA: Jones and Bartlett.

Butler, C. T. (2007). Pediatric skin care: Guidelines for assessment, prevention, and treatment. *Dermatology Nursing, 19*(5), 471–472, 447–482, 485.

Carter, C. (2005). Evaluation and treatment of brown recluse spider bites. *American Family Physician, 72*(7), 1372, 1376.

Centers for Disease Control and Prevention. (2006). Fast facts: Anthrax information for health care providers. Retrieved March 3, 2008, from http://emergency.cdc.gov/agent/anthrax/anthrax-hcp-factsheet.asp

Centers for Disease Control and Prevention. (2006). Ricin: Epidemiology overview for clinicians. Retrieved March 3, 2008, from http://emergency.cdc.gov.agent/ricin/clinicians/epidemiology.asp

Chambers, M. A., & Jones, S. (Eds.). (2007). *Surgical nursing of children.* Philadelphia: Elsevier.

Chernecky, C., & Berger, B. (2004). *Laboratory tests and diagnostic procedures* (4th ed.). Philadelphia: Saunders.

Chial, H. (2008). Somatic mosaicism and chromosomal disorders. *Nature Education Online.*

Coté, C. J., & Wilson, S. (2008). Guidelines for monitoring and management of pediatric patients during and after sedation for diagnostic and therapeutic procedures: An update. *Paediatric Anaesthesia, 18*(1), 9–10.

Cox, J. E. (2008). Teenage pregnancy. In L. S. Neinstein (Ed.), *Adolescent health care: A practical guide* (5th ed., pp. 565–569). Philadelphia: Wolters Kluwer Health/Lippincott Williams & Wilkins.

DeBaun, M. R., & Vichinsky, E. (2007). Hemoglobinopathies. In R. M. Kliegman, R. E. Behrman, H. B. Jenson, & B. F. Stanton (Eds.), *Nelson textbook of pediatrics* (18th ed.). Philadelphia: Saunders Elsevier.

Department of Health and Human Services, Centers for Disease Control and Prevention. (2005). Acute radiation syndrome. Retrieved August 25, 2010, from http://www.bt.cdc.gov/radiation/ars.asp

Dierssen, M., Ortiz-Abalia, J., & Arqué, G. (2006). Pitfalls and hopes in Down syndrome therapeutic approaches: In the search for evidence-based treatments. *Behavior Genetics, 36*(3), 454–468.

Drake Melander, S. (Ed.). (2004). *Case studies in critical care nursing: A guide for application and review* (3rd ed.). Philadelphia: Saunders.

Emergency Nurses Association & Newberry, L. (2003). *Sheehy's emergency nursing: Principles and practice* (5th ed.). St. Louis, MO: Mosby/Elsevier.

Fitzgerald Macksey, L. (2009). *Pediatric anesthetic and emergency drug guide.* Sudbury, MA: Jones and Bartlett.

Forbes-Duchart, L., Marshall, S., Strock, A., & Cooper, J. E. (2007). Determination of inter-rater reliability in pediatric burn scar assessment using a modified version of the Vancouver Scar Scale. *Journal of Burn Care & Research, 28*(3), 460–467.

Garretson, S., & Malberti, S. (2007). Understanding hypovolaemic, cardiogenic and septic shock. *Nursing Standard, 21*(50), 46–55; quiz 58.

Gasparis Vonfrolio, L., & Noone, J. (1999). *Critical care examination review* (3rd ed. revised). Staten Island, NY: Power Publications.

Glapa, M., Kourie, J. F., Doll, D., & Degiannis, E. (2007). Early management of gunshot injuries to the face in civilian practice. *World Journal of Surgery, 31*(11), 2104–2110.

Gora-Harper, M. (1998). *The injectable drug reference.* Princeton, NJ: Bioscientific Resources.

Gravholt, C. (2008). Epidemiology of Turner syndrome. *Lancet Oncology, 9*(3), 193–195.

Gregg, X. T., & Prchal, J. T. (2005). Red blood cell enzymopathies. In R. Hoffman, E. J. Benz, Jr., S. J. Shattil, B. Furie, & H. J. Cohen (Eds.), *Hematology: Basic principles and practice* (4th ed.). Philadelphia: Churchill Livingston Elsevier.

Hall, J. G. (2007). Single-gene and chromosomal disorders. In L. Goldman & D. Ausiello, *Cecil medicine* (23rd ed.). Philadelphia: Saunders Elsevier.

Hardin, S. R., & Kaplow, R. (Eds.). (2004). *Synergy for clinical excellence: The AACN Synergy Model for Patient Care.* Sudbury, MA: Jones and Bartlett.

Hay, W. W. Jr., Levin, M. J., Sondheimer, J. M., & Deterding, R. R. (Eds.). (2007). *Current diagnosis and treatment in pediatrics* (18th ed.). New York: McGraw-Hill.

Hickey, J. V. (2008). *The clinical practice of neurological and neurosurgical nursing* (6th ed.). Philadelphia: Lippincott Williams & Wilkins.

Hjerrild, B. E., Mortensen, K. H., & Gravholt, C. H. (2008). Turner syndrome and clinical treatment. *British Medical Bulletin, 86*(1), 77–93.

Hullett, B., Chambers, N., Preuss, J., Zamudio, I., Lange, J., Pascoe, E., & Ledowski, T. (2009). Monitoring electrical skin conductance: A tool for the assessment of postoperative pain in children? *Anesthesiology, 111*(3), 513–517.

Jones & Bartlett Learning (2011). *2011 nurse's drug handbook.* (10th ed.). Sudbury, MA: Jones & Bartlett Learning.

Jones, K. L. (2006). Smith's recognizable patterns of human malformation (6th ed.). Philadelphia: Elsevier.

Joulin, O., Petillot, P., Labalette, M., Lancel, S., & Neviere, R. (2007). Cytokine profile of human septic shock serum inducing cardiomyocyte contractile dysfunction. *Physiological Research, 56*(3), 291–297.

Lanie, A. D., Jayaratne, T. E., Sheldon, J. P., et al. (2004). Exploring the public understanding of basic genetic concepts. *Journal of Genetic Counseling, 13*(4), 305.

Levin, M. J., & Weinberg, A. (2009). Infections: Viral and rickettsial. In W. W. Hay, Jr., M. J. Levin, J. M. Sondheimer, & R. R. Deterding (Eds.), *Current diagnosis and treatment in pediatrics* (19th ed., p. 1087). New York: McGraw-Hill Medical.

Luthra, R., Abramovitz, R., Greenberg, R., Schoor, A., Newcorn, J., Schmeidler, J., & Chemtob, C. M. (2009). Relationship between type of trauma exposure and posttraumatic stress disorder among urban children and adolescents. *Journal of Interpersonal Violence, 24*(11), 1919–1927.

Mahindra, P., Guillen, C., & Glick, S. A. (2009). A 5-year-old girl with scarring. *Pediatric Annals, 38*(7), 359–364.

Martin, B. (2010). Family presence during resuscitation and invasive procedures: AACN practice alert. Retrieved from http://www.aacn.org

McDermott, B. M., Cobham, V. E., Berry, H., & Stallman, H. M. (2010). Vulnerability factors for disaster-induced child post-traumatic stress disorder: The case for low family resilience and previous mental illness. *Australian and New Zealand Journal of Psychiatry, 44*(4), 384–389.

Medina, J., & Puntillo, K. (2006). *AACN protocols for practice: Palliative care and end-of-life issues in critical care*. Sudbury, MA: Jones and Bartlett.

Mejías, A., Bustos, R., Ardura, M. I., Ramírez, C., & Sánchez, P. J. (2009). Persistence of herpes simplex virus DNA in cerebrospinal fluid of neonates with herpes simplex virus encephalitis. *Journal of Perinatology, 29*(4), 290–296.

Merhar, S. L., & Manning-Courtney, P. (2007). Two boys with 47, XXY and autism. *Journal of Autism and Developmental Disorders, 37*(5), 840–846.

Nguyen, B. T., & Zaller, N. (2009). Male access to over-the-counter emergency contraception: A survey of acceptability and barriers in Providence, Rhode Island. *Women's Health Issues, 19*(6), 365–372.

Overview of obstetrics. (2010). In F. G. Cunningham, K. J. Leveno, S. L. Bloom, J. C. Hauth, D. J. Rouse, & C. Y. Spong (Eds.), *Williams obstetrics* (23rd ed., pp. 10–11). New York: McGraw-Hill Medical.

Paschall, M. J., Grube, J. W., & Kypri, K. (2009). Alcohol control policies and alcohol consumption by youth: A multi-national study. *Addiction, 104*(11), 1849–1855.

Pasek, T. A., Geyser, A., Sidoni, M., Harris, P., Warner, J. A., & Spence, A. (2008). Skin care team in the pediatric intensive care unit: A model for excellence. *Critical Care Nurse, 28*(2), 125–135.

Prescribing reference. (2009, Summer). *NPPR: Nurse Practitioner's Prescribing Reference, 16*(2).

Purnell, L. D. (2009). *Guide to culturally competent health care* (2nd ed.). Philadelphia: F. A. Davis.

Rimmer, R. B., Foster, K. N., Bay, C. R., Floros, J., Rutter, C., & Bosch, J. (2007). The reported effects of bullying on burn-surviving children. *Journal of Burn Care & Research, 28*(3), 484–489.

Shavit, I., Kofman, M., Leder, M., Hod, T., & Kozer, E. (2008). Observational pain assessment versus self-report in paediatric triage. *Emergency Medical Journal, 25*(9), 552–555.

Shaw, B. A., & Hosalkar, H. S. (2002). Rattlesnake bites in children: Antivenin treatment and surgical indications. *Journal of Bone and Joint Surgery, 84*(9), 1624–1629.

Shields, A. L., Campfield, D. C., Miller, C. S., Howell, R. T., Wallace, K., & Weiss, R. D. (2008). Score reliability of adolescent alcohol screening measures: A meta-analytic inquiry. *Journal of Child & Adolescent Substance Abuse, 17*(4), 75–97.

Slota, M. C. (Ed.). (2006). *Core curriculum for pediatric critical care nursing* (2nd ed.). St. Louis, MO: Saunders.

Smeltzer, S., & Bare, B. G. (2003). *Brunner and Suddarth's textbook of medical–surgical nursing* (10th ed.). Philadelphia: Lippincott Williams & Wilkins.

Spratto, G. R., & Woods, A. L. (2001). *PDR: Nurse's drug handbook*. Montvale, NJ: Delmar & Medical Economics.

Taeusch, H. W., Ballard, R. A., & Gleason, C. A. (2005). *Avery's diseases of the newborn* (8th ed.). Philadelphia: Elsevier.

Takken, T., van Brussel, M., Engelbert, R. H., van der Net, J. J., Kuis, W., & Helders, P. P. (2008). Exercise therapy in juvenile idiopathic arthritis. *Cochrane Database of Systematic Reviews, 2*, CD005954.

Taylor, E. M., Boyer, K., & Campbell, F. A. (2008). Pain in hospitalized children: A prospective cross-sectional survey of pain prevalence, intensity, assessment and management in a Canadian pediatric teaching hospital. *Pain Research and Management, 13*(1), 25–32.

Thomas, D. R. (2010). Pressure ulcers. In E. T. Bope, R. E. Rakel, & R. Kellerman (Eds.), *Conn's current therapy 2010* (pp. 869–871). Philadelphia: Saunders Elsevier.

Trivits Verger, J., & Lebet, R. M. (Eds.). (2008). *AACN procedure manual for pediatric acute and critical care*. St. Louis, MO: Saunders.

Warniment, C., Tsang, K., & Glazka, S. S. (2010). Lead poisoning in children. *American Family Physician, 81*(6), 751–757.

Warwick, A. M., Goonewardene, K., Burton, P. R., Usatoff, V., & Evans, P. M. (2007). HP38P management of the traumatic pancreatic injury. *ANZ Journal of Surgery, 77*(s1), A48.

SECTION 11

Behavioral

1. Nadine, a 14 year old, was admitted to the pediatric ICU after fainting at school due to bradycardia. She is 67 inches tall but weighs only 87 pounds. You find her crying in her room. She tells you that she is worried the intravenous fluid will make her gain weight. What is the most effective way to manage this problem?

A. Have her mother talk to her

B. Ask Nadine if she wants to speak to her minister

C. Ask the physician for a dietary consult

D. Ask for a patient conference with the healthcare team and the family

2. You are assisting Madison, a 17 year old, with oral care when you notice multiple rotted teeth. You suspect that she has bulimia nervosa. Madison tells you that she regularly purges after meals so she can meet the weight standards for the cheer-leading squad. Which family dynamics would you expect to find associated with bulimia nervosa?

A. No significant family dynamics are noted with bulimia nervosa

B. A family history of drug abuse or psychiatric disorders

C. A strong sense of ego

D. Poor school performance

3. Asperger's syndrome is considered to be which of the following types of disorders in the United States?

A. Developmental delay disorder

B. Autistic spectrum disorder

C. Pervasive developmental disorder

D. Attention-deficit disorder

4. Kelly is a 15 year old girl in the pediatric ICU after a suicide attempt. She took more than 60 500mg acetaminophen tablets with alcohol. While caring for her, you notice multiple 3–4 inch thin scars on her thighs and abdomen. What is your best response to this discovery?

A. Tell her parents so they can deal with it

B. Ask her what happened in a nonjudgmental way

C. Tell her how lucky she is to be alive

D. Tell her this behavior is not acceptable

5. **Ted is a 13 year old boy who was admitted to the pediatric ICU after ingesting about 80 extra-strength acetaminophen tablets. Until now he has refused to say why he ingested the drug. In the middle of the night, you find him crying. When you ask him why he is crying, he tells you he was sexually assaulted by a neighbor 3 weeks ago and he is afraid this will make him a homosexual. Which of the following responses is the most therapeutic?**
   A. "Don't worry, you'll get over this and be okay"
   B. "Let me get the psychologist to come talk with you tomorrow"
   C. "Why do you think this will make you a homosexual?"
   D. "What is wrong with being a homosexual?"

6. **Luann was at a party with some friends where she consumed alcohol and a mix of over the counter and prescription medications. She is now comatose and on life support, and is not expected to survive. Her parents are devastated and angry. They challenge everything you say and keep copious notes about her care. You are concerned they may plan to sue you or the hospital. What should be your first action?**
   A. Try to get a hold of their notebook and make copies of it
   B. Contact the nursing supervisor or your nurse manager with your concerns
   C. Contact your malpractice carrier for advice
   D. Ask to change assignments

7. **Depression in children often devastates families and often goes undiagnosed and misunderstood by families, the public, and the medical community. Which of the following statements is also true regarding depression in children?**
   A. Depression is seen only in maltreated children
   B. Childhood depression is easy to diagnose
   C. Children do not respond to antidepressant therapy
   D. Childhood depression is recurrent and may increase in severity

8. **Alcohol abuse may lead to a deficiency in micronutrients, which in turn may cause depression and suicidal behavior in children and adolescents. One of the micronutrients affected in this way by alcohol abuse is**
   A. Potassium
   B. Copper
   C. Sodium
   D. Selenium

9. **Heather is a 7 year old with sickle cell anemia who is frequently admitted to your unit. You were told in report that Heather's parents were escorted out of the unit for arguing in the hallway about financial difficulties and responsibilities. During your assessment, Heather appears to have difficulty concentrating on your questions and is withdrawn and restless. When attempting to engage her in activities, she refuses and states that she "wants to be alone." You should**
   A. Respect her wishes and go care for your other patients
   B. Leave the room to contact her mother
   C. Clean her room while looking for sharp objects or potential dangers
   D. Leave the room to contact the child life specialist and the doctor

10. DJ is a 5 year old admitted to the unit after an appendectomy. She is grimacing and will not allow you to assess her incision. The physician ordered IM Demerol for pain. Approximately 10 minutes after administration of the Demerol, DJ is combative, has pulled her IV out, has torn off her dressing, and is screaming at the staff and her parents. You should

A. Apply restraints by yourself, as she is only 5 years old and additional staff may scare her
B. Wear personal protective equipment to enter her room to apply restraints
C. Call security to help subdue DJ
D. Use a Posey restraint system to subdue DJ

11. A patient intoxicated with methamphetamine would exhibit which of the following conditions?

A. Elevated liver enzymes
B. Bradycardia
C. Hypothermia
D. Hypotension

12. Letisha is a 15 year old admitted for observation after fighting at a rave party. She has a fractured humerus, mild concussion, and right orbital fracture. When paramedics arrived, she was found talking to herself, resisted medical care, and stated she could heal herself. During your assessment, you find that Letisha is withdrawn, irritable, fatigued, and indecisive about what to order for breakfast. You should

A. Request a drug screen
B. Request a psychologist evaluation for schizophrenia
C. Request a social worker to assess Letisha's home life
D. Evaluate Letisha for feelings of suicide

13. Lithium is used as an antipsychotic medication to treat bipolar disorder. Lithium toxicity is deadly. Which of the following statements is true regarding lithium toxicity?

A. Toxicity may occur if blood levels reach 1 mEq/L
B. Signs of lithium toxicity include constipation, hypertonicity, and giddiness
C. Untreated lithium toxicity may lead to seizures, coma, and cardiac dysrhythmias
D. Lithium toxicity may be treated safely on a medical–surgical floor

14. Mary is a 14 year old who gave birth two months ago to a healthy baby boy. She has been suffering from postpartum depression. She was admitted with hallucinations, agitation, ventricular arrhythmias, and a possible seizure (witnessed by her mother). She has been taking a tricyclic antidepressant. Which of the following drugs is classified as a tricyclic antidepressant?

A. Amitriptyline
B. Gentamicin
C. Clonidine
D. Fluvastatin

15. Mary's mother said the last time Mary took one of prescribed doses of her Amitriptyline was last evening. A blood level was drawn in the PICU and considered a trough level. Mary's treatment should include

A. Hemodialysis
B. Sodium bicarbonate
C. Syrup of Ipecac
D. Trazodone

16. Binge eating, mutilation, obesity, drug abuse, and alcoholism are all examples of

A. Self-destructive behavior
B. Psychotic behavior
C. Neurosis
D. Immaturity

17. Amy is the lone survivor of a car crash that killed her parents and two siblings. She is recovering from a pneumothorax, hemothorax, and bilateral broken legs. She has been extremely depressed and withdrawn. You are discussing medications, psychiatric therapy, and the increased risk of suicide and suicidal behavior with Amy's distant relatives. The family makes each of the following statements. Which of these statements is inaccurate and needs to be corrected?

A. "If Amy is considering suicide, she will make statements or give warnings of suicide"
B. "We should trust our instincts if we feel if Amy is in danger"
C. "As she recovers from her depression, she is at greater risk of suicide"
D. "If she talks about suicide or asks about pills, then she is just voicing the thought and will not attempt suicide"

18. Kyle is a 15 year old admitted to the PICU after being bullied and beaten at school. He is angry and verbally assaultive with the staff. The goal of anger management for Kyle is to not

A. Confront Kyle directly with whatever made him angry
B. Discuss what most in the current situation makes Kyle angry
C. Discuss with Kyle alternative and positive ways to express his feelings
D. Decide on positive ways for Kyle to express his feelings when confronted with frustrating situations in the future

19. As the educator for a busy PICU, you note an increased frequency of patients with underlying mental disorders being admitted. You overhear some negative comments regarding nursing assignments for these patients. You ask the nurses to complete a self-awareness survey regarding their beliefs and understanding of mental health issues. You will use this information to

A. Determine which nurses should never care for patients with mental health issues
B. Change nursing assignments immediately
C. Determine which nurses should be written up and counseled
D. Create an education program for the nurses that will increase understanding of mental health issues and ways to access resources

20. **You are discussing post-discharge psychiatric resources with the patient's family. You note that they are using the terms "psychological emergency" and "crisis" interchangeably. To clarify this issue, you tell the family that**
    A. A crisis is an immediate danger to someone else, and an emergency is a suicide attempt
    B. A crisis develops over time as a result of a psychological stressor and an emergency is an immediate situation that, if not corrected, will result in violence
    C. A crisis occurs when no intervention will be effective and an emergency is when interventions have the greatest impact
    D. A crisis is sudden and precedes a psychological emergency in which lives may be threatened

21. **While passing your terminally ill patient's room, you see his mother crying at the bedside. She is unkempt, tired, and unable to focus during conversations. You believe that she is in the middle of a situational crisis. Your best action is to**
    A. Call your charge nurse to cover your other patient while you initiate a conversation with the mother to identify stressors and develop a list of resources
    B. Call the appropriate spiritual advisor for this patient
    C. Let the mother continue to sit with the patient and do not interfere
    D. Call the social worker to speak with the mother

22. **Your staff in the PICU has just completed a code lasting 2 hours for a 13 year old rape and trauma victim. Due to overwhelming injuries, the patient did not survive. Chaplain services are called in to assist with a nursing staff debriefing. Staff members experiencing which of the following emotions are at highest risk for psychological stress?**
    A. Anger
    B. Fear
    C. Anxiety
    D. Denial

23. **You are talking to your 16 year old patient about his newly diagnosed type II diabetes. He states that he is fine with the diagnosis and knows that he will need to make some changes. His speech is rapid and pressured, he is making frequent jokes, and he talks about playing football with the guys when he is discharged. You would still be concerned about this patient's psychological health because of his**
    A. Talk about social activities
    B. Frequent jokes
    C. Rapid, pressured speech
    D. Failure to acknowledge his dietary restrictions

24. Abel, a 13 year old drug abuser with cirrhosis, has returned again to the PICU after failing rehabilitation. Although you previously had a friendly and open relationship, he will not look at you and gives only minimal answers to your questions. You tell him

A. "I can't believe you wasted the opportunity at the rehabilitation center"
B. "I know you want to stay drug free but now you will have a permanent criminal record"
C. "Why don't we work together to find new resources for you to utilize when you are tempted to take one of these drugs"
D. "I am proud of how long you stayed sober. Let's try again"

25. You are caring for a 16 year old patient who was the driver in a motor vehicle accident in which a child was killed. She is combative and restless, hyperventilating, tachycardic, and has an elevated blood pressure. She states, "I've got to leave here. . .they'll arrest me. . .they'll lock me up. . .I can't believe this. . .there is no way out." You should tell her

A. "They should arrest you, you killed a child"
B. "Calm down. It wasn't your fault"
C. "Stop it. You are working yourself up. Look at me and focus on what I am telling you to do"
D. "Just relax. They can't arrest you because you are a minor"

26. Mike is a 15 year old gang member and heavy alcohol abuser. During a fight approximately 20 hours ago, Mike was shot in the leg. He was restrained after being verbally and physically abusive to the staff. You see Mike thrashing around in the bed and he is suddenly awake when you enter the room. He is shaking, has vomited, and is tachycardic, hypertensive, and talking to people not in the room. You suspect he is

A. Exhibiting signs of paranoid schizophrenia
B. Experiencing delirium tremens
C. Experiencing sepsis
D. Experiencing drug withdrawal

27. During discharge teaching, you notice multiple bruises on the arms and reddened areas on the neck of the patient's older sister. You suspect she is being physically abused. Which other indicator would support your assessment?

A. Extroverted behavior
B. Denial of abuse when asked directly
C. Volunteering of information
D. Hesitance to discuss home situation

28. Within a Chinese family, cultural values and practices may include which of the following beliefs?

A. Chi is an external energy
B. Disease is caused by disharmony with society
C. Medicinal herbs are important
D. Family involvement is limited

29. Zoe and Parker are the 16 year old parents of a 13 month old infant with leukemia. Initially the parents say little while visiting and have a glazed expression while at their baby's bedside. As a PICU nurse, you recognize their response as

A. Adaptation to the PICU environment
B. The initial steps of coping
C. The initial response to a crisis
D. Normal and does not need to be addressed

30. The PICU unit director has asked you to represent the PICU in a risk management task force. The purpose of risk management is to

A. Identify healthcare staff who are negligent
B. Collect and store records regarding potential and actual injuries in the hospital
C. Monitor staff competency
D. Determine scope of practice within the hospital based on financial liability

31. To provide consistent and complete transfer of care from one healthcare professional to another, regulating bodies recommend standardized report-off or hand-off documentation or reports. An example of this practice is

A. RBAR
B. SOAR
C. SBAR
D. DBAR

32. Sally is the sole survivor of a plane crash that killed her immediate family. While recovering from massive injuries, her behavior and moods rapidly change. Which of the following behaviors is of most concern to the staff and indicates suicidal behavior?

A. Yelling at her distant relatives and the staff
B. Withdrawal from conversation and interactions with others
C. Drug seeking with multiple requests for pain medications and sedatives
D. Crying and statements about feeling helpless

33. Signs and symptoms of anorexia nervosa may include

A. Tachycardia
B. Absent menses
C. Hyperthermia
D. Hyperactivity

34. Which of the following statements is true about posttraumatic stress disorder in children?

A. Children react better to stress than adults
B. Children simply withdraw after a traumatic event
C. Multiple traumatic events heighten the risk of PTSD
D. Children become less aggressive

35. **Which of the following statements is untrue regarding a child's response to posttraumatic stress disorder?**
    A. Children exhibit decreased vigilance and decreased reflexes
    B. Children may have decreased ability to complete homework
    C. Children may become irritable and hostile
    D. Children may exhibit regressive behaviors

36. **Karl is recovering after emergency surgery for a fractured femur and tibia. He continually demands to have his phone and a computer in his room. His mother says Karl spends too much time on the computer at home. Karl insists he only spends about an hour after school on the computer and texting his friends. Karl probably suffers from**
    A. Internet addiction
    B. Bipolar disorder
    C. Depression anxiety
    D. Separation anxiety

37. **You are assessing Michelle's understanding regarding her daughter's ability to hear and react to sounds. Which of the following statements by Michelle is accurate and indicates realistic goals for her daughter?**
    A. Hearing will continue to mature until 4 years old
    B. By 1 month old, an infant can recognize all sounds
    C. A 1 month old should be turning toward the voices of family members when addressed
    D. It is okay if her 1 month old does not respond to sudden, loud noises

38. **At 3 months of age, Aaron should be exhibiting which of the following muscular movements?**
    A. Transfers toys from hand to hand
    B. Supports the upper body when lying prone
    C. Rolls to both prone and supine positions independently
    D. Pinches objects dangled in front of his face

39. **Full color vision occurs around what age?**
    A. 1 month
    B. 3 months
    C. 7 months
    D. 12 months

40. **Alexa is 4 months old. Which of the following behaviors is cause for concern and requires further evaluation?**
    A. Alexa does not smile at parents or visitors
    B. Alexa supports her head when sitting
    C. Alexa does not roll over independently
    D. Alexa babbles and imitates sounds

41. A toy with a mirror-like surface would be appropriate for a child at
   A. 3 months old
   B. 7 months old
   C. 12 months old
   D. 13 years old

42. Micki is 8 months old. During your assessment, you attempt to play peek-a-boo. Micki does not respond or interact with the play. Which statement is true about Micki's reluctance to play peek-a-boo?
   A. Micki is not responding because of boredom
   B. Micki is too old to play peek-a-boo
   C. Micki is too young to play peek-a-boo
   D. Micki will need further assessment

43. You are observing Jacob playing with his 3 month old son Harry. When Jacob stops playing with Harry to answer a phone call, Harry begins crying. Jacob calls you into the room to treat Harry for possible pain. You would
   A. Treat Harry with the prescribed medication
   B. Tell Jacob that pain medications are not indicated
   C. Play peek-a-boo with Harry
   D. Provide a sucrose pacifier to Harry

44. Which of the following is an indicator of normal development for a 12 month old?
   A. When the infant drops a toy, he says, "Oh-oh"
   B. The child must be assisted to stand
   C. The child responds only to "no"
   D. The child follows complex instructions

45. Which reflex normally disappears when an infant reaches 9 to 12 months of age?
   A. Moro reflex
   B. Rooting reflex
   C. Palmar grasp
   D. Plantar grasp

46. Millie is 6 months old. Which reflexes should no longer be elicited?
   A. Palmar grasp and rooting
   B. Moro reflex and stepping reflex
   C. Rooting and tonic grasp
   D. Palmar and plantar grasps

47. At which developmental age should an infant be able to find a hidden object under multiple layers of blankets, clothes, or covers?
   A. 9 months
   B. 12 months
   C. 24 months
   D. 36 months

48. Joseph works in the environmental services department. He asks your opinion as to what he should buy for his 12 month old nephew's birthday. With your understanding of motor and social developmental milestones, which of the following options should you recommend?

A. A bucket of blocks
B. Crayons and coloring books
C. A mirrored play pad
D. Lincoln logs

49. Michu questions why you constantly talk to his infant daughter while you are providing care. Which response is the most correct?

A. "She doesn't mind the stimulation"
B. "It lets her know what time of the day it is"
C. "Word repetition and speech improve language development."
D. "So she isn't afraid of me"

50. Sarah is nervous for her son, who is about to reach the "terrible twos." She asks you if defiant behavior can be avoided. Your best response is

A. "Yes, set strong limits and punish immediately"
B. "Yes, keep him away from other children for at least 6 months"
C. "No, it happens to everyone"
D. "No, some defiant behavior is a good thing"

51. What is the normal minimum word repertoire expected of an 18 month old?

A. 5 words
B. 10 words
C. 15 words
D. 20 words

52. Which of the following statements is true regarding home safety?

A. The toilets should have locks when a 2 year old is present
B. Plug covers should be installed when the infant reaches 12 months old
C. Knick-knacks on coffee tables can remain until the infant reaches 18 months
D. Stair gates should be used until the child reaches 3 to 4 years old

53. Clara tells you that she cannot wait to share with her niece her favorite paper doll cut-outs from when she was a girl. At what age is it appropriate to introduce this type of toy?

A. When the niece is 12 months old
B. When the niece is 24 months old
C. When the niece is 2 years old
D. When the niece is 3 years old

54. Which of the following children requires further evaluation?

A. 2 year old Jake, who cannot push a wheeled toy
B. 18 month old Allie, who has a language vocabulary of 20 words
C. 4 year old Madison, who tells rambling stories
D. 12 month old Jose, who cannot walk heel-toe after walking for 2 weeks

55. **"Monster" fears are normally seen at what age?**
    A. 1 to 2 years old
    B. 2 to 3 years old
    C. 3 to 4 years old
    D. 4 to 6 years old

56. **Which type of play is appropriate for a 3 year old?**
    A. Gymnastics with parallel bars
    B. Dress-up
    C. Board games
    D. Hopscotch

57. **According to Erikson's stages of psychosocial development, autonomy vs. doubt and shame should be developed in individuals at the age of**
    A. Birth to 12 months
    B. 1 to 3 years
    C. 3 to 5 years
    D. 2 to 7 years

58. **Piaget believed that a child has a vivid imagination and can communicate through play. During this preoperational stage of development, the child is incapable of seeing anyone else's point of view. This cognitive stage occurs at the age of**
    A. 12 months to 2 years
    B. 1 to 3 years
    C. 3 to 5 years
    D. 2 to 7 years

59. **When schoolchildren begin to see another person's point of view, Piaget believed these children had entered which stage of development?**
    A. Anal stage
    B. Concrete operational stage
    C. Formal operational stage
    D. Conceptual stage

60. **Freud believed that at a certain point children developed a sense of right and wrong and that their superegos continued to develop. According to Freud's theory of personality development, this ability is developed at age**
    A. 2 years
    B. 2 to 3 years
    C. 3 to 5 years
    D. 6 to 12 years

61. **Erikson believed that at a certain age children understood the concept of right and wrong and were developing the superego. What did Erikson call this stage?**
    A. Industry vs. inferiority stage
    B. Initiative vs. guilt stage
    C. Identity vs. role confusion stage
    D. Trust vs. mistrust stage

62. **Ketamine would be contraindicated in a child with**
   A. Bronchospasm
   B. Altered intracranial pressure
   C. Barbiturate overdose
   D. Opioid overdose

63. **Which of the following statements is true regarding the administration of propofol?**
   A. Propofol is used for long-term procedures
   B. Propofol is not indicated for use in a patient with bronchospasm
   C. Propofol is made from eggs and soybeans
   D. Propofol increases cerebral blood flow

64. **Your nephew is being evaluated for ADHD. Which of the following conditions or abnormalities would be expected to be present if he has ADHD?**
   A. A cousin with hyperthyroidism
   B. Eye problems
   C. A heart murmur
   D. None

65. **Methamphetamine is officially classified as a(n)**
   A. Stimulant
   B. Euphoric
   C. Hallucinogen
   D. Antidepressant

66. **The specific antidote for methamphetamine is**
   A. Desipramine
   B. Alkalinizing agents
   C. There is no antidote
   D. Naloxone

SECTION 11

Behavioral Answers

1. **Correct answer: D**
   Nadine has anorexia. It is very difficult to treat anorexia nervosa and often requires a team approach. This patient and her family may need psychological counseling as well as medical and nutritional assistance. The important concern for the pediatric ICU nurse is the impact anorexia has on the body and the patient's recovery. The typical anorexic may have multiple complications of one or more body systems. She may have symptoms such as cardiac arrhythmias, EKG abnormalities, amenorrhea, esophagitis, anemia, dehydration, electrolyte imbalances, peripheral neuropathy, hematuria, and osteopenia.

2. **Correct answer: B**
   Family dynamics you would expect to find associated with bulimia nervosa include a strong family history of similar disorders, drug abuse, and psychiatric disorders. Bulimia nervosa is often seen in teens who are overachievers, trying to please those around them. These children often do very well in school and have above average intelligence. They also have poor self-esteem or self-image problems.

3. **Correct answer: C**
   Asperger's syndrome is a pervasive developmental disorder. Children affected by this disorder are eccentric in their behavior and social interactions. Boys are most often affected by this disorder, by a 4:1 ratio over girls. There is no known cause of Asperger's syndrome, but it often occurs with fragile X syndrome, hypothyroidism, and neurofibromatosis. The condition is generally diagnosed when the child is between 3 and 11 years of age. Approximately one-fourth of those affected by Asperger's syndrome grow out of their condition by adulthood.

4. **Correct answer: B**
   When suspect scars are noted on patients who have attempted suicide, it is important to ask what happened in a nonjudgmental way. This approach allows the patient the option of discussing her feelings or the cause of her self-abuse. She should also be receiving psychiatric help, and both the physician and the psychologist/psychiatrist need to know about the cutting. Many teens cut themselves to relieve perceived pain and stress in their lives. Telling her parents so they can deal with it, telling the patient how lucky she is to be alive, and telling her that this behavior is not acceptable negates her feelings and may lead to further cutting and suicide attempts.

5. **Correct answer: C**
   This child has opened up to you, and it is important to maintain the communication. Finding out why he feels homosexuality is bad gives insight to the suicide attempt. There are many other legal and ethical issues that have to be handled with this case. It

is obvious he will need psychological counseling. After your conversation, you must follow your hospital's policy/procedure manual about reporting such incidents. "Don't worry, you'll get over this and be okay" and "Let me get the psychologist to come talk with you tomorrow" are not therapeutic and they negate his feelings. Asking, "What is wrong with being a homosexual?" could be perceived as threatening by Ted.

6. **Correct answer: B**
   Whenever you have concerns about a patient's or family's behavior, it is best to notify administration as soon as possible. Note taking does not necessarily mean a lawsuit is forthcoming. Taking the family's notebook is illegal. Contacting your malpractice carrier is possibly overreacting to a situation where a lawsuit has not been considered. Changing assignments may give the parents more anxiety and lead them to suspect that something is wrong with the care you have already provided. The best defense is to keep the family fully informed about their daughter's condition. Another valid response to this situation would be to have a patient conference and involve the family with the entire healthcare team.

7. **Correct answer: D**
   Childhood depression is recurrent and may increase in severity. After having their first depressive episode, as many as 40% of children and teens will experience another episode within 2 years. Often these children are diagnosed with multiple psychiatric disorders, such as anxiety disorder, dysthymic disorders, disruptive behavior, or substance abuse. Depression may be seen in any child or teen, although environmental factors such as maltreatment can contribute to risk of depression. A child with chronic illness, infection, or biochemical factors is also a risk for depression. Depression is difficult to diagnose unless there is an understanding of depression and risk factors. Unfortunately, depression can be just as severe in children and teens as in adults, and is associated with approximately 80% of childhood and teen suicides. Undiagnosed and untreated depression can continue into adulthood, affecting the individual's personal and professional relationships and ability to function successfully in society.

8. **Correct answer: D**
   Alcohol abuse may cause a loss of selenium. Selenium is a trace element necessary for brain function. Research has shown that selenium deficiency in children and adolescents who abuse alcohol may contribute to the development of depression and suicidal behavior.

9. **Correct answer: C**
   Heather is exhibiting signs of depression and should not be left alone until you have determined that she is not a danger to herself or to others. While cleaning her room, you should note any potential items that could be used by Heather to harm herself or others. If the items can be removed, do so. If not, attempt to lessen the danger. Heather's depression may have been brought on by many factors, such as her prolonged and recurrent illness, family financial and emotional stress, and feelings of guilt or anger regarding her hospitalization. Only after ensuring Heather's safety should the nurse leave the room to contact the physician, child life specialist, social worker, case manager, charge nurse, and manager. Should Heather's mental health continue to deteriorate, she may need constant observation for suicide or restraints applied. Heather's parents will need to be contacted and updated on the situation, but it is important that the staff have a clear

plan of action when speaking with the parents. This plan of action should include family support, financial guidance, specialist support, and most important, a plan for improving Heather's mental and physical health.

10. **Correct answer: B**
When entering DJ's room (or any patient's room) to apply restraints, wear appropriate personal protective equipment to protect yourself against exposure to bodily fluids. DJ most likely has had a psychotic reaction to the Demerol and has exposed her wound and removed her IV, a potential for exposure to bodily fluids. When attempting to place restraints on a combative patient, regardless of the age, at least four staff members should be present, one for each limb. The parents should not be asked to participate in placement of the restraints as they are untrained and it may be seen as a betrayal by the patient. Instead, parents should remain at a safe distance to avoid injury or interference with healthcare providers. A Posey would not be the best choice, as it will leave the patient's hands free to continue pulling on lines and her dressing. Whenever restraints are in use, be vigilant to document continued need of restraints, type used, time placed, vital signs including airway, breathing, and circulation prior to and after restraints are placed, time of removal and reassessments. Be sure to follow your facility's restraint protocols and policies. Patient and staff safety is paramount.

11. **Correct answer: A**
A patient intoxicated with methamphetamine would exhibit elevated liver enzymes, tachycardia, hyperthermia, and hypertension.

12. **Correct answer: D**
You should first evaluate Letisha's feelings, paying close attention to any statements indicating a risk for suicide or injury to staff. Letisha is now exhibiting signs of depression after a manic episode. Patients with psychotic elements exhibited with mania or depression, or both, may be misdiagnosed with schizophrenia, anxiety disorder, or drug abuse. Patients with bipolar disorder may swing between moods over the course of minutes, hours, or days. Symptoms include hallucinations, delusions, and aggressive or violent behavior. A careful history may reveal a trend of manic and depressive episodes that would clarify Letisha's true condition and lead to faster and correct treatment. A social worker should be involved, but ensuring immediate patient and staff safety is the primary concern.

13. **Correct answer: C**
Untreated lithium toxicity may lead to seizures, coma, and cardiac dysrhythmias when levels exceed 2.5 mEq/L. Toxicity usually occurs with levels of 2 mEq/L, but symptoms may be observed at even lower blood levels with certain body chemistries. Initial toxicity is noted when the patient experiences diarrhea, vomiting, drowsiness, muscular weakness, and disorientation. As toxicity and symptoms worsen, nystagmus, ataxia, giddiness, tinnitus, confusion, and blurred vision may be present. Patients must be managed in the PICU by close monitoring and immediate intervention in case of dysrhythmias and electrolyte imbalances.

14. **Correct answer: A**
Amitriptyline is classified as a tricyclic antidepressant. Tricyclic antidepressants act by blocking norepinephrine and serotonin uptake in the central nervous system. They also have anticholinergic properties. The really interesting thing about this group of

drugs is that each is metabolized in the liver into one of the other tricyclics. Given this fact, you must test for levels of all the tricyclic agents, because the one you are testing for may have been metabolized and exacerbated the effects in the patient.

15. **Correct answer: B**
Mary's treatment should include sodium bicarbonate. ABG results should guide the amount to be given. Hemodialysis will not remove amitriptyline from the patient's system. Syrup of Ipecac is not indicated, especially given that the patient ingested the medication last evening. You may administer hypertonic saline for hypotension.

16. **Correct answer: A**
Binge eating, mutilation, obesity, drug abuse, and alcoholism are all examples of self-destructive behavior. Self-destructive behaviors are those that, if continued over time, will shorten or threaten length and quality of life.

17. **Correct answer: D**
Careful consideration and observation should be given to any person voicing any thought or plan regarding suicide. Many individuals will provide warnings about their suicidal thoughts providing family members or other persons in proximity the opportunity to intervene. Warnings are often cries for help and intervention. Family members should pay close attention to any impression or instinct that the person is considering suicide. As individuals enter and exit depression, they are at greatest risk for suicide, as they have sufficient mental focus at this point to form a plan and energy or motivation to carry it out.

18. **Correct answer: A**
Direct confrontation with the object of anger may further exacerbate the situation and limit the person's ability to deal positively with the situation. Instead, engage Kyle in a conversation regarding the stressor and assist him in identifying his feelings and options.

19. **Correct answer: D**
Surveys can be used to anonymously identify staff perceptions and determine educational opportunities. Mental health issues will affect almost every person at some point in their lives. Whether patients' distress is due to a catastrophic event or ongoing psychological issues, it is important that nurses understand their own biases regarding mental health and be able to identify resources when caring for this population. If the nurses believe the survey will be used punitively, then data may be skewed toward what the staff believe the surveyor is looking for, not the truth. Instead of changing assignments immediately, it is best to use the opportunity for education and professional growth.

20. **Correct answer: B**
Although there is no specific definition for either term, accepted criteria for both are a crisis is a less immediate situation that has developed over time in the presence of a psychological stressor and an emergency is an immediate situation that if not corrected will result in violence. Coping mechanisms may be partially effective, but do not address the situation directly to lead to a conclusion of the problem. A crisis may develop into an emergency if coping mechanisms fail or additional stressors appear. A psychological emergency has four basic elements: a sense of urgency that if the situation is not resolved, that anxiety may be intolerable and may lead to feelings of being

overwhelmed. Coping skills have completely failed, and the patient recognizes the need for help to alleviate the stressors. Suicide calls, notes, and messages meet these criteria.

21. **Correct answer: A**
The mother may need time to open up to you. Even though the social worker and the spiritual advisor may need to be called, it is important not to overwhelm the mother until the stressor and situation are fully understood.

22. **Correct answer: C**
Anger, fear, and denial are normal emotions in this situation; those staff members who feel anxiety are at greater risk. Anxiety is an emotion commonly experienced in psychological emergencies. Anxiety involves uncertainty of the unknown and may limit the person's ability to identify resources or initiate appropriate coping mechanisms. Debriefings after codes, both successful and unsuccessful, are therapeutic and allow staff to verbalize their emotions in a safe and stable environment. As a team, the staff may identify ways to support families and one another during crisis and emergency situations.

23. **Correct answer: C**
Rapid and pressured speech are signs of tension and indicate that the patient needs further support and assistance in coping with his diagnosis. Humor and social activities can be positive coping techniques as long as they are not used to avoid the stressful situation. The patient will need assistance and education regarding his diagnosis to effectively identify positive lifestyle changes.

24. **Correct answer: C**
The patient may feel as if he has failed the nurse by not remaining sober and that assistance may be withdrawn. This statement does not judge the patient and shows him that the help is still available by initiating communication and encouraging the patient to talk about his struggles with staying away from drugs.

25. **Correct answer: C**
The goal at this point is to regulate the patient's breathing and stabilize her vital signs. Using a firm and quiet voice with simple sentences can help the severely anxious patient focus and diffuse the anxiety. Severely anxious individuals are less able to see options and cope at this stage. Goals should include decreasing unnecessary stress and remaining available to the patient for communication. The other answers speak to facts not known or are judgmental and may either increase fear or lead to false hope.

26. **Correct answer: B**
The timing of Mike's symptoms is consistent with alcohol withdrawal or delirium tremors (DTs). DTs usually are seen 12 to 24 hours after last ingestion of alcohol, as blood alcohol levels drop. Effects may peak up to 15 days after DTs begin. Fluids, vitamins, nutrition, and short-term pharmacological treatments are appropriate. The severity of symptoms is affected by the amount and duration of alcohol ingestion as well as the patient's underlying physical health, use of other drugs, and existing psychological status. There are no indications at this time that the patient is septic or has schizophrenia. There may be underlying drug withdrawal symptoms, but the patient history does not provide an indication of such history.

27. **Correct answer: B**
Abuse may be suspected if the sister denies abuse in the presence of bruising, including injury to bones and around the throat. Many abused women and children tell stories of a positive home life and cite clumsiness as an excuse to explain injuries. Due to the likely introverted personalities of abused individuals, it is important to establish a safe zone and build trust to encourage honest communication and initiate assistance to help these persons escape the abuse.

28. **Correct answer: C**
Many cultures have beliefs and practices that may influence medical management of the neonate in the intensive care setting. Persons who belong to Chinese culture will often use medicinal herbs and religious beliefs regarding internal energy, known as a person's chi, to manage health. Cultural beliefs must be acknowledged as influential in patient care regardless of staff beliefs.

29. **Correct answer: C**
In the face of the severe illness of their child, these young parents are experiencing the initial response to a crisis. The situation is sudden, unexpected, and involves an environment and circumstances beyond the parents' experience or ability to cope. The crisis may last for weeks depending on available support systems, the healthcare team, parent education, culture, and spiritual intervention.

30. **Correct answer: B**
Risk management plays a role in the collection, analysis, and storage of records regarding potential and actual injuries in the hospital, as well as court filings. It also identifies situations or actions of potential liability and analyzes techniques to prevent future injuries, medication errors, and accidents.

31. **Correct answer: C**
SBAR is an abbreviation for situation, background, assessment, and recommendation for use when reporting patient care to another healthcare professional. SBAR is used to organize information succinctly to provide rapid report and recommendations for actions to physicians, advanced practice personnel, another nurse, social services, and ancillary departments. Situation refers to information that is most important or critical to patient care at the time. Background provides the necessary history that has brought the patient into the unit. Assessment includes objective and subjective data relevant to the patient situation. Recommendation refers to the course of action that the reporting staff member believes should occur to improve the patient's situation.

32. **Correct answer: D**
Feelings of helplessness or hopelessness and crying indicate psychotic emergencies. Extreme anxiety and an inability to recognize options should alert staff and family to a greater risk of suicide, as the patient may see suicide as the only option, and are a warning of suicide. The other statements indicate depression or levels of grief and emotional expression.

33. **Correct answer: B**
Patients with anorexia nervosa may have a diminished or absent menses. Other signs and symptoms may include bradycardia, hypothermia, fatigue, GERD, electrolyte abnormalities, hair loss, and loss of tooth enamel.

34. **Correct answer: C**
Posttraumatic stress disorder in children may result in many different symptoms. If the child experiences multiple traumatic events, the risk for developing PTSD increases. Additional causes of PTSD can include physical or sexual abuse, neglect, bullying, death of a significant other, accidents, war, terrorist attacks, disasters, life-threatening illnesses, or injuries. PTSD may also be caused by witnessed domestic violence, suicide, or murder.

35. **Correct answer: B**
Children may have diminished concentration and are unable to concentrate on homework. Children often regress, have increased anxiety, become aggressive, suffer panic attacks, avoid family, and reenact the event with drawings and stories. Children with PTSD are six times more likely to attempt suicide than their peers without PTSD.
The Children's Posttraumatic Stress Disorder Inventory or the Clinician-Administered PTSD Scale for Children and Adolescents measures PTSD symptoms. These tests may be administered by a licensed mental health practitioner.

36. **Correct answer: A**
There is actually a diagnosis of Internet addiction. The American Psychiatric Association is currently developing criteria for this diagnosis. Criteria that are recognized are lying about time spent on the Internet, avoiding friends or family to be on the Internet, anxiety when the Internet is not available, and increasing hours spent on the Internet. Academic performance often suffers. IA rehabilitation centers are becoming more prevalent. Karl needs a referral to a mental health practitioner.
At present, it is believed that approximately 9 million Americans fulfill the criteria for IA and 30% of those with IA have one or more comorbid psychiatric disorders.

37. **Correct answer: C**
A 1 month old should be turning toward the voices of family members when addressed. By 1 month old, an infant's hearing is fully matured and he or she should be able to recognize some sounds and respond to sudden, loud noises. It is important that infants be monitored in the first month of life for any hearing deficits to allow for early diagnosis and treatment of auditory compromise. Most parents, especially first-time parents, may not understand or follow up with healthcare professionals to monitor hearing. Treatment with certain medications, such as gentamicin, will require close monitoring for auditory toxicity.

38. **Correct answer: B**
By 3 months of age, Aaron should be able to support his upper body when lying prone. Additional motor movements for a 3 month old include swiping movements at objects, shaking a rattle, stretching legs and kicking when supine or prone, and raising the head and chest when prone. Hand coordination to pinch objects, hand-to-hand transfers, and rolling to both prone and supine positions independently occur later in development.

39. **Correct answer: C**
Full color vision is achieved around 7 months of age. Until a child is 7 months old, visual stimulation should focus on shades of gray, texture, and patterns.

40. Correct answer: A

At 3 months old, Alexa should be further evaluated if not smiling at parents or visitors. This may indicate complications with vision or facial muscle control. At 3 months, she should not be able to roll over independently—this is a 7 month old milestone. An infant of 3 months old should be babbling and imitating sounds.

41. Correct answer: B

Although teens may love mirrors, a reflective surface is an appropriate toy beginning at 7 months of age, when infants are able to visually cue in on partially obstructed objects and recognize familiar people.

42. Correct answer: D

At 8 months of age, an infant's visually acuity and developmental milestones should allow for play such as peek-a-boo. Micki's failure to interact or respond to the play indicates need for further developmental assessment. Illness may alter the normal response, but interest in play should be present with an infant who is awake and alert.

43. Correct answer: B

Pain medications are not indicated at this time. Harry began crying only when play ceased, which suggests he has reached a normal developmental milestone of social interaction and communication with facial expressions and body movement. The nurse should complete an assessment, but the likely indication of Harry's crying is displeasure when play stopped. Peek-a-boo is too advanced a concept for play at 3 months old and a sucrose pacifier is no longer indicated. Pain medications should not be administered until the patient has been assessed.

44. Correct answer: A

When the infant drops a toy, he says "oh-oh" is an indicator of normal development of a 12 month old. Additional indicators include an ability to stand by pulling up on objects, walking while holding on to furniture, crawling easily, and sitting independently. Language should include several single-word exclamations such as "oh-oh," "mama," and "dada" and response to several simple words and phrases.

45. Correct answer: D

The plantar grasp will normally disappear when an infant reaches 9 to 12 months.

46. Correct answer: B

The Moro and stepping reflexes should not be present once an infant is older than 2 months of age. The rooting reflex should disappear at 4 months. The tonic reflex should not be seen after 5 to 7 months. The palmar grasp is not normally seen past 5 to 6 months. The last reflex to disappear is the plantar grasp, at 9 to 12 months.

47. Correct answer: C

At 24 months of age, an infant should be able to find a hidden object under multiple layers of blankets, clothes, or covers. Other observations of appropriate development include sorting objects by color and shapes, and play using imagination.

48. Correct answer: A

An appropriate toy for a 12 month old infant would be a bucket of blocks. The blocks would exercise pincer grasps and allow for minor and major motor practice by pouring out the blocks and putting the blocks in the container. Although infants at 12 months mimic scribbling motions, the relationship and control for coloring are not complete.

The crayons also pose a choking risk. A mirrored play pad is appropriate for a 7 month old. Lincoln logs are more appropriate for a toddler (2 to 3 years old).

49. **Correct answer: C**
It is important to provide word repetition and speech to infants and toddlers to improve their language development. Infants and toddlers learn language through mimicry. Although conversation with infants tends to be one-sided, the infant is learning language patterns, tones, emotion, and inflection. Vocalization or babbling is the beginning of speech and should be encouraged through repetition. Encourage parents to use normal speech with infants and to avoid "baby-talk" to build language development.

50. **Correct answer: D**
Some defiant behavior seen during the "terrible twos" indicates normal social and emotional milestones. As Sarah is asking questions about development, it is vital that you follow the statement with teaching. At 2 years of age, the toddler is testing for social behavior limits and learning how to respond in certain situations. Increasing self-awareness and interrelationships lead to situational learning. The toddler will imitate behaviors, speech, and attitudes of persons around him or her without fully understanding the meaning of those actions. Punishment should not be used, but rather praise for appropriate behaviors. Child interactions are important for building and practicing language and emotions. Saying that the "terrible twos" happen to everyone does not provide any information or build parent understanding of normal development.

51. **Correct answer: C**
The minimum word repertoire of an 18 month old is typically 15 words. These words may be said singularly or in two-word phrases.

52. **Correct answer: D**
Home safety is important at every age. Stair gates should be used until the child reaches 3 to 4 years old. At this age, the child should have sufficient motor development to traverse stairs without support. By the time the child is 7 months of age, plug covers should be in place, knick-knacks moved to higher ground, and toilet lids have locks installed to prevent injuries during development. By 12 months of age, infants should be mobile and able to pull themselves up on furniture.

53. **Correct answer: D**
When a child reaches approximately 3 years of age, it is appropriate to introduce scissors (blunt cut) with supervision to play with paper doll cut-outs. This practice would stimulate and encourage appropriate fantasy play.

54. **Correct answer: A**
At 2 years old, Jake should be able to push a wheeled toy. Inability to accomplish this motor movement should be further evaluated. At 18 months old, Allie is meeting the minimum language vocabulary of 15 words and is developing language normally. Storytelling is normal cognitive and language development at 4 years old. Walking heel-toe is not expected until the child has been walking for several months and by age 2.

55. **Correct answer: C**
Children who are 3 to 4 years old will develop "monster" fears as fantasy and imagination develop. Primarily related to unfamiliar images and situations, the cognitive

inability to separate fantasy and reality makes these fears very real and they should not be ignored. The hospital setting may further increase fears and increase distress at night.

56. **Correct answer: B**
Playing dress-up is an appropriate activity for a 3 year old. Tumbling, board games with rules, and hopscotch are appropriate play activities for a 4 to 5 year old. Parallel bars should not be encouraged until the child has sufficient upper body strength and coordination to avoid injury.

57. **Correct answer: B**
The stage of autonomy vs. doubt and shame should occur when a toddler is 1 to 3 years old. They start to seek independence and gain control over their bodies. If the toddler perceives that this independence is not satisfying, the toddler will become frustrated and exhibit negative behaviors.

58. **Correct answer: D**
At 2 to 7 years old, the child is in the preoperational stage, according to Piaget. Piaget believed that a child has a vivid imagination and can communicate through play. During this stage of development, the child is incapable of seeing anyone else's point of view.

59. **Correct answer: B**
When schoolchildren begin to see another person's point of view, use logic, and solve problems, Piaget classified this as the concrete operational stage.

60. **Correct answer: D**
According to Freud's theory of personality development, during the latency period (6 to 12 years), children develop a sense of right and wrong and their superegos continue to develop.

61. **Correct answer: B**
According to Erikson, in the initiative versus guilt stage, children recognize the concept of right and wrong and develop the superego.

62. **Correct answer: B**
Ketamine would be contraindicated in a child with altered intracranial pressure because it increases ICP and cerebral blood flow.

63. **Correct answer: C**
Propofol is made from egg phosphates and soybeans. It is incumbent on the nurse to determine if the patient has allergies or sensitivities to these ingredients.

64. **Correct answer: D**
In the majority of cases, no additional abnormalities are found in patients diagnosed with ADHD. However, if there is a family history of ADHD, there is a higher probability of an individual having ADHD.

65. **Correct answer: C**
Methamphetamine is officially classified as a hallucinogen by The Diagnostic and Statistical Manual of Mental Disorders. The World Health Organization (WHO) published a list that shows methamphetamine as the second most abused chemical substance.

The drug may be ingested, smoked, injected, inserted into the anus or urethra, or snorted. Street names include crystal meth, big blue, base, and ice. The base of the drug is pseudoephedrine or ephedrine mixed with common ingredients. The mixture is often highly explosive, and the first warning a meth lab is nearby is when it blows up.

66. **Correct answer: C**
There is no specific antidote for methamphetamine. It is only possible to treat symptoms as they appear. Desipramine may cause sustained activity of amphetamines in the brain. Alkalinizing agents may potentiate the actions of amphetamines.

BEHAVIORAL REFERENCES

Aehlert, B. (Ed.). (2005). *Comprehensive pediatric emergency care*. St. Louis, MO: Mosby.

Allen, S. F., Pfefferbaum, B., Cuccio, A., & Salinas, J. (2008). Early identification of children at risk for developing posttraumatic stress symptoms following traumatic injuries. *Journal of Psychological Trauma, 7*(4), 235–252.

American Academy of Pediatrics. (2009). Caring for your baby and young child: Birth to age 5. Retrieved from http://www.healthychildren.org

Baker, A. L., Kavanagh, D. J., Kay-Lambkin, F. J., Hunt, S. A., Lewin, T. J., Carr, V. J., & Connolly, J. (2010). Randomized controlled trial of cognitive-behavioural therapy for coexisting depression and alcohol problems: short-term outcome. *Addiction, 105*(1), 87–99.

Bruni, V., Dei, M., Peruzzi, E., & Seravalli, V. (2010). The anorectic and obese adolescent: Best practice and research. *Clinical Obstetrics & Gynaecology, 24*(2), 243–258.

Buxton, J. A., & Dove, N. A. (2008). The burden and management of crystal meth use. *Canadian Medical Association Journal, 178*(12), 1537–1539.

Chambers, M. A., & Jones, S. (Eds.). (2007). *Surgical nursing of children*. Philadelphia: Elsevier.

Chernecky, C., & Berger, B. (2004). *Laboratory tests and diagnostic procedures* (4th ed.). Philadelphia: Saunders.

Cruickshank, C. C., & Dyer, K. R. (2009). A review of the clinical pharmacology of methamphetamine. *Addiction, 104*(7), 1085–1099.

Czincz, J., & Hechanova, R. (2009). Internet addiction: Debating the diagnosis. *Journal of Technology in Human Services, 27*(4), 257–272.

Diagnostic and safety issues critical for bipolar disorder in young children. (2009). *Brown University Child and Adolescent Psychopharmacology Update, 11*(7), 1–3.

Drake Melander, S. (Ed.). (2004). *Case studies in critical care nursing: A guide for application and review* (3rd ed.). Philadelphia: Saunders.

Du, Y. S., Jiang, W., & Vance, A. (2010). Longer term effect of randomized, controlled group cognitive behavioral therapy for Internet addiction in adolescent students in Shanghai. *Australian and New Zealand Journal of Psychiatry, 44*(2), 129–134.

Faden, V. B., Ruffin, B., Newes-Adeyi, G., & Chen, C. (2010). The relationship among pubertal stage, age, and drinking in adolescent boys and girls. *Journal of Child & Adolescent Substance Abuse, 19*(1), 1–15.

Fitzgerald Macksey, L. (2009). *Pediatric anesthetic and emergency drug guide*. Sudbury, MA: Jones and Bartlett.

Fortson, B. L., Scotti, J. R., Chen, Y.-C., Malone, J., & Del Ben, K. S. (2007). Internet use, abuse, and dependence among students at a Southeastern regional university. *Journal of American College Health, 56*(2), 137–144.

Fuh, J.-L., Wang, S.-J., Juang, K.-D., Lu, S.-R., Liao, Y.-C., & Chen, S.-P. (2010). Relationship between childhood physical maltreatment and migraine in adolescents. *Headache, 50*(5), 761–768.

Gora-Harper, M. (1998). *The injectable drug reference*. Princeton, NJ: Bioscientific Resources.

Hay, W. W. Jr., Levin, M. J., Sondheimer, J. M., & Deterding, R. R. (Eds.). (2007). *Current diagnosis and treatment in pediatrics* (18th ed.). New York: McGraw-Hill.

Hernandez, L., Eaton, C. A., Fairlie, A. M., Chun, T. H., & Spirito, A. (2010). Ethnic group differences in substance use, depression, peer relationships, and parenting among adolescents receiving brief alcohol counseling. *Journal of Ethnicity in Substance Abuse, 9*(1), 14–27.

Hudson, J. L., Rapee, R. M., Deveney, C., Schniering, C. A., Lyneham, H. J., & Bovopoulos, N. (2009). Cognitive-behavioral treatment versus an active control for children and adolescents with anxiety disorders: A randomized trial. *Journal of the American Academy of Child and Adolescent Psychiatry, 48*(5), 533–544.

Jones & Bartlett Learning (2011). *2011 nurse's drug handbook.* (10th ed.). Sudbury, MA: Jones & Bartlett Learning.

Klein, R. G. (2009). Anxiety disorders. *Journal of Child Psychology and Psychiatry, and Allied Disciplines, 50*(1–2), 153–162.

Lemstra, M., Bennett, N., Nannapaneni, U., Neudorf, C., Warren, L., Kershaw, T., & Scott, C. (2010). A systematic review of school-based marijuana and alcohol prevention programs targeting adolescents aged 10–15. *Addiction Research and Theory, 18*(1), 84–96.

Lindrigan, P. J. (2010). What causes autism? Exploring the environmental contribution. *Current Opinion in Pediatrics, 22*(2), 219–225.

McDermott, B. M., Cobham, V. E., Berry, H., & Stallman, H. M. (2010). Vulnerability factors for disaster-induced child post-traumatic stress disorder: The case for low family resilience and previous mental illness. *Australian and New Zealand Journal of Psychiatry, 44*(4), 384–389.

National Institute of Mental Health. (2009). How is bipolar disorder treated? Retrieved August 18, 2010, from http://www.nimh.nih.gov/health/publications/bipolar-disorder/how-is-bipolar-disorder-treated.shtml

National Institute on Drug Abuse. (2010). *NIDA InfoFacts: Methamphetamine.* Retrieved July 7, 2010, from http://www.nida.nih.gov/infofacts/methamphetamine.html

Rouget, B. W., & Aubry, J. M. (2007). Efficacy of psychoeducational approaches on bipolar disorders: A review of the literature. *Journal of Affective Disorders, 98*(1–2), 11–27.

Saraceno, L., Munafó, M., Heron, J., Craddock, N., & van den Bree, M. B. (2009). Genetic and non-genetic influences on the development of co-occurring alcohol problem use and internalizing symptomatology in adolescence: A review. *Addiction, 104*(7), 1100–1121.

Shakespeare-Finch, J., & De Dassel, T. (2009). Exploring posttraumatic outcomes as a function of childhood sexual abuse. *Journal of Child Sexual Abuse, 18*(6), 623–640.

Sher, L. (2008). Depression and suicidal behavior in alcohol abusing adolescents: Possible role of selenium deficiency. *Minerva Pediatrica, 60*(2), 201–209.

Slota, M. C. (Ed.). (2006). *Core curriculum for pediatric critical care nursing* (2nd ed.). St. Louis, MO: Saunders.

Snyder, D. M., Goodlin-Jones, B. L., Pionk, M. J., & Stein, M. T. (2008). Inconsolable night-time awakening: Beyond night terrors. *Journal of Developmental & Behavioral Pediatrics, 29*(4), 311–314.

Spratto, G. R., & Woods, A. L. (2001). *PDR: Nurse's drug handbook.* Montvale, NJ: Delmar & Medical Economics.

Stice, E., Rohde, P., Gau, J., & Shaw, H. (2009). An effectiveness trial of a dissonance-based eating disorder prevention program for high-risk adolescent girls. *Journal of Consulting and Clinical Psychology, 77*(5), 825–834.

Stores, G. (2009). Aspects of parasomnias in childhood and adolescence. *Archives of Disease in Childhood, 94*(1), 63–69.

Tao, R., Huang, X., Wang, J., Zhang, H., Zhang, Y., & Li, M. (2010). Proposed diagnostic criteria for Internet addiction. *Addiction, 105*(3), 556–564.

Tolou-Shams, M., Ewing, S. W. F., Tarantino, N., & Brown, L. K. (2010). Crack and cocaine use among adolescents in psychiatric treatment: Associations with HIV risk. *Journal of Child & Adolescent Substance Abuse, 19*(2), 122–134.

Treasure, J., Claudino, A. M., & Zucker, N. (2010). Eating disorders. *Lancet, 375*(9714), 583–593.

Trivits Verger, J., & Lebet, R. M. (Eds.). (2008). *AACN procedure manual for pediatric acute and critical care.* St. Louis, MO: Saunders.

U.S. Drug Enforcement Administration. (n.d.). Drug abuse prevention and control. Retrieved July 7, 2010, from http://www.usdoj.gov/dea/pubs/csa.html

Yacoubian, G. S. Jr., & Peters, R. J. (2007). An exploration of recent club drug use among rave attendees. *Journal of Drug Education, 37*(2), 145–161.

Young, K. (2009). Understanding online gaming addiction and treatment issues for adolescents. *American Journal of Family Therapy, 37*(5), 355–372.

5Th of exam

CV
Pulm
Neurology
Multisystem